Oral Anticoagulation Therapy

Kathryn Kiser
Editor

Oral Anticoagulation Therapy

Cases and Clinical Correlation

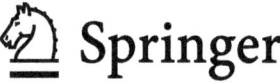

Editor
Kathryn Kiser
South College School of Pharmacy
Knoxville, Tennessee
USA

ISBN 978-3-319-54641-4   ISBN 978-3-319-54643-8 (eBook)
DOI 10.1007/978-3-319-54643-8

Library of Congress Control Number: 2017942960

© Springer International Publishing AG 2017

This work is subject to copyright. All rights are reserved by the Publisher, whether the whole or part of the material is concerned, specifically the rights of translation, reprinting, reuse of illustrations, recitation, broadcasting, reproduction on microfilms or in any other physical way, and transmission or information storage and retrieval, electronic adaptation, computer software, or by similar or dissimilar methodology now known or hereafter developed.

The use of general descriptive names, registered names, trademarks, service marks, etc. in this publication does not imply, even in the absence of a specific statement, that such names are exempt from the relevant protective laws and regulations and therefore free for general use.

The publisher, the authors and the editors are safe to assume that the advice and information in this book are believed to be true and accurate at the date of publication. Neither the publisher nor the authors or the editors give a warranty, express or implied, with respect to the material contained herein or for any errors or omissions that may have been made. The publisher remains neutral with regard to jurisdictional claims in published maps and institutional affiliations.

Printed on acid-free paper

This Springer imprint is published by Springer Nature
The registered company is Springer International Publishing AG
The registered company address is: Gewerbestrasse 11, 6330 Cham, Switzerland

Thank you to all the authors for providing their insight, dedication, and time to each chapter of this book. This series of cases reflects the contribution that these talented authors have made to add more clarity and safety to the management of anticoagulants and to the care of our patients. Thank you to all my mentors, colleagues, and friends for your tremendous support both professionally and personally. Thank you to my loving husband, Matt, and daughters, Sophia, Olivia, and Emma, for sharing this amazing journey of life with me.

Contents

Part I Introduction

1. **Introduction** 3
   Kathryn Kiser

Part II Atrial Fibrillation

2. **CHA$_2$DS$_2$-VASc and HAS-BLED Risk Stratification Tools** 7
   Lea E. dela Pena

3. **Male with Priority of Ischemic Stroke Reduction** 15
   David Parra and Augustus Hough

4. **Choosing an Anticoagulant in an Elderly Patient** 19
   Jena I. Burkhart

5. **Patient with Prior History of GI Hemorrhage** 25
   Michael Brenner and David Parra

6. **Patients with a History of Intracranial Hemorrhage** 31
   Jordan D. Long and Douglas C. Anderson

7. **Concerns with Anticoagulant Adherence** 37
   David Parra and Michael Brenner

8. **Oral Anticoagulants in Stable Moderate Chronic Kidney Disease** 43
   James C. Lee

9. **Oral Anticoagulants in Severe Renal Dysfunction** 53
   Jennifer Babin

10. **Oral Anticoagulants in Patients with Variable Renal Function** 61
    James C. Lee

11	**Patient with Concomitant Stable Coronary Artery Disease** Michael Brenner and Augustus Hough	69
12	**Patient with Concomitant Acute Venous Thromboembolism** Lea E. dela Pena	75
13	**Patient with Concomitant Mitral Valve Stenosis** Augustus Hough and Michael Brenner	81
14	**Patient with Concomitant Aortic Valve Stenosis** Augustus Hough and David Parra	87

Part III Warfarin Management

15	**Best Practice for Switching Stable Warfarin Patients** Dave L. Dixon	93
16	**Patient-Centered Strategies for Improving Warfarin Management** James C. Lee	101

Part IV Venous Thromboembolism (VTE)

17	**Provoked Versus Unprovoked Venous Thromboembolism** Jasmine M. Pittman	111
18	**Venous Thromboembolism (VTE) Prophylaxis in Hip and Knee Replacement Surgery** Mary G. Amato and Danielle Carter	121
19	**Venous Thromboembolism (VTE) Prophylaxis in the Intensive Care Unit (ICU)** Dillon Elliott	127
20	**VTE and Recent Drug Eluting Stent (DES) Placement** Wendy M. Gabriel	135
21	**Acute VTE in a Patient with Moderate Chronic Kidney Disease** Brenda Pahl and Douglas Anderson	143
22	**Oral Anticoagulation and Duration in Recurrent Venous Thromboembolism (VTE)** Regina Arellano	151
23	**Pulmonary Embolism (PE) with Thrombolytic Therapy** Justin M. Schmidt	159

Part V Acute Coronary Syndrome (ACS)

24 Patient on Oral Anticoagulant Presenting with ACS............ 167
Craig J. Beavers

25 Oral Anticoagulant Therapy Post-Percutaneous Coronary Intervention.. 173
Craig J. Beavers

26 ST-Segment Elevation Myocardial Infarction (Lytic Candidate) on Oral Anticoagulant 181
Craig J. Beavers

27 ACS with Bypass Surgery 187
Craig J. Beavers

Part VI Drug Interactions

28 Anticoagulant Drug-Drug Interactions with CYP 3A4 Inhibitors... 195
Lea E. dela Pena

29 Significance of P-glycoprotein (P-gp) Drug-Drug Interactions 201
Dave L. Dixon

30 Considerations with Pharmacodynamic Drug-Drug Interactions... 207
Jill S. Borchert

31 Management of Direct Oral Anticoagulants with Mixed P-gp/3A4 Drug-Drug Interactions........................... 213
Kathryn Wdowiarz

32 Pharmacokinetic Drug-Drug Interactions with Warfarin 221
Rachel C. Ieuter

Part VII Special Populations

33 Chronic Pain Management with Anticoagulation 231
Leah Sera

34 Anticoagulation Management in Atrial Fibrillation Catheter Ablation 239
Brian Cryder

35 Anticoagulation Management Considerations for Mechanical Valves... 245
Denise M. Kolanczyk

36	**Management of Antiphospholipid Antibody Syndrome**	253
	Margaret A. Felczak	
37	**Venous Thromboembolism and Pregnancy**	259
	Erika L. Hellenbart	
38	**Venous Thromboembolism in Active Malignancy**	269
	Margaret A. Felczak	
39	**Anticoagulation Management in Patients Undergoing Gastric Bypass Procedures**.	277
	Brian Cryder	
40	**Patient Presenting with Minor Bleeding**.	283
	Daniel M. Witt	
41	**Patient Presenting with Major, Life-Threatening Bleeding**	289
	Daniel M. Witt	
42	**Overdose of Dabigatran**	295
	Alicia Potter DeFalco	

Index. 305

Part I
Introduction

Chapter 1
Introduction

Kathryn Kiser

Keywords warfarin • direct oral anticoagulants • international normalized ratio (INR) • drug drug interactions • diet • heparin • low molecular weight heparins • fondaparinux • antiplatelets

Warfarin and other coumarin derivatives have long been the mainstays of oral anticoagulant therapy. While evidence has proven them effective for treating and decreasing the risk of thromboembolism, these agents also have many burdensome traits for use for both the clinician and patient. As narrow therapeutic index drugs, the therapeutic window between efficacy and toxicity is small with little correlation between dose and therapeutic effect. Genetic factors and other interpatient variability, such as diet and drug-drug interactions, also contribute to the wide dose range and need for frequent monitoring of the international normalized ratio (INR). The alternative therapies to oral anticoagulants used to only include injectable anticoagulants which were often utilized in place of or in addition to warfarin. These injectable agents limitations were mainly in cost and route of administration, and thus lack of patient acceptance. Fortunately, we have entered an era where several viable oral anticoagulant alternatives exist. These direct oral anticoagulants have much more predictable

K. Kiser, PharmD, BCACP
Assistant Professor of Pharmacy Practice,
Ambulatory Care Clinical Specialist - NHC Farragut,
South College School of Pharmacy,
400 Goody's Lane, Knoxville, TN 37922, USA
e-mail: kkiser@southcollegetn.edu

© Springer International Publishing AG 2017
K. Kiser (ed.), *Oral Anticoagulation Therapy*,
DOI 10.1007/978-3-319-54643-8_1

dose-response profiles thus eliminating the need for frequent monitoring. In addition, they have few dietary precautions and much less drug-drug interactions. However, these agents are not benign, not interchangeable, and not entirely characterized in regards to drug-drug interactions, reversibility, or use in populations outside of those in the pivotal clinical trials. Dosing, although more predictable in response, does have limitations including various doses and renal doses based on indication. As such, management of all the anticoagulants, whether warfarin, injectable, or the direct oral anticoagulants, is complicated and very patient specific. A need for extensive education of health care professionals is required.

Given the amount and complexity of information surrounding the use of anticoagulants, a lengthy didactic educational format has the potential to be overwhelming to the reader and difficult to translate and apply to direct patient care. This casebook is designed to provide clinical cases to simultaneously develop the readers' knowledge base, problem-solving skills, and practically apply their knowledge to a variety of clinical situations. These cases will be short focused case presentations that provide critical information and pose questions to the reader at key points in the decision making process. The cases will be relevant to what clinicians will encounter on a daily basis and focus on a variety of disease states for which anticoagulants are used. Cases will also focus on scenarios that clinicians may not encounter as often, but are equally important to be able to act upon such as a bleeding patient, patient scheduled for elective or emergent procedure, patient with changing renal function, or new drugs that may have a drug-drug interaction with an anticoagulant.

Included in the case studies will be evidence-based discussions that provide context and support for the process of selecting or managing the different anticoagulant treatment options. The case studies will be designed to instruct the reader how to select and effectively utilize the most appropriate agent for a given clinical scenario. They will focus on key features of warfarin, injectable anticoagulants such as heparin, low molecular weight heparins, or fondaparinux, the direct oral anticoagulants, and antiplatelets, as applicable. At the end of each case there are self-assessment questions to aid in reinforcement of main case concepts and application of knowledge.

Part II
Atrial Fibrillation

Chapter 2
CHA$_2$DS$_2$-VASc and HAS-BLED Risk Stratification Tools

Lea E. dela Pena

Abstract When deciding on appropriate therapy for stroke prevention in patients with atrial fibrillation, clinicians should calculate a CHA$_2$DS$_2$-VASc score as well as a HAS-BLED score in order to determine the patient's risk for stroke and risk for bleeding, respectively; higher scores indicate increased risk for stroke and/or bleed. Medication options include aspirin plus clopidogrel, warfarin, dabigatran, rivaroxaban, apixaban, or edoxaban; patient-specific factors must be taken into account when deciding the best option for a patient, which include cost, adherence, drug interactions, monitoring, and patient preference.

Keywords Atrial fibrillation • Stroke prevention • CHA$_2$DS$_2$-VASc • HAS-BLED • Aspirin plus clopidogrel

Case Introduction

A 67 year old female patient with past medical history significant for hypertension, type 2 diabetes, dyslipidemia, obesity, and GERD presents to the emergency room with a 2 day complaint of racing heartbeat, shortness of breath, dizziness, and fatigue. Her vital signs are as follows: BP 152/86 mmHg, pulse 132 bpm, respiratory rate 24 breaths per minute, and O$_2$ saturation 99% on room air. Twelve lead EKG reveals atrial fibrillation. Lab work is otherwise unremarkable. Her home medications include lisinopril, metformin, glipizide, atorvastatin, ranitidine, MVI, and calcium + vitamin D. She denies any history of tobacco or alcohol use. She is started on IV metoprolol for rate control.

L.E. dela Pena, PharmD, BCPS
Midwestern University Chicago College of Pharmacy,
555 W 31st Street, Downers Grove, IL 60515, USA
e-mail: ldelap@midwestern.edu

© Springer International Publishing AG 2017
K. Kiser (ed.), *Oral Anticoagulation Therapy*,
DOI 10.1007/978-3-319-54643-8_2

Case Discussion

What factors need to be considered when developing a medication regimen to prevent stroke in this patient?

Risk of Stroke

There are multiple ways of stratifying a patient's risk for stroke. Current AHA/ACC/HRS guidelines suggest using the CHA_2DS_2-VASc score [1]. This score is calculated based on the risk factors a patient has for stroke, with a possible maximum score of 9. The factors that go into a CHA_2DS_2-VASc score are included in Table 2.1. The higher the CHA_2DS_2-VASc score the higher the patient's annual risk for stroke as shown in Table 2.2 [1]. The treatment options, based on overall score includes no therapy, antiplatelet therapy, or anticoagulant therapy as shown in Table 2.3.

Table 2.1 CHA_2DS_2-VASc score

Risk factor for stroke	Score
Congestive heart failure/left ventricular dysfunction	1
Hypertension	1
Age ≥ 75 years old	2
Diabetes mellitus	1
Stroke/transient ischemic attack/arterial thromboembolism	2
Vascular disease	1
Age 65–74 years old	1
Sex category (female)	1

Table 2.2 Annual risk of stroke based on CHA_2DS_2-VASc score

CHA_2DS_2-VASc score	Adjusted stroke rate per year (%)
0	0
1	1.3
2	2.2
3	3.2
4	4.0
5	6.7
6	9.8
7	9.6
8	6.7
9	15.2

Table 2.3 Stroke prevention therapy based on CHA_2DS_2-VASc score

Score	Treatment
0	No therapy or aspirin
1	Aspirin or oral anticoagulant
≥2	Oral anticoagulant

According to current guidelines, oral anticoagulant indicates one of the following medications: warfarin, dabigatran, rivaroxaban, or apixaban [1]; edoxaban was not yet approved when the most recent guidelines were published, but it is commonly included in this group as well. This patient has a CHA_2DS_2-VASc score of 4—one point each for hypertension, diabetes, age 65–74 years old, and female sex—so she is indicated for oral anticoagulation.

Risk of Bleeding

One major drawback to anticoagulation in stroke prevention is the potential for bleeding, including major bleeding such as intracranial hemorrhage and gastrointestinal bleeding, which can be fatal. The HAS-BLED score is one way to stratify a patient's risk for bleeding. Similar to the CHA_2DS_2-VASc score, the higher the HAS-BLED score, the higher the risk for bleeding. The maximum possible HAS-BLED score is 9, and is calculated based on many factors illustrated in Table 2.4 [2].

A HAS-BLED score of ≥ 3 indicates that a patient is at high risk of developing a bleed. However, it is important to note that a score of ≥ 3 does not mean oral anticoagulants are contraindicated or that therapy should be discontinued. Instead, clinicians should use this score to see if there are any factors that could be modified to help decrease this risk such as controlling blood pressure or decreasing alcohol intake, as well as regularly re-evaluating patients on oral anticoagulants to make sure the benefits still far outweigh the risks. There are also other risk factors that are not part of the HAS-BLED score that can put a patient at increased risk of bleeding, such as patients with a history of falls or other risk factors for falls, such as balance problems, vision problems, or medications such as sedatives. This patient has a HAS-BLED score of 1 (elderly). Together with her CHA_2DS_2-VASc score of 4, this indicates that the benefits of oral anticoagulation outweigh the risks of bleeding for

Table 2.4 HAS-BLED score

Risk factor for bleeding	Score
Hypertension (uncontrolled, SBP >160 mmHg)	1
Abnormal renal and/or liver function • Renal: dialysis, renal transplantation, serum creatinine >2.3 mg/dL (≥ 200 µmol/L) • Liver: chronic hepatic disease, bilirubin >2× upper limit of normal, AST/ALT/Alk Phos >3× upper limit of normal	1 or 2
Stroke	1
Bleeding (history or predisposition to bleeding)	1
Labile INRs (time in therapeutic range < 60%)	1
Elderly (> or = 65 years old)	1
Drugs (concomitant antiplatelet or non-steroidal anti-inflammatory agents) or alcohol (> or = 8 drinks per week)	1 or 2

our patient. The risk versus benefit of initiating anticoagulation therapy becomes a bit more blurred when the CHA_2DS_2-VASc score is ≥2 and the HAS-BLED score is ≥3, indicating that a patient is indicated for oral anticoagulation, but is also at high risk of developing a bleed. In situations like this, it is prudent to look at other risk factors for stroke and bleeding, as well as discussing the potential benefits and drawbacks of the different medications.

How Does a Clinician Choose Among the Various Agents for Stroke Prevention?

The ACTIVE-A trial showed that clopidogrel plus aspirin reduced the rate of major vascular events, including stroke, compared to aspirin monotherapy in patients with atrial fibrillation; however, an increase in major bleeding was found in the clopidogrel plus aspirin group [3]. The ACTIVE-W trial showed that warfarin is superior to clopidogrel plus aspirin in preventing strokes in patients with atrial fibrillation [4]. The overall rate of major bleeding was similar between the two groups in ACTIVE-W; however there was an increased number of intracranial bleeds in the warfarin group [4]. Aspirin monotherapy or aspirin plus clopidogrel combination therapy should be considered in patients at low risk for stroke or in patients in whom oral anticoagulation is contraindicated or where the risks outweigh the benefits. A discussion with the patient and family members/caregivers may yield useful information that can help distinguish which patients are better suited for a particular medication; this can include the patient or family's preference, a history of non-adherence with medications or appointments, and/or patients with a history of falls/bleeds.

When choosing between warfarin and the direct oral anticoagulants (DOACs) (dabigatran, rivaroxaban, apixaban, edoxaban), it should be noted that the DOACs are not indicated if a patient has valvular atrial fibrillation or extremely poor renal function; additionally, edoxaban should not be used if a patient has a CrCl >95 mL/min [5]. Warfarin does not have these limitations. However, there are also other factors to assess including cost, adherence, drug interactions, monitoring, and patient preference. For our patient, she would be eligible for either warfarin or one of the DOACs; the exact drug could only be chosen after a thorough discussion with the patient. This discussion can include the following points:

- The patient's risk for stroke using their individual CHA_2DS_2-VASc score
- The patient's risk for major bleed using their HAS-BLED score
- The possible medication options for the patient based on the above scoring systems
- Patient-specific factors that may make one or more medications more preferable compared to others. Table 2.5 discusses some key points that the clinician can use when deciding between options. While certain medications may be preferable due to patient-specific characteristics, ultimately the final decision comes down to shared decision making between the clinician and patient/family.

Table 2.5 Considerations for clinical decision making with oral anticoagulation therapy [5–9]

Issue/concern	Drugs to consider	Drugs to avoid	Comments
Non-adherence to medication doses	Warfarin	Dabigatran Rivaroxaban Apixaban Edoxaban	The DOACs in general are not ideal medications if patients cannot reliably adhere to the prescribed regimen as even one missed dose can put the patient at risk for stroke. Both dabigatran and apixaban are dosed twice daily which can further decrease adherence
Non-adherence to medical appointments	Dabigatran Rivaroxaban Apixaban Edoxaban	Warfarin	
Cost	Warfarin	Dabigatran Rivaroxaban Apixaban Edoxaban	Since the DOACs are relatively new to the market, there are no generic equivalents currently available
GI bleed	Warfarin	Dabigatran	
Renal dose adjustments	Warfarin	Dabigatran Apixaban Rivaroxaban Edoxban	For apixban, if patients have at least two of the following characteristics, a dose adjustment is warranted: age $\geq$ 80 years old, weight $\leq$ 60 kg, or SCr $\geq$ 1.5 mg/dL. In addition to renally adjusting doses due to reduced kidney function, do not use edoxaban in patients with CrCL > 95 mlm/min
Availability of an antidote	Warfarin Dabigatran	Rivaroxaban Apixaban Edoxaban	
Less laboratory monitoring	Dabigatran Rivaroxaban Apixaban Edoxban	Warfarin	
Drug interactions	Dabigatran Rivaroxaban Apixaban Edoxaban	Warfarin	Although the DOACs do not interact with as many medications as warfarin, caution should still be exercised when using these medications, especially if medications go through certain pathways (see cases 28–31 for more information). There are several examples of drug interactions with warfarin that may make DOACs preferable such as amiodarone or frequent antibiotic use

Key Points

- Calculate a CHA_2DS_2-VASc score in order to assess a patient's annual risk for stroke.
- Calculate a HAS-BLED score in order to assess a patient's risk for bleeding.

- A HAS-BLED score of ≥3 does not preclude a patient from starting or continuing oral anticoagulation. Modify any risk factors for bleeding if possible.
- Medication options for stroke prevention include aspirin, aspirin plus clopidogrel, warfarin, dabigatran, rivaroxaban, apixaban, or edoxaban.
- Take into account patient-specific factors when deciding between warfarin and the DOACs, including cost, adherence, drug interactions, monitoring, and patient preference.

Self-Assessment Questions

1. A 66 year old male patient just got out of surgery for bioprosthetic aortic valve replacement. He has a past medical history of atrial fibrillation, hypertension, gout, and BPH. Prior to this hospital admission and surgery, his medications included apixaban, lisinopril, HCTZ, and tamsulosin. His labs and renal function are all within normal limits. Which of the following medications is the best for this patient's anticoagulation needs?

   (a) Apixaban
   (b) Warfarin with goal INR 2.0–3.0
   (c) Warfarin with goal INR 2.5–3.5
   (d) Aspirin plus clopidogrel

   The correct answer is B. The patient's CHA_2DS_2-VASc score is 2 (1 point each for age and hypertension) which indicates that anticoagulation is still needed in this patient. His HAS-BLED score is 1 for being over 65 years old which indicates that his risk of a major bleed is not high. The patient now has valvular atrial fibrillation due to the aortic valve replacement so he will not be able to continue on apixaban or start any of the other DOACs, which makes answer A incorrect. He does not have mechanical mitral valve replacement which makes answer C incorrect. Warfarin was shown to be superior to aspirin plus clopidogrel in preventing strokes in patients with atrial fibrillation, so answer D is also incorrect.

2. A 54 year old female patient with newly diagnosed non-valvular atrial fibrillation is ready to start on a medication for stroke prevention. She would ideally like something that is taken once a day with minimal appointments needed as she works full time. Her past medical history is significant for hypertension, type 2 diabetes, GERD, and seasonal allergies. Her medications include metformin XR, omeprazole, and loratadine. Her estimated CrCl is >100 mL/min; all other labs and vitals are within normal limits. Which of the following medications would be best suited for this patient?

   (a) Warfarin
   (b) Apixaban
   (c) Dabigatran
   (d) Edoxaban
   (e) Rivaroxaban

The correct answer is E. Her CHA_2DS_2-VASc score is 3 (hypertension, diabetes, female sex) which indicates that oral anticoagulation is needed. This patient prefers once daily medications which would make answers B and C incorrect; if she is unable to adhere to a twice daily regimen, she may miss a dose which would put her at risk for stroke. Additionally she has a CrCl >95 mL/min which would make answer D incorrect. Answer A is incorrect since the patient states she would like a medication that required minimal appointments due to her work schedule.

References

1. January CT, Wann LS, Alpert JS, et al. 2014 AHA/ACC/HRS guideline for the management of patients with atrial fibrillation: a report of the American College of Cardiology/American Heart Association task force on practice guidelines and the Heart Rhythm Society. J Am Coll Cardiol. 2014;64:e1–e76.
2. Pisters R, Lane DA, Nieuwlaat R, et al. A novel user-friendly score (HAS-BLED) to assess 1-year risk of major bleeding in patients with atrial fibrillation: the euro heart survey. Chest. 2010;138:1093–100.
3. Connolly SJ, Pogue J, Hart RG, et al. Effect of clopidogrel added to aspirin in patients with atrial fibrillation. N Engl J Med. 2009;360:2066–78.
4. Connolly SJ, Pogue J, Hart R, et al. Clopidogrel plus aspirin versus oral anticoagulation for atrial fibrillation in the Atrial fibrillation Clopidogrel Trial with Irbesartan for prevention of Vascular Events (ACTIVE W): a randomised controlled trial. Lancet. 2006;367:1903–12.
5. Savaysa [package insert]. Parsippany, NJ: Daiichi Sankyo, Inc; 2015.
6. Coumadin [package insert]. Princeton, NJ: Bristol-Myers Squibb Company; 2015.
7. Pradaxa [package insert]. Ridgefield, CT: Boehringer-Ingelheim Pharmaceuticals, Inc; 2015.
8. Xarelto [package insert]. Titusville, NJ: Janssen Pharmaceuticals, Inc; 2016.
9. Eliquis [package insert]. Princeton, NJ and New York, NY: Bristol-Myers Squibb Company and Pfizer, Inc; 2016.

Chapter 3
Male with Priority of Ischemic Stroke Reduction

David Parra and Augustus Hough

Abstract Although all direct oral anticoagulants compare equally or favorably versus warfarin in the prevention of stroke or systemic embolism in patients with non-valvular atrial fibrillation examination of stroke components in the pivotal trials with direct oral anticoagulants may influence selection.

Keywords Atrial fibrillation • Ischemic stroke • Hemorrhage • Risk stratification • Risk-benefit • Shared decision making

A 77-year-old male presents to office for initiation of oral anticoagulation for non-valvular atrial fibrillation. He has a past medical history of hypertension (controlled with an average of previous months readings of 136/72 mmHg), type 2 diabetes, osteoarthritis of the knees, benign prostatic hypertrophy, and insomnia. His $CHADS_2$ score is 3, with a CHA_2DS_2-VASc score of 4. Pertinent laboratory values include CrCl estimated by Cockcroft-Gault equation 105 mL/min and CBC within normal limits. Current medications include aspirin, simvastatin, lisinopril, amlodipine, terazosin, metformin, and zolpidem as needed. The patient reports his mother had a disabling stroke and after caring for her for year he wanted to avoid one "at all costs". After a discussion of the benefits and risks of oral anticoagulation he indicates a preference for the greatest possible stroke risk reduction, and places a lower priority on minimizing bleeding risk.

D. Parra, PharmD, FCCP, BCPS (✉)
Veterans Integrated Service Network 8 Pharmacy Benefits Management, Veterans Health Administration, Bay Pines, FL, USA

Department of Experimental and Clinical Pharmacology, University of Minnesota College of Pharmacy, Minneapolis, MN 55455, USA
e-mail: David.Parra@va.gov

A. Hough, PharmD, BCPS
West Palm Beach VA Medical Center,
7305 N. Military Trial, West Palm Beach, FL 33410-6400, USA
e-mail: Augustus.Hough@va.gov

© Springer International Publishing AG 2017
K. Kiser (ed.), *Oral Anticoagulation Therapy*,
DOI 10.1007/978-3-319-54643-8_3

Based on the above history, patient preferences, laboratory values, and current medications, what is the most appropriate oral anticoagulant to reduce ischemic stroke for this patient?

1. Apixaban
2. Dabigatran
3. Edoxaban
4. Rivaroxaban
5. Warfarin

Discussion

Although it is well accepted that oral anticoagulation is superior to antiplatelet therapy in reducing stroke and systemic embolism in patients with non-valvular atrial fibrillation it is less clear which oral anticoagulant, if any, is superior in reducing what is considered by many to be the most feared complication of atrial fibrillation; ischemic stroke. While each direct oral anticoagulant has been compared directly to warfarin there are no comparative data between the direct oral anticoagulants, and each of the pivotal trials comparing each individual agent to warfarin differed in regards to the degree of warfarin control, and thromboembolic risk of the patient populations studied. Nonetheless, since the primary endpoint of each of these pivotal trials was the same (stroke or systemic embolism) examination of the effects on the primary endpoint and its sub-components can provide general observations that may be useful in guiding selection of an agent in a patient whose primary objective is reducing ischemic stroke over other outcomes.

In the ROCKET AF trial rivaroxaban was demonstrated to be non-inferior when compared to warfarin with respect to stroke or systemic embolism [1]. An evaluation of the stroke components revealed no statistical difference between rivaroxaban or warfarin with respect to ischemic stroke. Similarly, in the ENGAGE AF-TIMI 48 trial both high dose (60 mg once daily adjusted to 30 mg once daily based on renal function) and low dose (30 mg once daily adjusted to 15 mg once daily based on renal function) edoxaban were demonstrated to be non-inferior when compared to warfarin with respect to stroke or systemic embolism [2]. However, an evaluation of the stroke components revealed that while there was no statistical difference between high dose edoxaban or warfarin with respect to ischemic stroke there was a statistically significant higher rate of ischemic stroke with low dose edoxaban versus warfarin. In contrast, in the ARISTOTLE trial apixaban was demonstrated to be superior when compared to warfarin with respect to stroke or systemic embolism [3]. Despite this, evaluation of the stroke components revealed no statistical difference between apixaban or warfarin with respect to ischemic or uncertain type of stroke (ischemic stroke was not reported individually). In the RE-LY trial high dose dabigatran (150 mg twice daily) was superior to warfarin and lower dose (110 mg twice daily) non-inferior to warfarin with respect to stroke or systemic embolism [4]. In addition, dabigatran 150 mg twice daily was superior to both warfarin and dabigatran

Table 3.1 Summary of clinical trial endpoint data for oral anticoagulants in atrial fibrillation

Trial	Drug	Primary endpoint result (stroke and systemic embolism) versus warfarin	Ischemic stroke endpoint[a] versus warfarin
ARISTOTLE	Apixaban	Superior	No difference
ENGAGE AF-TIMI 48	Edoxaban high dose	Non-inferior	No difference
	Edoxaban low dose	Non-inferior	Statistically higher with edoxaban low dose
RE-LY	Dabigatran 150 mg twice daily	Superior	Statistically lower with dabigatran 150 mg twice daily
	Dabigatran 110 mg twice daily	Non-inferior	No difference
ROCKET AF	Rivaroxaban	Non-inferior	No difference

[a]In the Aristotle and RE-LY this included ischemic or uncertain/unspecified type of stroke

110 mg twice daily with respect to ischemic or unspecified stroke. See Table 3.1 for summary of the results from these trials.

Given these findings and that the patient places reducing ischemic stroke as his highest priority with oral anticoagulation it would appear dabigatran 150 mg twice daily would be the most reasonable agent. Careful review of his renal function and concurrent medications do not provide any concerns with the selection of dabigatran. In the United States edoxaban would not be indicated per product labeling based upon his renal function (CrCl > 95 ml/min). He should be advised to discontinue aspirin when dabigatran is initiated as there is no additional benefit of aspirin in addition to oral anticoagulation in reducing stroke or systemic embolism in patients with non-valvular atrial fibrillation. Exceptions to this may be in patients with recent acute coronary syndromes, or coronary artery stenting.

Key Points

- All direct oral anticoagulants compare equally or favorably versus warfarin in the prevention of stroke or systemic embolism in patients with non-valvular atrial fibrillation.
- Direct comparison between direct oral anticoagulants in the prevention of stroke or systemic embolism in patients with non-valvular atrial fibrillation are not available.
- Examination of stroke components in the pivotal trials with direct oral anticoagulants reveals that only dabigatran 150 mg twice daily had statistically significant fewer cases of ischemic stroke versus warfarin.
- Dabigatran 150 mg twice daily may be preferred in patients whose primary priority is to reduce ischemic stroke and whom place lesser value on bleeding risks.

Self-Assessment Questions

1. Which of the following have been shown to be superior to warfarin in reducing the risk of stroke or systemic embolism in patients with non-valvular atrial fibrillation (select all that apply)?

    (a) apixaban at dose appropriate based on weight, renal function and age
    (b) dabigatran 150 mg twice daily
    (c) dabigatran 110 mg twice daily
    (d) edoxaban 60 mg once daily
    (e) rivaroxaban at dose appropriate based on renal function

    Correct answers: a (abixaban) and b (dabigatran 150 mg twice daily).

    Rationale: Both apixaban and high dose dabigatran (150 mg twice daily) demonstrated superiority to warfarin in reducing stroke or systemic embolism in patients with non-valvular atrial fibrillation (ARISTOTLE and RE-LY trials respectively). Rivaroxaban, dabigatran 110 mg twice daily, and edoxaban (high and low doses) all demonstrated non-inferiority to warfarin in reducing stroke or systemic embolism in patients with non-valvular atrial fibrillation (ROCKET AF, RE-LY, and ENGAGE AF-TIMI 48 trials respectively).

2. In a patient who places the greatest value in reducing ischemic stroke which of the following oral anticoagulants would be most appropriate for non-valvular atrial fibrillation?

    (a) apixaban at dose appropriate based on weight, renal function and age
    (b) dabigatran 150 mg twice daily
    (c) edoxaban 60 mg once daily
    (d) rivaroxaban at dose appropriate based on renal function

    Correct answer: b (dabigatran 150 mg twice daily).

    Rationale: When reviewing stroke endpoints in the pivotal trials comparing each direct oral anticoagulant with warfarin in patients with non-valvular atrial fibrillation only dabigatran 150 mg twice daily revealed a statistically significant difference (lower) in rates of ischemic stroke (RE-LY trial).

Disclaimer The views expressed in this chapter reflect those of the authors, and not necessarily those of the Department of Veterans Affairs

References

1. Patel MR, Mahaffey KW, Garg J, et al. For the ROCKET AF investigators. Rivaroxaban versus warfarin in non-valvular atrial fibrillation. N Engl J Med. 2011;365:1557–9.
2. Giugliano RP, Ruff CT, Braunwald E, et al. Edoxaban versus warfarin in patients with atrial fibrillation. N Engl J Med. 2013;369:2093–104.
3. Granger CG, Alexander JH, McMurray JJV, et al. For the ARISTOTLE Committees and Investigators. Apixaban versus warfarin in patients with atrial fibrillation. N Engl J Med 2011;365:981–92.
4. Connolly SJ, Ezekowitz MD, Yusuf S, et al. on behalf of the RE-LY Steering Committee and Investigators. Dabigatran versus warfarin in patients with atrial fibrillation. N Engl J Med. 2009;361:1139–51.

Chapter 4
Choosing an Anticoagulant in an Elderly Patient

Jena I. Burkhart

Abstract Elderly patients pose a difficult treatment dilemma for clinicians in terms of deciding upon an anticoagulant to minimize the patient's risk for thromboembolism, stroke or death, with the potential for increasing the risk of a potentially serious bleeding event (e.g., a recurrent GI bleed or intracerebral hemorrhage). Validated clinical tools exist to assess embolic vs. bleeding risk and these tools can assist clinicians in deciding upon the most appropriate anticoagulant choice in this special patient population.

Keywords Elderly • Atrial fibrillation • Thromboembolism • Stroke • Bleeding • Practical considerations

Case Introduction

Lucy is an 88-year-old female with a long history of hypertension, heart failure (HF), CKD stage 4 (last CrCl estimated 20 mL/min), and hypothyroidism. She also has a history of hospitalization for gastrointestinal (GI) bleeding due to *H. pylori* infection 1.5 years ago. She was discharged from the hospital several days ago after being admitted for a TIA and new onset atrial fibrillation (AF). The patient was referred to her PCP after discharge from the hospital for further evaluation of her AF and anticoagulation treatment options. The patient is currently taking esomeprazole for h/o *H. pylori*, as well as furosemide, metoprolol, lisinopril, levothyroxine, calcitriol, and acetaminophen. Which anticoagulant treatment is most appropriate given the patient's age and medical history?

J.I. Burkhart, PharmD, BCPS, CPP
Geriatrics Specialty Clinic, UNC Medical Center,
6011 Farrington Rd, Bldg 100, Suite 101, Chapel Hill, NC 27517, USA
e-mail: jena.ivey@unchealth.unc.edu

Case Discussion

There are several main concerns to take into consideration when treating patients of this nature with anticoagulants. These include recurrence of GI bleed or other bleeding event, recent TIA and risk for a subsequent event, and worsening of Afib leading to worsened HF.

This patient, an elderly woman with newly diagnosed atrial fibrillation and recent TIA, is at risk for both recurrent stroke and bleeding. This case represents a common challenge frequently faced by clinicians, who must weigh the benefits of beginning treatment with an anticoagulant to minimize the patient's risk for thromboembolism, stroke or death from atrial fibrillation, with the potential for increasing the risk of a potentially serious bleeding event (e.g., a recurrent GI bleed or intracerebral hemorrhage). The decision is difficult, and in many cases concerns about bleeding may lead to the decision not to prescribe an anticoagulant. Therefore, many patients who are appropriate candidates for an anticoagulant may not be treated [1, 2]. To further complicate the therapeutic decision, there is also consideration warranted for initiation of antiplatelet therapy with aspirin after a TIA/ischemic stroke. In a recent study by Rothwell and colleagues, pooled data from all randomized trials of aspirin versus control in secondary prevention after TIA or ischemic stroke demonstrated that intervention with aspirin substantially reduced the risk of recurrent stroke particularly when given in the first 6 weeks after the initial event [3]. So at this juncture, would aspirin or warfarin, or both be warranted? This decision is not exactly clear and warrants careful consideration based on the patient's unique characteristics, balancing risks vs. benefits of combination therapy vs. warfarin alone.

Data indicates that only about 50% of patients with AF in either hospital or ambulatory care settings who are at high risk for stroke receive a vitamin K antagonist (VKA) [4]. This "underanticoagulation" represents a critical need, and is a major public health issue, as it leaves many patients at risk for thromboembolism or stroke. Regarding patients who are treated with VKAs, it is important to clarify a common concern related to the risk for bleeding when the INR is elevated. It is widely accepted that an INR range of 2.0–3.0 is the appropriate goal for most patients with nonvalvular AF. An INR below 2.0 may lead to ischemic stroke of death; conversely, an INR above 4.0 is associated with an increased risk for intracranial bleeding [5].

What is the patient's CHA_2DS_2-VASc risk stratification score, and given this, what is her risk for stroke (low vs. moderate vs. high)?

Tools for assessing stroke risk, such as $CHADS_2$ or CHA_2DS_2-VASc are options for use in clinical practice. The CHA_2DS_2-VASc tool is similar to the $CHADS_2$ tool, however is also includes the risk factors of female gender and vascular disease, and age-related risk begins at the age of 65 years [6]. The CHA_2DS_2-VASc tool has been shown to improve stroke risk prediction and help identify more patients who may be ideal for anticoagulation therapy for stroke reduction. The CHA_2DS_2-VASc score is based on a point system, with 1 point assigned for each of the following:

female sex, CHF, HTN, Age 65–74 years, diabetes, and vascular disease (history of MI, PAD, or aortic atherosclerosis); 2 points are assigned for prior stroke/TIA and age ≥ 75 years. This patient's CHA_2DS_2-VASc score is 7 (maximum possible score 9), placing her at high risk for stroke, with an estimated unadjusted ischemic stroke rate of approximately 11.2% per year [6]. Based on the 2012 focused updates for the management of AF developed by the American College of Cardiology, the American Heart Associated and the European Society of Cardiology, treatment with a VKA is indicated [7].

What do you think her risk of bleeding is based on the HAS-BLED score?

Older patients are generally at high risk for thromboembolism, yet they are also at increased risk for anticoagulant-related bleeding [8]. Therefore, a balanced assessment should also include the patient's bleeding risk.

There are several clinical prediction tools available to evaluate bleeding risk in patients on an anticoagulant [8]. One tool, HAS-BLED, has been incorporated into the 2010 ESC guidelines, and the Canadian guidelines for managing AF. Based on the information in the case, the patient's HAS-BLED score is ≥3, meaning she is a "high risk" for bleeding [9, 10].

What are the anticoagulant treatment options that exist for Lucy and how do you decide on the most appropriate one?

Given Lucy is deemed at high risk for an embolic event, if sole therapy with an anticoagulant is preferred, her anticoagulant treatment options would be: warfarin treated with an INR goal of 2.0–3.0, or one of the direct oral anticoagulants (DOACs)—dabigatran, apixaban, rivaroxaban, and edoxaban. Warfarin has long been considered the cornerstone of anticoagulant therapy for prevention of stroke in patients with atrial fibrillation. The benefits of warfarin over aspirin in older patients with atrial fibrillation is well validated [11]. However, warfarin can pose challenges in its use given its multitude of drug-drug, drug-food interactions, and the necessity for close monitoring of INR values. Since the DOACs do not require routine laboratory monitoring, may be less susceptible to dietary and drug interactions, and do not have warfarin's narrow therapeutic window, their use may be attractive for the older adult patient who has limited ability to attend anticoagulation clinics, is taking multiple medications, and is at increased risk for bleeding and/or thrombosis. Anticoagulation with each of these DOACs led to similar or lower rates both of ischemic stroke and major bleeding compared to adjusted dose warfarin (INR of 2.0–3.0) in patients with nonvalvular AF in large randomized trials [12].

Despite the DOACs looking like extremely attractive options for an older adult, several practical considerations must be considered when weighing whether to use one versus warfarin in elderly patients. Two of the DOACs (dabigatran and apixaban) require twice daily dosing, and dabigatran's package insert recommends that is be stored in the original dispensed bottle only to protect from light [13]. Twice daily dosing is often not practical in older patients and the inability of dabigatran to be placed in a weekly pillbox may render its administration unreliable [14]. Cost is also a very important consideration, with the DOACs costing considerably more than warfarin for a 30-day supply. Finally, renal function status must be taken into account when deciding on a DOAC vs. warfarin. Most of the DOACs are contraindicated in patients with chronic severe kidney disease whose estimated glomerular filtration rate is less than 30 mL/min. Warfarin can be safely and effectively used in severe kidney disease with close follow-up and monitoring. Other disadvantages of the DOACs include lack of easily available monitoring of blood levels and compliance, lack of FDA-approval as an anticoagulant option for those patients with prosthetic valves, and the potential that unanticipated side effects becoming evident with long-term use.

In conclusion, when deciding on an appropriate anticoagulant treatment for an older individual, it is extremely important to be aware of both stroke and bleeding risk assessment tools, and that the clinician weighs the risks vs. the benefits of the individual agents to ensure the safest, most appropriate option is chosen for the unique patient.

Key Points

- Clinicians are often faced with the challenge of weighing the benefits of beginning treatment with an anticoagulant to minimize the patient's risk for thromboembolism, stroke or death, with the potential for increasing the risk of a potentially serious bleeding event (e.g., a recurrent GI bleed or intracerebral hemorrhage), especially in extremely elderly individuals.
- The CHA_2DS_2-VASc tool as well as the HAS-BLED tool are validated, easy to use clinical tools that can help in assessing risk for embolic event vs. risk for bleeding.
- There are several treatment options available for the prevention of stroke in patients with atrial fibrillation and when treating elderly patients, each option must be given careful consideration when deciding upon the best agent for that individual patient.
- When deciding on an appropriate anticoagulant treatment for an older individual, it is extremely important to be aware of both stroke and bleeding risk assessment tools.

Self-Assessment Questions

1. Which of the following patients would be the BEST candidate for DOAC therapy?
    (a) A 80yo patient with AF, CHA_2DS_2-VASc score = 5, severe hepatic dysfunction, and mitral valve stenosis
    (b) A 88yo patient with AF, CHA_2DS_2-VASc score = 7, and has had a prior GI bleed requiring transfusion and ICU stay

(c) A 77yo patient with recurrent stroke and afib, and INR is highly variable on warfarin due to non-adherence with the medication

(d) A 72yo patient with CHA_2DS_2-VASc score of 6, with afib and a new onset DVT, is homebound, and a CrCl of 50 mL/min

Correct answer: c.

Answer a. although risk score is high enough to warrant anticoagulation, not a candidate for a DOAC because of the patient's hepatic dysfunction.

Answer b. not the best candidate for a DOAC due to prior history of GIB requiring transfusion, at high risk for recurrence and minimal reversal options at this time.

Answer c. is likely not a candidate as patient has problems with adherence. Adherence is still crucial with the DOACs for them to be optimally effective.

Answer d. is the BEST options as patient has an appropriate FDA indication for a DOAC, has adequate renal function to safely take a DOAC, and the homebound status makes monitoring warfarin a challenge.

2. Which is the preferred oral anticoagulant for patients with a prosthetic valve?

   (a) Warfarin
   (b) Dabigatran
   (c) Rivaroxaban
   (d) Apixaban
   (e) Edoxaban

Correct answer: a. warfarin is the only agent mentioned in the list that is also FDA indicated for stroke prevention in patients with a prosthetic valve.

References

1. Lane DA, Lip GYH. Maintaining therapeutic anticoagulation: the importance of keeping "within range". Chest. 2007;131:1277–9.
2. Wittkowsky AK. Effective anticoagulation therapy: defining the gap between clinical studies and clinical practice. Am J Manag Care. 2004;10:S297–306.
3. Rothwell P, Algra A, Chen Z, et al. Effects of aspirin on risk and severity of early recurrent stroke after transient ischemic attack and ischemic stroke: time-course analysis of randomized trials. Lancet. Published online May 18, 2016. doi:10.1016/S0140-6736(16)30468-8.
4. Waldo AL, Beck RC, Tapson VF, et al. For the NABOR steering committee. Hospitalized patient with atrial fibrillation and a high risk for stroke are not being provided with adequate anticoagulation. J Am Coll Cardiol. 2005;46(9):1729–36.
5. Fuster V, Rydén LE, Asinger RW, et al. ACC/AHA/ESC guidelines for the management of patients with atrial fibrillation: executive summary. J Am Coll Cardiol. 2001;38(4):1231–66.
6. Lip GHY, Nieuwlaat R, Pisters R, et al. Refining clinical risk stratification for predicting stroke and thromboembolism in atrial fibrillation using a novel risk factor based approach: The Euro Heart Study on Atrial Fibrillation. Chest. 2010;137(2):263–72.
7. Friberg L, Rosenqvist M, Lip GYH. Evaluation of risk stratification schemes for ischemic stroke and bleeding in 182,678 patients with atrial fibrillation: the Swedish Atrial Fibrillation cohort study. Eur Heart J. 2012;33(12):1500–10.

8. You JJ, Singer DE, Howard PA, et al. Antithrombotic therapy for atrial fibrillation. Chest. 2012;141(2 Suppl):e531S–75S.
9. Lip GYH, Andreotti F, Fauchier L, et al. Bleeding risk assessment and management in atrial fibrillation patients: a position document from the European Heart Rhythm Association, endorsed by the European Society of Cardiology Working Group on Thrombosis. Europace. 2011;13:723–46.
10. Camm JA, Kirchoff P, Lip GYH, et al. The Task Force for the Management of Atrial Fibrillation of the European Society of Cardiology. Eur Heart J. 2010;31:2369–29.
11. Cairns JA, Connolly S, McMurtry S, et al. CCS Atrial Fibrillation Guidelines Committee. Canadian Cardiovascular Society atrial fibrillation guidelines 2010: prevention of stroke and systemic thromboembolism in atrial fibrillation and flutter. Can J Cardiol. 2011;27:74–90.
12. van Walraven C, Hart RG, Connolly S, et al. Effect of age on stroke prevention therapy in patients with atrial fibrillation: the atrial fibrillation investigators. Stroke. 2009;40(4):1410–6.
13. Ruff CT, Giugliano RP, Braunwald E, et al. Comparison of the efficacy and safety of new oral anticoagulants with warfarin in patients with atrial fibrillation: a meta-analysis of randomised trials. Lancet. 2014;383(9921):955–62.
14. Dabigatran Package Insert. http://docs.boehringer-ingelheim.com/Prescribing%20Information/PIs/Pradaxa/Pradaxa.pdf. Accessed 29 Apr 16.

Chapter 5
Patient with Prior History of GI Hemorrhage

Michael Brenner and David Parra

Abstract The benefits of using anticoagulants for stroke prevention in atrial fibrillation patients with prior GI bleed can outweigh the risks. Selecting warfarin or a direct oral anticoagulant with a similar incidence of GI bleeding compared to warfarin should be considered to minimize the risk for bleeding.

Keywords Anticoagulation • GI hemorrhage • Atrial fibrillation • Direct oral anticoagulants • DOACs • Warfarin

Case Introduction

A 68 year old male is diagnosed with non-valvular atrial fibrillation. Past medical history consists of hypertension, type 2 diabetes, heart failure with reduced ejection fraction, (echocardiogram 1 year ago revealed LVEF of 35% and normal valvular function) and upper gastrointestinal (GI) bleed 2 months ago while on aspirin enteric-coated 81 mg per day. At the time of the GI bleed the patient presented to the Emergency Room with hypotension and a hemoglobin of 6. He received 3 units of packed red blood cells and underwent esophagogastroduodenoscopy with successful sclerotherapy of a large peptic ulcer. Aspirin was discontinued and a proton pump inhibitor was initiated at that time. The patient has a CHA_2DS_2-VASc score of 4 and $CHADS_2$ score of 3 as well as a HAS-BLED score is 3. After discussion of

---

M. Brenner, PharmD, BCPS (✉)
VA Ann Arbor Healthcare System, 2215 Fuller Road, Ann Arbor, MI, USA
e-mail: Michael.Brenner@va.gov

D. Parra, PharmD, FCCP, BCPS
Veterans Integrated Service Network 8 Pharmacy Benefits Management, Veterans Health Administration, Bay Pines, FL, USA

Department of Experimental and Clinical Pharmacology, University of Minnesota College of Pharmacy, Minneapolis, MN, USA
e-mail: David.Parra@va.gov

the risks and benefits of anticoagulation he agrees to therapy. The patient has difficulty attending appointments due to lack of transportation and relies on his brother who works full-time. His medications consist of lisinopril, metoprolol succinate, omeprazole and metformin. A review of the patient's medication refill history reveals good compliance. He reports no known drug allergies. He denies alcohol, tobacco, and illicit drug use. All labs are within normal limits. The patient's estimated CrCl based on Cockcroft-Gault equation is 85 mL/min.

Based on the case description, what is the preferred anticoagulant for this patient?

1. Warfarin
2. Apixaban
3. Dabigatran
4. Edoxaban
5. Rivaroxaban

Case Discussion

Given a diagnosis of atrial fibrillation with a CHA_2DS_2-VASc risk score of 4 (age, hypertension, heart failure, and type 2 diabetes) and $CHADS_2$ score of 3 (hypertension, heart failure, and diabetes mellitus), anticoagulation should be considered in this patient to reduce the risk for stroke. The patient's HAS-BLED score of 3 indicates the patient is at high risk for major bleeding which should be taken into account when selecting an agent. Other considerations that factor into selecting an appropriate anticoagulant are presence of valvular disease, age, bleeding risk, drug-drug and drug-food interactions, renal and hepatic function, complete blood count, medication adherence, patient preference, financial considerations, and ability and willingness to attend appointments.

Given that this patient has a history of a GI bleed on aspirin, choosing an anticoagulant must be done with thoughtful consideration. A history of GI bleeding does not eliminate the use of anticoagulants if the benefits outweigh the risk. However, the cause, length of time since the bleed, severity and risk of recurrence of the bleed, as well as concomitant aggravating (e.g. additional antiplatelet or non-steroidal anti-inflammatory agents) and protective (e.g. proton pump inhibitors) factors at the time of the bleed must all be given thoughtful consideration prior to initiation of anticoagulation. For example, GI bleeding secondary to arteriovenous malformations, esophageal varices, ulcerative colitis, or an unidentified source may influence the decision differently than bleeding due to a source with a known cause (e.g. NSAIDs, infectious diarrhea, colon polyps, hemorrhoids, or anal fissures) that can be successfully treated. Consultation with specialty services (e.g. gastroenterology/hepatology) may be warranted to fully estimate risk of recurrence. If a GI bleed occurs while on an anticoagulant, consideration to resume therapy should be done once the patient is hemodynamically stable. A cohort study revealed that not restarting warfarin after a GI bleed was associated with an increased risk for thrombosis and death compared to patients who were restarted. Resuming warfarin between

5 Patient with Prior History of GI Hemorrhage   27

Table 5.1 Summary of clinical trial data for oral anticoagulants incidence of GI bleeding

Trial	Drug	Incidence of GI bleeding versus warfarin
ARISTOTLE	Apixaban	No difference
ENGAGE AF-TIMI 48	Edoxaban LD	Statistically lower with edoxaban LD
	Edoxaban HD	Statistically higher with edoxaban HD
RE-LY	Dabigatran 110 mg	No difference
	Dabigatran 150 mg	Statistically higher with dabigatran 150 mg
ROCKET AF	Rivaroxaban	Statistically higher with rivaroxaban

days 1 and 7 (median time for resumption was 4 days) after a GI bleed was associated with a lower risk of thrombosis. Although recurrent GI bleed was higher with resumption of warfarin, the risk was modest and nonsignificant [1]. This type of study has not been done with DOACs, but it may be reasonable to withhold therapy closer to 7 days after the bleed given their attainment of therapeutic anticoagulation is much quicker (within hours) than warfarin (days). Landmark trials studying DOACs have reported the incidence of GI bleeding as compared to warfarin (see Table 5.1 for summary of these results). In the RE-LY trial, the rate of major bleeding compared to warfarin was similar with dabigatran 150 mg twice daily and lower with dabigatran 110 mg twice daily. With regards to GI bleeding, dabigatran 150 mg had a higher incidence compared to warfarin, while dabigatran 110 mg had a similar incidence of GI bleeding to warfarin. Dabigatran 110 mg is not approved for use in the United States, but is available in other countries. [2]. Approximately 50% of the major GI bleeding events on both doses of dabigatran met the criteria for life-threatening bleeding, but the incidence was lower than warfarin. Criteria for life-threatening bleeding per the International Society on Thrombosis and Haemostasis (ISTH) is defined as fatal bleeding, symptomatic intracranial bleeding, bleeding with decrease of hemoglobin of ≥5 g/dL, bleeding requiring inotropic support, bleeding requiring surgery, or transfusion of ≥4 units of packed red blood cells. In the ROCKET-AF trial, rivaroxaban demonstrated a similar incidence of major and non-major clinically relevant bleeding compared to warfarin. However, the incidence of GI bleeding was significantly higher with rivaroxaban compared to warfarin, although the incidence of life-threatening GI bleeding was not different. Gastrointestinal bleeding included upper, lower, and rectal sites [3]. Of the GI bleeds that occurred, 87% did not meet criteria for life-threatening bleeds which was defined as transfusion of ≥4 g/dL of red blood cells. In the ENGAGE-AF-TIMI 48 trial the rate of major bleeding was significantly higher with warfarin compared with edoxaban high dose (HD) and edoxaban low dose (LD). Edoxaban HD was defined as 60 mg (adjusted to 30 mg based on renal function) and LD was defined as 30 mg (adjusted to 15 mg based on renal function). The rate of GI bleeding was higher with edoxaban HD and lower with edoxaban LD in comparison to warfarin, and both met statistical significance [4]. In the ARISTOTLE trial, the rate of major bleeding was significantly lower with apixaban compared to warfarin. Unlike dabigatran, edoxaban and rivaroxaban, apixaban displayed a lower incidence of GI bleeding compared to warfarin, but was not statistically significant [5]. There is no published data that reports whether any of the GI bleeds met the ISTH criteria for life-threatening bleeding.

There are no drug-drug interactions that exist between the patient's current medication list and anticoagulants. Renal and hepatic function and complete blood count are normal. Transportation is a concern since the patient does not have a car and relies on his brother. Since the patient's sibling has full-time job, appointment compliance may not be optimal, which can affect routine INR monitoring with warfarin. DOACs do not require frequent monitoring, unlike warfarin; making these medications more advantageous in a situation where a patient cannot reliability attend regular appointments.

Dabigatran 150 mg, edoxaban HD, and rivaroxaban are not preferred first line anticoagulants for this patient as they have higher rates of GI bleed at normal doses compared to warfarin. Patient has normal renal function and thus reduced doses of the DOACs are not indicated. Apixaban has similar rates of GI bleeding to warfarin. Since appointment compliance may be difficult, apixaban would be preferred over warfarin for this patient. Dabigatran 110 mg could also be considered outside of the United States as a treatment option as this dose has similar rates of GI bleeding to warfarin.

Key Points

- In patients with non-valvular atrial fibrillation the CHA_2DS_2-VASc score should be used in conjunction with a bleeding risk score (e.g. HAS-BLED) to guide therapeutic decisions.
- The decision to anticoagulate a patient with non-valvular atrial fibrillation and a history of GI bleeding should incorporate the patients thromboembolic risk as well as patient specific factors surrounding the bleed such as location, cause, and risk of recurrence.
- Rivaroxaban and higher doses of dabigatran and edoxaban increase the risk of GI bleeding compared to warfarin in patients with non-valvular atrial fibrillation.
- In patients with a history of GI bleeding apixaban, lower dose dabigatran, or warfarin should be considered when a decision has been made to anticoagulate.

Self-Assessment Questions

1. Which of the following anticoagulant(s) did not have a higher incidence of GI bleeding compared to warfarin in patients with non-valvular atrial fibrillation?

    (a) Apixaban
    (b) Dabigatran 150 mg twice daily
    (c) Edoxaban HD once daily
    (d) Rivaroxaban

    Correct Answer: A (Apixaban)

Rationale: In the RE-LY, ENGAGE AF TIMI 48, and ROCKET-AF trial, both dabigatran and rivaroxaban respectively demonstrated a higher incidence of GI bleeding compared to warfarin. In the ARISTOTLE trial, the incidence of GI bleeding was similar between apixaban and warfarin.

2. Which anticoagulant has been shown to yield a higher rate of major bleeding than warfarin?

   (a) Apixaban
   (b) Edoxaban LD once daily
   (c) Dabigatran 150 mg twice daily
   (d) Rivaroxaban
   (e) None of the above

Correct Answer: C (Dabigatran 150 mg twice daily)

Rationale: Major bleeding was similar between dabigatran 150mg, rivaroxaban, edoxaban LD once daily, and warfarin whereas apixaban yielded a lower rate than warfarin.

Disclaimer The views expressed in this presentation reflect those of the authors, and not necessarily those of the Department of Veterans Affairs.

References

1. Witt DM, Delate T, Garcia D, et al. Risk of thromboembolism, recurrent hemorrhage, and death after warfarin therapy interruption for gastrointestinal tract bleeding. Arch Intern Med. 2012;172(19):1484–91.
2. Connelly SJ, Ezekowitz MD, Yusuf S, et al., for the RE-LY Steering Committee and Investigators. Dabigatran versus warfarin in patients with atrial fibrillation. N Engl J Med. 2009;361:1139–51.
3. Patel MR, Mahaffey KW, Garg J, et al. Rivaroxaban versus warfarin in nonvalvular atrial fibrillation (ROCKET AF). N Engl J Med. 2011;365(10):883–91.
4. Giugliano RP, et al. Edoxaban versus warfarin in patients with atrial fibrillation. N Engl J Med. 2013;369(22):2093–104.
5. Granger CB, Alexander JH, McMurray JJV, et al. Apixaban versus warfarin in patients with atrial fibrillation (ARISTOTLE). N Engl J Med. 2011;365:981–92.

Chapter 6
Patients with a History of Intracranial Hemorrhage

Jordan D. Long and Douglas C. Anderson

Abstract Patients with prior intracranial hemorrhage may have indications that warrant the initiation of anticoagulant therapy. The decision if therapy should be initiated, how long after the ICH should therapy be started, and what therapy to use is vital to patient care and safety.

Keywords Anticoagulation • Stroke • Hemorrhagic stroke • Intracranial hemorrhage • Intracerebral hemorrhage • Subarachnoid hemorrhage • Intraventricular hemorrhage • Anticoagulant reinitiation

Case Introduction

MS is a 47 year old female who presented to the anticoagulation clinic with a complaint of "the worst headache I've ever had," asking to get her INR checked because she believed, "My blood is too thick." On triage by the pharmacist she was found to have slurred speech, blurred vision, and right-sided face drooping. She had been woken up in the middle of the night with the headache which grew progressively worse. An INR was checked and was found to be 4.2 (target 2.0–3.0) and blood pressure 187/103 mmHg. She was sent to the emergency department to rule out stroke. The patient had a medical history of atrial fibrillation, hypertension, type 2 diabetes, and hyperlipidemia. Her home medication list on admission included lisinopril, hydrochlorothiazide, metformin, atorvastatin, and warfarin. She was reportedly compliant with all medications. Her INR the previous month was 2.4 and she had been well controlled on her warfarin therapy. Recreational drug use included moderate alcohol use (1–2 drinks per month), no tobacco or illicit drug use. In the emergency department, warfarin was held and she was treated with intravenous

---

J.D. Long, PharmD, MBA (✉) • D.C. Anderson, PharmD, DPh
Pharmacy Practice Department, Cedarville University School of Pharmacy,
251 North Main Street, Cedarville, OH 45314, USA
e-mail: jordanlong@cedarville.edu; andersond@cedarville.edu

© Springer International Publishing AG 2017
K. Kiser (ed.), *Oral Anticoagulation Therapy*,
DOI 10.1007/978-3-319-54643-8_6

vitamin K 10 mg and prothrombin complex concentrate to reverse the anticoagulation. CT confirmed intracranial hemorrhage.

In treatment of ICH in patients on VKA therapy, rapid reversal of anticoagulation is recommended [1]. Current recommendations are that rapid reversal be accomplished using 4-factor prothrombin complex concentrate (PCC) which contains factors II, VII, IX, and X and does not require cross matching [2]. Vitamin K 5–10 mg by slow IV infusion should be added to PCC therapy rather than used alone. Fresh frozen plasma (FFP) and cryoprecipitate both require cross-matching and pose the risk of infusion reactions and thus PCC is preferred.

Irreversible cerebral hemorrhage has been reported with direct oral anticoagulants (DOACs) [3]. There is limited data on reversing these agents in the presence of ICH. Supportive measures, activated PCC, 4-factor PCC, antifibrinolytic agents (e.g. tranexamic acid, aminocaproic acid), and hemodialysis (for dabigatran) have all been suggested. The monoclonal antibody fragment idarucizumab has been approved for reversal of dabigatran-induced anticoagulation. In the RE-VERSE AD study, patients with atrial fibrillation were given two doses of idarucizumab 2.5 g 15 min apart [4]. This resulted in complete reversal of dilute thrombin time and ecarin clotting time within 10–30 min. For the anti-Xa agents, reversal with 4-factor PCC should provide the factor Xa needed to reverse the coagulopathy, though no data exist to guide therapy [5].

Anticoagulation therapy in patients with prior or recent intracranial hemorrhage is a complicated therapeutic decision that includes a lot of medical variables. Since stroke risk independently varies from patient to patient and with many options for inpatient and outpatient anticoagulant therapy, it is important to know when to anticoagulate a patient and what anticoagulant is best to use. No matter what decision is made in regards to anticoagulant therapy, a holistic approach should be taken when making a treatment plan for patients with a history of intracranial hemorrhage.

Preventing recurrent ICH is important in all patients who have a prior history of ICH. General steps for secondary cardiovascular risk reduction should be implemented. Blood pressure should be aggressively controlled; a long term goal of <130/80 mmHg should be attained for the best prevention of recurrence [1]. Blood glucose should also be tightly controlled (between 80 and 110 mg/dL). ICH patients who have recurrence have been shown to have improved outcomes if blood glucose is within goal on admission. Patients should avoid alcohol consumption of >2 drinks per day, while also abstaining from tobacco and illicit drug use. Admitted patients should be frequently ambulated and intermittent pneumatic compression should be used.

Multiple factors should be considered before a decision is made on whether to anticoagulate a patient or not. Location of the prior ICH is an important factor to consider. Patients with prior lobar ICH are at a higher risk of recurrence compared to patients with a prior deep ICH [1]. Presence of micro-bleeds and patients of older age increases the risk of recurrence, especially if the hemorrhage was in the lobar location. It is recommended that anticoagulant therapy not be restarted in patients with a previous lobar ICH [1]. Anticoagulant therapy may be considered for patients with prior non-lobar ICH, however, the indication for anticoagulation should be considered [1]. Patients with a mechanical heart valve replacement (MVR) would be at a higher risk of ischemic stroke compared to patients without MVR. There is currently no recommended time after cessation of ICH to restart anticoagulation. It has been suggested that patients with a mechanical heart valve should wait at least 4 weeks after cessation of prior ICH to reduce the risk of recurrent ICH [1]. Of note, none of the DOACs are approved for use in patients with MVR because of lack of studies showing their efficacy and safety in patients with an MVR. When the decision is made that anticoagulation therapy is not appropriate for patients, antiplatelet therapy may be appropriate in patients regardless of location of prior ICH [1]. Studies have not shown efficacy of antiplatelet therapy in patients with MVR, but can be used alone in patient with prosthetic heart valves to reduce the risk of ischemic stroke [6]. Appropriateness of antiplatelet therapy should be assessed in patients with prior ICH to reduce the risk of recurrence.

When the decision is made that anticoagulation therapy is needed in a patient with prior ICH, the choice of therapy is important to maintain proper anticoagulation while minimizing the risk of ICH recurrence. For patients that need VTE prophylaxis after an ICH, including patients with Factor V Leiden, Lupus anticoagulant, recurrent VTE, massive pulmonary embolism, or a high CHA_2DS_2-VASc, LMWH is the most appropriate option for reduction and can be given 1–4 days after onset if the patient is immobile [1]. For long term anticoagulant therapy, there are limited head to head comparisons between therapies in patients with prior ICH. In one meta-analysis, it was shown that a pooled group of patients on DOACs (dabigatran, edoxaban, apixaban, rivaroxaban) had less occurrence of hemorrhagic stroke compared to patients being treated with warfarin, regardless of prior ICH or not, in patients with atrial fibrillation [7]. In comparison of warfarin versus dabigatran in patients with atrial fibrillation, patients on dabigatran showed less occurrence of hemorrhagic stroke [8]. Heparins and LMWHs have not been studied significantly in this patient population and their benefit of use should be weighed against the risks. Current ACC/AHA guidelines state that the usefulness of DOACs in patients with a history of ICH to reduce recurrence in uncertain [1].

The time to wait after ICH to restart anticoagulation therapy can vary among patients and depends on the risk factors of recurrent ICH and thromboembolism. In one study, the estimated optimal time to restart long-term anticoagulation therapy has been shown to be between 10 and 30 weeks after ICH [9]. In other reports, restarting long-term anticoagulation therapy between 1 and 3 weeks after ICH has been argued in patients with a high risk of thromboembolism and low risk of recurrent ICH. An evaluation of the patient is critical to ensure that the benefits heavily outweigh the risks of anticoagulation before restarting therapy so early after an ICH [5].

Key Points

- Preventative measures, such as tightly controlling blood pressure and glucose, limiting alcohol consumption, and abstaining from tobacco and alcohol, are important in patients that have a history of hemorrhagic stroke.
- In patients with a prior ICH and a mechanical heart valve, warfarin should be used with the appropriate INR goals because of proven efficacy.
- In patients with atrial fibrillation (without a mechanical heart valve) with a history of ICH who are at a high risk of thromboembolism, including patients with coagulopathies or a high CHA_2DS_2-VASc, can be restarted on warfarin, DOACs, or LMWHs.
- The time after ICH to restart anticoagulant therapy varies among patients, depending on thromboembolic risk and risk of ICH recurrence.
- Patients with prior ICH should be educated on the risks of restarting anticoagulant therapy, including the signs and symptoms of recurrent ICH.

Self-Assessment Questions

1. Which one of the following characteristics is most likely to increase the risk of recurrent intracerebral hemorrhage?

    (a) previous ICH without micro-bleeds
    (b) previous lobar ICH
    (c) previous TIA
    (d) controlled blood pressure

    Correct Answer: B. Previous lobar intracerebral hemorrhage.

    Answer B is correct. Patients with a lobar ICH have a high risk of recurrence. It is recommended that patients with a previous lobar ICH not be restarted on anticoagulant therapy. Answer A is incorrect because ICH without micro-bleeds has a decreased risk of recurrence compared to the presence of micro-bleeds. Answer C and D are incorrect because history of TIA and controlled blood pressure do not increase your risk of ICH over the other options.

2. What is the appropriate time to wait before restarting long-term anticoagulation (if indicated) after an intracerebral hemorrhage?

    (a) 1–3 days
    (b) 1 week
    (c) 10 and 30 weeks
    (d) After 40 weeks

    Correct answer: C. Between 10 and 30 weeks.

    Answer C is the correct answer. A retrospective study looking at the outcomes of patients restarted on long-term anticoagulation therapy showed that patients restarted on therapy between 10 and 30 weeks had better outcomes than other times. Patients needing VTE prophylaxis can be started on LMWH days after an ICH, but this is only for immobile patients and is at a prophylactic dose.

References

1. Hemphill JC, Greenberg SM, Anderson CS, et al. Guidelines for the management of spontaneous intracerebral hemorrhage. Stroke. 2015;46(7):2032–60. doi:10.1161/str.0000000000000069.
2. Holbrook A, Schulman S, Witt DM, et al. Evidence-based Management of Anticoagulant Therapy: antithrombotic therapy and prevention of thrombosis, 9th ed: American College of Chest Physicians evidence-based clinical practice guidelines. Chest. 2012;141(2):152–84. doi:10.1378/chest.11-2295.
3. Garber ST, Sivakumar W, Schmidt RH. Neurosurgical complications of direct thrombin inhibitors—catastrophic hemorrhage after mild traumatic brain injury in a patient receiving dabigatran. J Neurosurg. 2012;116(5):1093–6. doi:10.3171/2012.2.JNS112132.
4. Pollack CV, Reilly PA, Eikelboom J, et al. Idarucizumab for dabigatran reversal. N Engl J Med. 2015;373(6):511–20. doi:10.1056/nejmoa1502000.
5. Hankey GJ, Norrving B, Hacke W, et al. Management of acute stroke in patients taking novel oral anticoagulants. Stroke. 2014;9:627–32. doi:10.1111/ijs.12295.
6. Nishimura RA, Otto CM, Bonow RO, et al. 2014 AHA/ACC guideline for the management of patients with valvular heart disease: executive summary: a report of the American College of Cardiology/American Heart Association Task Force on Practice Guidelines. Circulation. 2014;129(23):2440–92. doi:10.1161/cir.0000000000000029.
7. Ruff CT, Gugliano RP, Braunwald E, et al. Comparison of the efficacy and safety of new oral anticoagulants with warfarin in patients with atrial fibrillation: a meta-analysis of randomized trials. Lancet. 2013;383(9921):955–62. doi:10.1016/s0140-6736(13)62343-0.
8. Hori M, Connolly SJ, Zhu J, et al. Dabigatran versus warfarin: effects on ischemic and hemorrhagic strokes and bleeding in Asians and non-Asians with atrial fibrillation. Stroke. 2013;44(7):1891–6.
9. Majeed A, Kim YK, Roberts RS, et al. Optimal timing of resumption of warfarin after intracranial hemorrhage. Stroke. 2010;41:2860–6.

Chapter 7
Concerns with Anticoagulant Adherence

David Parra and Michael Brenner

Abstract Non-adherence to oral anticoagulation increases the risk of thromboembolism underscoring the need for effective evaluation of adherence and implementation of strategies to improve adherence. Assessment of the patient's priorities and preferences, understanding of medical conditions and expectations of therapies, adverse effect concerns, affordability of therapy, and understanding of renewal/refill process should all be considered when selecting an oral anticoagulant.

Keywords Medication adherence • Medication compliance • Enhancing medication adherence • Patient adherence • Treatment adherence • Adverse outcomes • Dosing regimens • Shared decision making • Drug storage

A 65-year-old male presents to his primary care providers office for routine follow-up. He has a past medical history of non-valvular atrial fibrillation, coronary artery disease (history of myocardial infarction 2007 with subsequent four vessel coronary artery bypass grafting), history of transient ischemic attack, type 2 diabetes, hypertension, dyslipidemia, and mild cognitive impairment. Pertinent laboratory data includes CrCl as estimated by Cockcroft-Gault equation 118 mL/min, CBC within normal limits, and a low density lipoprotein cholesterol level of 185mg/dL (baseline 200mg/dL). Blood pressure in the office is 158/88 mmHg and he reports he does not measure it at home. Current medications include dabigatran 150 mg by mouth twice daily, losartan, hydrochlorothiazide, nifedipine, doxazosin, metoprolol tartrate,

---

D. Parra, PharmD, FCCP, BCPS (✉)
Veterans Integrated Service Network 8 Pharmacy Benefits Management, Veterans Health Administration, Bay Pines, FL, USA

Department of Experimental and Clinical Pharmacology, University of Minnesota College of Pharmacy, Minneapolis, MN 55455, USA
e-mail: David.Parra@va.gov

M. Brenner, PharmD, BCPS
VA Ann Arbor Healthcare System, 2215 Fuller Road, Ann Arbor, MI, USA
e-mail: Michael.Brenner@va.gov

© Springer International Publishing AG 2017
K. Kiser (ed.), *Oral Anticoagulation Therapy*,
DOI 10.1007/978-3-319-54643-8_7

maximal dose atorvastatin, metformin, and glipizide. He denies any chest pains, palpitations, dizziness or lightheadedness and has no complaints. After a thorough review of his medications he does admit he has "some trouble at times" in remembering to take his medications. He keeps all pill bottles on his kitchen counter, but will realize about one to two times a week that he has missed either his morning or evening doses. In addition, upon further questioning he states "I skip my pills at times as I think they cause me a lot of heartburn…when I skip them I feel better."

How critical is adherence with anticoagulants and can it be improved?

Adherence with oral anticoagulation is paramount in providing adequate prophylaxis from ischemic stroke in patients with atrial fibrillation. Unfortunately, many factors may lead to less than optimal adherence including poor patient understanding of benefits, risks, and goals of anticoagulation, side effects, inability to afford therapy, difficulty in obtaining renewal or refills, administration or storage requirements, medical and non-medical media coverage, among others. Assessment of adherence is critical in patients receiving oral anticoagulation and should be conducted regularly during all routine visits or upon suspicion of potential nonadherence (e.g., notification by insurer (or other mechanism) of poor refill history, occurrence of embolic event, erratic INR control if receiving therapy with warfarin). Suggested questions to assist in assessing patient adherence are included in Table 7.1. Non-adherence to anticoagulation with warfarin or direct oral anticoagulants (DOACs) is associated with an increase in adverse outcomes including stroke and all-cause mortality [1, 2]. In one study the risk of stroke with nonadherence increased with higher CHA_2DS_2-VASc scores and with greater duration of no anticoagulation [2]. Interestingly, in this study of over 64,000 patients adherence to therapy appeared to be most important in patients with CHA_2DS_2-VASc score ≥ 2, as time not taking anticoagulation was not associated with stroke in patients with a CHA_2DS_2-VASc score of 0–1. However, it should be noted that the median follow-up in this study was 1.1 years.

While certain characteristics of anticoagulation with warfarin such as need for regular lab-work, changing doses over time, numerous drug-drug and drug-dietary interactions may lend to nonadherence with warfarin, the requirement for frequent monitoring may allow for rapid identification of patients who are not adherent allowing early intervention. On the other hand, certain characteristics of the DOACs such as cost and lack of need for regular monitoring may increase the risk of nonadherence with them. Characteristics that may influence adherence to an oral anticoagulant that should be considered when selecting a therapy are shown in Table 7.2.

Table 7.1 Suggested questions when assessing medication adherence	
	1. What are you taking this medication for?
	2. How are you taking this medication?
	3. What problems have you had with this medication?
	4. How many days a week (a month) do you miss your medication?
	5. How do you refill this medication?

Table 7.2 Characteristics of oral anticoagulants that may influence adherence to consider when selecting therapy

- Monitoring requirements (frequency and type of lab-work or lack of requirement for regular monitoring)
- Dosing complexity (variable doses over time, or day to day)
- Frequency of administration
- Ability to crush tablets (e.g., patients with enteral feeding tubes or dysphagia who take medications in applesauce)
- Storage requirements (dabigatran must be kept in original container)
- Dietary requirements (consistency in vitamin K foods with warfarin, rivaroxaban administration with dinner, dabigatran administration with full glass of water)
- Side effect profile which may limit tolerability (patients with underlying esophageal conditions may be more prone to dyspepsia with dabigatran)
- Cost

Although specific adherence rates in the pivotal randomized controlled trials with the DOACs are not available, overall discontinuation rates were between 21–25% and not significantly different than discontinuation rates (17–27%) observed with warfarin [3]. How this compares to real-world experience and comparatively between different oral anticoagulants is only beginning to be described. In the previously referred retrospective cohort analysis [2] of 64,661 patients using a large US commercial insurance database, adherence (defined as the proportion of days covered ≥80%) was better for the DOACs than warfarin ($p < 0.001$), but still disappointingly sub-optimal at 58.9% (vs. 49.9% with warfarin). Interestingly the theoretical advantage in regards to adherence of once daily rivaroxaban was not reflected in the proportion of days covered ≥80% as it was very similar to dabigatran and apixaban (59.5% vs. 57.3% vs. 62.5% respectively; p value not provided).

So, while it is apparent that poor adherence with oral anticoagulation will increase adverse events, it is also apparent that greater utilization of DOACs will not solve the problem. As such, certain strategies need to be considered. Instrumental in this effort includes shared decision making between the clinician and patient at the time of therapy is initially being recommended. Patient priorities and preferences must be considered when developing a treatment strategy as well as a focus on patient education and understanding. Adherence is improved when patients understand their diagnosis and indication for therapy, believe in the therapy, and trust the provider [4]. In addition, adherence is also associated with female sex, regular users of cardiovascular drugs and CHA_2DS_2-VASc score ≥ 2 [5]. Specific interventions such as medication organizers (i.e. pill boxes) interactive voice response systems, compliance-linked financial incentives, and patient self-testing and monitoring have demonstrated promise with warfarin therapy [6]. With the DOACs it is becoming apparent that periodic monitoring is a necessary component in maintaining adherence. A specific study focusing on dabigatran revealed that appropriate patient selection (review to assure appropriate indication and assessment of patients adherence to prior warfarin therapy or other medications), provision of pharmacist-led monitoring, longer duration of monitoring, and more intensive care (tailoring of monitoring process, contacting patients) to non-adherent patients all were associated with a greater proportion of days covered of ≥80% [7]. Recent guidance focusing on the use of DOACs provide specific recommendations to regular monitoring and highlight the need for regular assessment of adherence as a component of this [8, 9].

In regards to our patient a careful review of current medications, vitals, and lab results reveal that he is probably poorly adherent to multiple therapies. Given his CHA_2DS_2-VASc of six, poor adherence with his oral anticoagulant is of particular concern. Poor response of his lipid panel to atorvastatin 80 mg, poor blood pressure control despite five anti-hypertensive agents, and failure to monitor his blood pressure at home, all independently of how he answered the initial question regarding medication adherence, should prompt a more detailed and personal discussion on adherence. Efforts should be made in regards to identifying his priorities and preferences, understanding (health literacy) of his medical conditions and expectations of therapies, adverse effect concerns, affordability with therapy, and understanding of renewal/refill process. His treatment strategy should then be adjusted accordingly and include a component of long-term monitoring. The patient's apparent "heartburn" may be contributing to nonadherence and may very well be related to dabigatran therapy. If the patient is interested in using a medication organizer, the storage requirements of dabigatran may complicate this modality to improve adherence. Although once-daily versus twice-daily doses of oral anticoagulants is not clearly associated with improvement of adherence as assessed by proportion of days covered ≥80%, this patient may put a high personal preference to once-daily dosing or perhaps even prefer twice-daily dosing over the requirement to take the once-daily medication (rivaroxaban) with a meal. In addition, anticoagulation with warfarin should also be reconsidered as the need for regularly scheduled visits and the ability to measure the degree of anticoagulation will provide greater objective insight into his adherence. Lastly, given that the patient has a diagnosis of mild cognitive impairment this should be monitored closely, and consideration given (after discussion with patient) to involving family members or health care surrogates with his medication management and monitoring.

Key Points

- The risk of stroke with nonadherence to oral anticoagulation increases with higher CHA_2DS_2-VASc scores and with greater duration of no anticoagulation.
- Although real-world adherence (defined as the proportion of days covered ≥80%) may appear better for the DOACs than warfarin it is still disappointingly sub-optimal.
- Once-daily versus twice-daily doses of oral anticoagulants is not clearly associated with improvement of adherence as assessed by proportion of days covered ≥80% and efforts to evaluate and improve adherence should be instituted regardless of the dosing regimen selected.

- Adherence is improved when patients understand their diagnosis and indication for therapy, believe in the therapy, and trust the provider.
- Efforts should be made in regards to identifying the patient's priorities and preferences, understanding (health literacy) of medical conditions and expectations of therapies, adverse effect concerns, affordability with therapy, and understanding of renewal/refill process. Treatment strategy should then be adjusted accordingly and include a component of long-term monitoring.

Self-Assessment Questions

1. Which of the following is not suitable for use in a medication organizer?
   (a) apixaban
   (b) dabigatran
   (c) edoxaban
   (d) rivaroxaban
   (e) warfarin

   Correct answer: b (dabigatran). Dabigatran must be stored in its original bottle to protect from moisture, and should not be put in pill boxes or pill organizers (PRADAXA Package Insert, 2015).

2. List 5 important things that may impact patient adherence thereby influencing the initial selection of an oral anticoagulant.

   Answer: Patient's priorities, patient's health literacy, patient's belief in therapy, patient's trust of provider, adverse effect concerns, affordability with therapy, ability to adhere to monitoring (e.g., regular lab-work with warfarin), patient's administration preferences (e.g., once daily, requirement to be taken with a meal or not, use of medication organizer), comorbidities (e.g., cognitive impairment) among other things may impact patient adherence thereby influencing selection of an oral anticoagulant.

Disclosure The views expressed in this chapter reflect those of the authors, and not necessarily those of the Department of Veterans Affairs.

References

1. Shore S, Carey EP, Turakhia MP, Jackevicius CA, Cunningham F, Pilote L, Bradley SM, Maddox TM, Grunwald GK, Barón AE, Rumsfeld JS, Varosy PD, Schneider PM, Marzec LN, Ho PM. Adherence to dabigatran therapy and longitudinal patient outcomes: insights from the veterans health administration. Am Heart J. 2014;167(6):810–7.

2. Yao X, Abraham NS, Alexander GC, Crown W, Montori VM, Sangaralingham LR, Gersh BJ, Shah ND, Noseworthy PA. Effect of adherence to oral anticoagulants on risk of stroke and major bleeding among patients with atrial fibrillation. J Am Heart Assoc. 2016;5(2). pii:e003074. doi:10.1161/JAHA.115.003074
3. Sanfélix-Gimeno G, Rodríguez-Bernal CL, Hurtado I, Baixáuli-Pérez C, Librero J, Peiró S. Adherence to oral anticoagulants in patients with atrial fibrillation-a population-based retrospective cohort study linking health information systems in the Valencia region, Spain: a study protocol. BMJ Open. 2015;5(10):e007613. doi:10.1136/bmjopen-2015-007613.
4. Ewen S, Rettig-Ewen V, Mahfoud F, Bohm M, Laufs U. Drug adherence in patients taking oral anticoagulation therapy. Clin Res Cardiol. 2014;103:173–82.
5. Gorst-Rasmussen A, Skjøth F, Larsen TB, Rasmussen LH, Lip GY, Lane DA. Dabigatran adherence in atrial fibrillation patients during the first year after diagnosis: a nationwide cohort study. J Thromb Haemost. 2015;13(4):495–504. doi:10.1111/jth.12845.
6. Kneeland PP, Fang MC. Current issues in patient adherence and persistence: focus on anticoagulants for the treatment and prevention of thromboembolism. Patient Prefer Adherence. 2010;4:51–60.
7. Shore S, Ho PM, Lambert-Kerzner A, Glorioso TJ, Carey EP, Cunningham F, Longo L, Jackevicius C, Rose A, Turakhia MP. Site-level variation in and practices associated with dabigatran adherence. JAMA. 2015;313(14):1443–50.
8. Hedibuchel H, Verhamme P, Alings M, Antz M, Diener H-C, Hacke W, Oldgren J, Sinnaeve P, Camm AJ, Kirchof P. Updated European Heart Rhythm Association practical guide on the use of non-vitamin K antagonist anticoagulants in patients with non-valvular atrial fibrillation. Europace. 2015;17:1467–507.
9. Gladstone DJ, Geerts WH, Douketis J, Ivers N, Healey JS, Leblanc K. How to monitor patients receiving direct oral anticoagulants for stroke prevention in atrial fibrillation: a practice tool endorsed by Thrombosis Canada, the Canadian Stroke Consortium, the Canadian Cardiovascular Pharmacists Network, and the Canadian Cardiovascular Society. Ann Intern Med. 2015;163:382–6.

Chapter 8
Oral Anticoagulants in Stable Moderate Chronic Kidney Disease

James C. Lee

Abstract Although renal dosing recommendations are available for direct oral anticoagulants (DOAC), their use in atrial fibrillation patients with stable renal function bordering the recommended functional criteria for dose adjustments complicates dose selection and safe long-term use. Increased monitoring and assessment of the benefits and risks of direct oral anticoagulation therapy are required to mitigate poor outcomes resulting from clinical status changes requiring DOAC dose adjustments.

Keywords Stable chronic kidney disease • Rivaroxaban • Direct oral anticoagulants • Renal dosing • Atrial fibrillation • Direct oral anticoagulant management • Direct oral anticoagulant monitoring • Drug interactions

Case Introduction

LJ is a generally healthy and independent 70-year-old African-American female with a prior medical history significant for atrial fibrillation, hypertension, congestive heart failure, dyslipidemia, and recurrent urinary tract infections (UTI). Her baseline creatinine clearance (CrCl) is 55 mL/min, and serum creatinine (SCr) of 1.3 mg/dL for the past several years. LJ has been on warfarin therapy for 15 years with an International Normalized Ratio (INR) time in therapeutic range (TTR) of 90%. Her anticoagulation is managed by an anticoagulation specialty clinic. LJ's niece assists her with picking up medications (lisinopril, metoprolol succinate, atorvastatin, warfarin, calcium/vitamin D—all with reasonable Medicaid copays) and reliably drives LJ to all of her clinic appointments. LJ utilizes a weekly pillbox and

---

J.C. Lee, PharmD, BCACP
University of Illinois Hospital & Health Sciences System, University of Illinois at Chicago College of Pharmacy, 833 S Wood St, MC 886, Chicago, IL 60612, USA
e-mail: jamlee1@uic.edu

organizes her own medications. She cooks for herself and is consistent with her weekly dietary vitamin K intake, although she does occasionally have an extra serving of broccoli.

During her cardiology appointment today, LJ inquired about the "new blood thinners that are on TV." Her cardiologist is now contemplating if warfarin should be continued or if LJ should be transitioned to a direct oral anticoagulant (DOAC).

Case Discussion

Background

Chronic kidney disease (CKD) Stage III is defined as a moderately decreased glomerular filtration rate (GFR) of 30–59 mL/min for 3 or 4 months with or without kidney damage [1]. Stage III CKD is further subdivided into two states: IIIa (45–59 mL/min) and IIIb (30–44 mL/min). Individuals with CKD are at increased risk of cardiovascular events and death, with marked increase in all-cause cardiovascular mortality at Stage IIIb and greater [2, 3]. Kidney disease is also known to be a risk factor for venous thrombosis as a result of the overall hypercoagulable state arising from abnormally elevated clotting factor activity and decreased endogenous anticoagulant activity [4].

Although overall control and safety of warfarin therapy is complicated by various clinical factors and genetic factors, the therapeutic activity of warfarin is not significantly altered by changes in renal function as compared to DOACs due to its extensive metabolism into inactive metabolites prior to renal elimination. Decreased anticoagulation stability and dose requirements, however, have been observed in warfarin-treated patients with CKD [5, 6]. Despite this, warfarin has still been suggested as the oral anticoagulant of choice in patients with severe renal impairment [7].

Evidence for DOAC use in the setting of moderate chronic kidney disease is lacking. Renally-based DOAC dose modifications exist for atrial fibrillation, but not with venous thromboembolism treatment or prophylaxis (with the exception of edoxaban). DOAC avoidance is recommended in those with severely reduced renal function, and it should be noted that renal function criteria are agent-specific (Table 8.1) Although DOACs do not require routine monitoring of their therapeutic activity due to their predictable pharmacokinetic and pharmacodynamics profiles in

Table 8.1 Renal function criteria for direct oral anticoagulant discontinuation or avoidance [8–11]

Indication	Dabigatran (CrCl mL/min)	Rivaroxaban (CrCl mL/min)	Apixaban	Edoxaban (CrCl mL/min)
Atrial fibrillation	<15	<15	NR	<15 or >95
DVT/PE treatment	<30	<30	NR	<15
DVT prophylaxis	<30	<30	NR	N/A

CrCl creatinine clearance, *NR* no recommendation provided, *N/A* not an FDA-approved indication

normal renal function, DOAC use and dosing in the setting of stable moderate CKD should be approached with added caution due to DOAC reliance on renal elimination and possible potential DOAC accumulation.

What Factors Should be Considered When Selecting an Oral Anticoagulant for Patients with Stable Moderate Renal Function?

- Oral anticoagulant characteristics
  - **Warfarin**: Affordable as a generic medication, but requires regular monitoring of therapeutic activity. Anticoagulation control is influenced by various clinical and lifestyle factors such as dietary vitamin K intake. Dietary vitamin K intake is likely to be limited in those with CKD due to the high potassium content found in a wide variety of vegetables, thereby reducing the impact of diet on INR stability [12]. Anticoagulation intensity is easily monitored and reversible agents are readily accessible. Therapeutic activity is not dependent on renal function.
  - **DOAC**: All currently available agents are brand medications, potentially impacting patient affordability and accessibility based on individual insurance plans. Concomitant use of strong or dual CYP3A4 and p-glycoprotein inhibitors are contraindicated with most DOACs or require dose reduction. Due to the differences in the degree of renal clearance of each DOAC (Table 8.2), renal function criteria for dose modification are agent and indication-specific. DOACs do not require regular monitoring of therapeutic activity, but regular assessment of renal function and a complete blood count (CBC) is recommended to monitor for bleeding and distinguish between expected versus acute changes in renal function. Due to DOAC dependence on renal elimination, more frequent monitoring should be considered in those with reduced or variable renal function and in scenarios where impaired baseline function may be further acutely altered. Monitoring of therapeutic activity is agent-specific and less well established. Although common coagulation assays such as INR and aPTT may detect DOAC presence, assays correlating therapeutic activity with drug concentration are not currently widely available or approved [13]. Although INR may become elevated with DOAC use, it should not be considered a reliable marker of DOAC therapeutic activity.

Table 8.2 Degree of renal elimination of DOACs [8–11]

	Renal elimination (%)
Dabigatran	80
Rivaroxaban	36
Apixaban	27
Edoxaban	50

- Patient considerations
    - **Baseline renal function**: Assess if baseline function is reduced to CKD stage III or below where DOAC dose reduction may be potentially required (broadly, 50 mL/min or less). Although potentially more convenient, the risk for DOAC accumulation and supratherapeutic activity in worsened renal insufficiency is greater than with warfarin. Assess baseline function and variability over a selected time period. Is renal function stable or suddenly and unexpectedly decreased compared to 3 months ago, 6 months, or one to 2 years ago? Is the etiology unknown or have new medications (e.g., vancomycin, long-term non-steroidal anti-inflammatory drug use, chemotherapy) or recently diagnosed medical conditions (e.g., acute kidney injuries, systemic lupus nephritis, uncontrolled hypertension or diabetes, etc.) become part of the picture? LJ's renal function is moderately reduced and appears stable based on the given information. Her provider should be aware of the agent-specific indications for DOAC dose reduction, especially as LJ has borderline renal function that may require a dose reduction sometime in the future (Table 8.3).
    - **Comorbid illnesses**: Will comorbid or history of acute illnesses lead to a higher likelihood of treatment with drugs that significantly interact with warfarin or DOACs? LJ's history of recurrent UTI may result in regular use of antibiotics (e.g., ciprofloxacin, sulfamethoxazole/trimethoprim, etc.) that require warfarin dose reduction. Although drug–drug interactions with common medications may require warfarin dose adjustments, anticoagulation intensity can be monitored and adjusted for. LJ's long-term medications appear to be streamlined and without significant drug–drug interactions (Table 8.4). This makes either warfarin or a DOAC viable options.
    - **Adherence and control with warfarin therapy**: Evaluate if the existing anticoagulation regimen is well-controlled and monitoring parameters are acceptable to the patient. Has the patient "failed" warfarin therapy? Is the patient willing to adhere to regular monitoring or do other daily activities and responsibilities pose a barrier to appropriate monitoring frequency? LJ

Table 8.3 Renal function criteria for reduced direct oral anticoagulant dosing [8–11]

Indication	Dabigatran	Rivaroxaban	Apixaban	Edoxaban
Atrial fibrillation	CrCl 15–30 mL/min	CrCl 15–50 mL/min	SCr >1.5 mg/dL[a]	CrCl 15–50 mL/min
DVT/PE treatment	NR	NR	NR	CrCl 15–50 mL/min[b]
DVT prophylaxis	NR	NR	NR	—

NR no recommendation provided, *CrCl* creatinine clearance, *SCr* serum creatinine
[a]Age (80 years and older) and weight (60 kg or less) must also be assessed. Two of the three criteria must be met for dose reduction
[b]Weight (60 kg or less) and concomitant use of certain P-gp inhibitors (verapamil, quinidine, azithromycin, clarithromycin, erythromycin, oral itraconazole, oral ketoconazole) must also be considered

Table 8.4 Significant drug–drug interactions with direct oral anticoagulants [8–11]

	DOAC dose reduction required	Avoid DOAC with concurrent use
Dabigatran	**P-gp inhibitors + CrCl 30–50 (AF)**: Reduce dose to 75 mg BID • Dronedarone • Ketoconazole	**P-gp inducers (any indication)** • Rifampin **P-gp inhibitors + CrCl < 30 (AF)** • Dronedarone • Ketoconazole **P-gp inhibitors + CrCl < 50 (VTE treatment, VTE prophylaxis)** • Dronedarone • Ketoconazole
Rivaroxaban	N/A	**Combined P-gp + strong CYP3A4 Inhibitors (any indication)** • Conivaptan • Indinavir • Itraconazole • Ketoconazole • Lopinavir/ritonavir • Ritonavir **Combined P-gp + strong CYP3A4 Inducers (any indication)** • Carbamazepine • Phenytoin • Rifampin • St. John's wort **CrCl 15–80 + combined P-gp + moderate CYP3A4 inhibitors (any indication)** • Diltiazem • Dronedarone • Erythromycin • Verapamil
Apixaban	**Combined Dual Strong P-gp + CYP3A4 inhibitors (on 5 mg/10 mg original dose/any indication)**: Reduce dose by 50% to 2.5 mg/5 mg • Clarithromycin • Itraconazole • Ketoconazole • Ritonavir	**Combined Dual Strong P-gp + CYP3A4 inhibitors (on 2.5 mg original dose/any indication)** • Clarithromycin • Itraconazole • Ketoconazole • Ritonavir
Edoxaban	Reduce dose to 30 mg daily **(VTE)** • Azithromycin • Clarithromycin • Erythromycin • Itraconazole (oral) • Ketoconazole (oral) • Quinidine • Verapamil	**P-gp inducers** • Rifampin

AF atrial fibrillation, *CrCl* creatinine clearance, *P-gp* P-glycoprotein, *VTE* venous thromboembolism

appears capable of independently managing her medical affairs and diet, and does not appear to have any barriers to routine clinic follow-up. Her TTR indicates excellent control (TTR >60%) with warfarin. Additionally, the nature and tone of her inquiry about DOACs may not necessarily be indicative of a strong desire to discontinue her current regimen.
 - **Affordability**: Consult with the patient's pharmacy or insurance drug formulary to ensure that the selected DOAC is covered by the insurance plan. LJ should be made aware that an increased copayment or coinsurance is possible as DOACs may be assigned to a higher medication formulary tier (e.g., Tier 2 or Tier 3) with higher out-of-pocket cost compared to warfarin (typically a Tier 1 medication). Non-preferred DOACs likely require full out-of-pocket payment. The potential increase to out-of-pocket cost should be acceptable to the patient before transitioning from warfarin, especially for those who are likely to have fixed or limited incomes.
 - **Patient decision-making capacity**: Is the patient capable of reliably communicating health status changes with providers and pursuing care when necessary? Considerations may include medical conditions worsening cognition or neurological deficits, limited transportation access, poor adherence to appointments, frequent emergency department visits, etc. Patients with poor cognition who also have difficulty adhering to complex warfarin dosing instructions or providing good self-care, but possess adequate social support may benefit from DOAC treatment simplicity. Conversely, a patient with poor understanding and social support may be unable to adequately assess treatment-related complications that warrant further assessment. LJ appears to be functionally independent and has good social support available if needed.
- Provider considerations
 - **Routine monitoring is required regardless of anticoagulant**: Annual assessment of renal function and complete blood count are recommended for all DOACs. With moderate CKD or worsening insufficiency, more frequent laboratory monitoring should be performed. Continuing DOAC use should be reconsidered or discontinued if renal function has demonstrated a consistent or accelerating decline. LJ appears to have stable moderate CKD.
 - **Weigh the benefits and risks of continuing current therapy**: Providers should assess their capacity for safely managing all modes of anticoagulation therapy. If existing warfarin therapy is well controlled and acceptable to the patient, increasing INR monitoring interval should be considered. Transition to a DOAC may not necessarily lead to improved patient adherence, especially if systematic provider follow-up is lacking [14].

The Outcome

LJ's cardiologist decided to start rivaroxaban 20 mg daily with dinner based on the convenience of once daily dosing and LJ's CrCl > 50 mL/min. LJ agreed to the transition as well as regular assessment of her renal function every 6 months. The cardiologist informed the anticoagulation clinic of the therapy change and requested the clinic to manage the transition. The anticoagulation clinic verified a copay of $15 per month for rivaroxaban, which LJ found acceptable compared to her $5 copay for warfarin. LJ filled her rivaroxaban prescription and brought it with her to her anticoagulation clinic appointment. LJ's INR was 2.7; warfarin was stopped and rivaroxaban was initiated that evening as her INR was less than 3, as recommended by the FDA-approved Prescribing Information. LJ was informed that the clinic would follow-up with her by phone in 3 months to assess ongoing rivaroxaban therapy.

Key Points

- DOAC use in the setting of stable moderate CKD should be considered carefully due to the risk of drug accumulation if renal function worsens or an inappropriate dose is selected. Renal function criteria for dose modifications are available for all DOACs for the indication of atrial fibrillation. If existing warfarin therapy is well-controlled and acceptable to the patient, consider continuing with warfarin therapy.
- More frequent assessment of renal function and CBC should be performed with DOAC therapy. Those with borderline moderate renal function should be closely monitored to ensure the appropriate DOAC dosing is selected to avoid underanticoagulation (e.g., using renally-adjusted dose in normal renal function) or overanticoagulation (e.g., using standard dose or contraindication to use with reduced renal function). If renal function deteriorates further, transition to warfarin should be considered due to the limited evidence, interpretation, and access to useful coagulation assays for measuring ongoing DOAC therapeutic activity.
- When considering DOAC therapy in moderate CKD, consider all relevant factors in addition to patient and provider convenience. These include but are not limited to baseline renal function, patient affordability, overall medication adherence, logistical barriers affecting monitoring adherence, acceptance of routine laboratory monitoring, patient decision-making capacity, barriers to timely provider care, and prior anticoagulation control with warfarin.

Self-Assessment Questions

1. Which of the following patients being anticoagulated for atrial fibrillation is dosed appropriately?

    (a) A 32 year old 62 kg male with a CrCl of 20 mL/min taking edoxaban 30 mg daily
    (b) A 41 year old, 76 kg female with a CrCl of 55 mL/min taking rivaroxaban 15 mg daily

(c) A 53 year old, 55 kg male with a CrCl of 25 mL/min taking dabigatran 150 mg twice daily
(d) A 60 year old, 80 kg female with a SCr of 1.7 mg/dL taking apixaban 2.5 mg twice daily

Rationale for Question #1

(a) Correct. Edoxaban requires a dose reduction if CrCl 15–50 mL/min. The non-adjusted dose is 60 mg daily for those with CrCl 50–95 mL/min. Edoxaban should also be avoided in those with CrCl greater than 95 mL/min when anticoagulating for atrial fibrillation.
(b) Incorrect. This dose is the renally-adjusted dose. Reducing rivaroxaban dose is required if CrCl 15–50 mL/min. The non-adjusted dose is 20 mg daily. The patient is thus at risk for underanticoagulation.
(c) Incorrect. Dabigatran requires a dose reduction if CrCl 15–30 mL/min. This patient is currently on the non-adjusted dose. The renally-adjusted dose is 75 mg twice daily. This patient is thus at risk for overanticoagulation.
(d) Incorrect. Apixaban requires a dose reduction in those who have at least two of the following three criteria: age 80 years or older, body weight 60 kg or less, or SCr 1.5 mg/dL or greater. This patient only fulfills one criterion (elevated serum creatinine). The non-adjusted dose is 5 mg twice daily. This patient is thus at risk for underanticoagulation.

2. Which of the following patients with atrial fibrillation and moderate chronic kidney disease would transitioning to the proposed alternative anticoagulation therapy be the most appropriate?

(a) (Transitioning from warfarin to DOAC): A 76 year old female on warfarin for 15 years with a 90% INR time in therapeutic range (TTR) who is on an antiretroviral regimen that includes lopinavir/ritonavir.
(b) (Transitioning from warfarin to DOAC): A 61 year old male on warfarin for 3 years with a 65% TTR with Tier 3 copays for all DOACs, and consistently forgets to take his warfarin once a week.
(c) (Transitioning from DOAC to warfarin): A 55 year old male on rivaroxaban 15 mg daily for 3 years who has exhibited a steady decline in CrCl from 35 mL/min to 20 mL/min over the past 2 years.
(d) (Transitioning from DOAC to warfarin): A 40 year old female on apixaban 2.5 mg twice daily for 2 years with affordable Tier 1 copays for apixaban and exhibits adherence with twice-daily therapy.

Rationale for Question #2:

(a) Incorrect. Continuing warfarin is favorable due to the concomitant use of a strong dual inhibitor of CYP3A4 and P-glycoprotein. Concomitant use of strong CYP3A4 and P-glycoprotein inhibitors (i.e., ritonavir) with DOACs should be avoided. Additionally, the patient has demonstrated excellent anticoagulation control with her existing warfarin therapy.

(b) Incorrect. Although the patient's TTR is lower than the patient described in answer choice A, high DOAC copays and regular medication non-adherence are issues that may lead to underanticoagulation. DOACs have shorter half-lives compared to warfarin, and regularly missed DOAC doses would expose the patient to periods of no anticoagulation. Warfarin is also likely to be more acceptable due to lower out-of-pocket costs.

(c) Correct. This patient is exhibiting declining renal function and is approaching the renal functional threshold where most DOACs would be contraindicated. If rivaroxaban is continued, renal function should be assessed more frequently due to the recommendation for discontinuation should CrCl decrease below 15 mL/min. Considering the patient's age and life expectancy, it is likely he would need to transition to warfarin eventually. The need for regular monitoring with warfarin versus more frequent laboratory draws should be discussed with the patient when determining when to discontinue rivaroxaban and initiate warfarin.

(d) Incorrect. Despite the requirement for twice-daily dosing, the patient is able to afford apixaban and is adherent to a more frequent dosing interval compared to once-daily warfarin. Although warfarin elimination is not dependent on renal function, patient acceptability of relatively more frequent monitoring should be discussed with the patient prior to discontinuing existing DOAC therapy.

References

1. Kidney Disease: Improving Global Outcomes (KDIGO) CKD Work Group. KDIGO 2012 clinical practice guideline for the evaluation and management of chronic kidney disease. Kidney Int Suppl. 2013;3:1–150.
2. Sarnak MJ, Levey AS, Schoolwerth AC, et al. Kidney disease as a risk factor for development of cardiovascular disease: a statement from the American Heart Association councils on kidney in cardiovascular disease, high blood pressure research, clinical cardiology, and epidemiology and prevention. Circulation. 2003;108:2154–216.
3. Go AS, Chertow GM, Fan D, et al. Chronic kidney disease and the risks of death, cardiovascular events, and hospitalization. N Engl J Med. 2004;351(13):1296–305.
4. Capodanno D, Angiolillo DJ. Antithrombotic therapy in patients with chronic kidney disease. Circulation. 2012;125:2649–61.
5. Kleinow ME, Garwood CL, Clemente JL, Whittaker P. Effect of chronic kidney disease on warfarin management in a pharmacist-managed anticoagulation clinic. J Manag Care Pharm. 2011;17(7):523–30.
6. Limdi NA, Limdi MA, Cavallari L, et al. Warfarin dosing in patients with impaired kidney function. Am J Kidney Dis. 2010;56(5):823–31.
7. Ageno W, Gallus AS, Wittkowsky A, et al. Oral anticoagulant therapy: antithrombotic therapy and prevention of thrombosis, 9th ed: American College of Chest Physicians evidence-based clinical practice guidelines. Chest. 2012;141(2 Suppl):e44S–88S.
8. Pradaxa (dabigatran) package insert. Ridgefield, CT: Boehringer Ingelheim Pharmaceuticals, Inc; 2015.
9. Xarelto (rivaroxaban) package insert. Titusville, NJ: Janssen Pharmaceuticals, Inc; 2016.

10. Eliquis package insert. Princeton, NJ: Bristol-Myers Squibb Company; 2016.
11. Savaysa (edoxaban) package insert. Parsippany, NJ: Daiichi Sankyo, Inc; 2016.
12. National Kidney Foundation. Potassium and your CKD Diet. https://www.kidney.org/atoz/content/potassium. Accessed 20 June 2016.
13. Cuker A, Siegal DM, Crowther MA, Garcia DA. Laboratory measurement of the anticoagulant activity of the non-vitamin K oral anticoagulants. J Am Coll Cardiol. 2014;64(11):1128–39.
14. Shore S, Ho PM, Lambert-Kerzner A, et al. Site-level variation in and practices associated with dabigatran adherence. JAMA. 2015;313(14):1443–50.

Chapter 9
Oral Anticoagulants in Severe Renal Dysfunction

Jennifer Babin

Abstract When choosing an anticoagulant for a patient with chronic kidney disease (CKD), consider that patients with CKD were excluded from landmark direct oral anticoagulant (DOAC) trials if their creatinine clearance (CrCl) was <25–30 mL/min, but use of these agents has been approved in patients with a CrCl as low as 15 mL/min based on extrapolated data. Limited data suggests that warfarin is beneficial and relatively safe in patients with CKD and atrial fibrillation.

Keywords Non-dialysis dependent chronic kidney disease • Severe chronic kidney disease • Atrial fibrillation • Anticoagulation • Direct oral anticoagulant • Warfarin Stroke risk • Bleeding risk

Case Introduction

TC is a 58 year old Caucasian female with a history of hypertension and non-dialysis dependent chronic kidney disease (CKD) who has been diagnosed with atrial fibrillation. Her weight today in clinic is 62 kg, height is 168 cm, serum creatinine (SCr) is 2.0 mg/dL, and creatinine clearance (CrCl) is 30 mL/min based on the Cockcroft-Gault equation. Estimated glomerular filtration rate (GFR) is 26 mL/min based on the MDRD equation and 27 mL/min based on the CKD-EPI equation. Her baseline SCr is consistently around 2.0 mg/dL. She has health insurance through her employer and has no difficulty paying for her medications. She also reports good

---

J. Babin, PharmD, BCPS
Department of Pharmacotherapy, University of Utah College of Pharmacy,
30 South 2000 East, Salt Lake City, UT 84112, USA
e-mail: jennifer.babin@hsc.utah.edu

adherence with her current anti-hypertensive prescriptions. Her physician must decide on the most appropriate anticoagulation plan for TC.

Case Discussion

What Is this Patient's Risk of Stroke and Bleeding?

Risk of stroke and bleeding must be weighed when deciding whether to start anticoagulation, especially in patients with CKD. Stroke risk in atrial fibrillation is commonly estimated using the CHA_2DS_2-VASc score, which evaluates congestive heart failure, hypertension, age, diabetes, history of stroke or transient ischemic attack, vascular disease, and sex as risk factors. This patient's CHA_2DS_2-VASc score is 2 since she has hypertension and is a female, indicating she is at high risk of having an ischemic stroke [1]. It is important to note that CKD also contributes to stroke risk, although it is not included as a factor in the CHA_2DS_2-VASc score [2, 3]. Likewise, bleeding risk can be estimated using the HAS-BLED score (Table 9.1), which lists hypertension, abnormal renal or liver function, stroke, bleeding history, labile INRs, age, and concomitant use of alcohol or drugs with bleeding risk as risk factors. Although this patient has a history of hypertension and CKD, her HAS-BLED score is 0 since systolic blood pressure must be >160 mmHg and SCr must be ≥2.26 mg/dL in order to qualify as risk factors. However, as with stroke risk, CKD also increases bleeding risk, although it is not included as a factor in the HAS-BLED score [2]. In this patient with newly diagnosed atrial fibrillation and CKD, the risk of stroke appears to outweigh the risk of bleeding.

Table 9.1 The HAS-BLED score for assessment of one year major bleeding risk in patients with atrial fibrillation [2]

Hypertension[a]	1 point
Abnormal renal[b] or liver function[c]	1 point each
Stroke	1 point
Bleeding history or predisposition	1 point
Labile INRs[d]	1 point
Elderly[e]	1 point
Drugs[f] or alcohol concomitantly	1 point each

INR international normalized ratio
[a]Uncontrolled hypertension with systolic blood pressure >160 mmHg
[b]Presence of long-term dialysis, kidney transplantation, or serum creatinine ≥2.26 mg/dL
[c]Chronic hepatic disease (i.e. cirrhosis) or biochemical evidence of significant hepatic derangement (i.e. bilirubin >2 times the upper limit of normal in association with aspartate or alanine aminotransferase or alkaline phosphatase level >3 times the upper limit of normal)
[d]Time in therapeutic range <60%
[e]Age >65 years or frail condition
[f]Antiplatelet agents or nonsteroidal anti-inflammatory agents

What Is the Evidence for Use of Direct Oral Anticoagulants (DOACs) in Severe CKD?

This patient's estimated GFR places her into the severely decreased renal function category according to KDIGO guidelines, although her CrCl, which tends to overestimate renal function, is slightly higher [4, 5]. The landmark studies for dabigatran, rivaroxaban, apixaban, and edoxaban included few patients with CKD, and an even smaller number with severe CKD. Of note, studies examining all four of the DOACs used the Cockcroft-Gault equation to estimate renal function in participants [5, 6]. Use of actual body weight in the equation, as opposed to ideal or adjusted body weight, was specified in the dabigatran and rivaroxaban trials [5]. The weight selected may significantly impact the accuracy of the calculated creatinine clearance. Some studies have found that using actual instead of ideal body weight for normal-weight patients can falsely elevate estimated creatinine clearance using the Cockcroft-Gault equation [7, 8].

The RE-LY trial, which compared dabigatran with warfarin in patients with atrial fibrillation, excluded patients with a CrCl <30 mL/min. Patients with a CrCl 30–50 mL/min comprised about 19% of the study population [9]. However, even though patients with severe renal dysfunction were not included in the study, the Food and Drug Administration (FDA) approved a lower dose (75 mg twice daily) for patients with a CrCl 15–30 mL/min based on pharmacokinetic modeling, which estimated that in patients with impaired renal function, the lower dose would result in drug exposure comparable to that of the approved higher dose in patients with normal renal function [10].

The ROCKET AF trial compared rivaroxaban with warfarin and also excluded patients with a CrCl <30 mL/min. The median CrCl of study participants was 67 mL/min. Patients with moderate renal dysfunction received a reduced dose of rivaroxaban (15 mg daily), and were found to have increased stroke and bleeding rates compared to patients with mild renal dysfunction, although rates remained similar to warfarin [11].

The landmark trial for apixaban, ARISTOTLE, excluded patients with SCr >2.5 mg/dL or CrCl <25 mL/min. Of the patients who were enrolled, 1.5% had a CrCl ≤30 mL/min. The apixaban dose was reduced to 2.5 mg twice daily if patients had a SCr ≥1.5 mg/dL and met one additional criterion, either age ≥80 years or weight ≤60 kg [12]. A sub-group analysis found that apixaban reduced stroke and bleeding risk more effectively than warfarin even with declining renal function, although stroke and bleeding risk both became more elevated as renal function declined [13].

As with the landmark dabigatran and rivaroxaban studies, the landmark edoxaban trial excluded patients with a CrCl <30 mL/min. The trial also specified a reduced anticoagulant dose for patients with a CrCl 30–50 mL/min (about 19% of participants) [6]. However, according to the manufacturer, 30 mg daily can be used in patients with a CrCl 15–50 mL/min, which includes patients who were not represented in the study [14].

Table 9.2 DOAC data in patients with CKD and atrial fibrillation [6, 9, 11, 12, 14–18]

	Dabigatran	Rivaroxaban	Apixaban	Edoxaban
Landmark trial, publication year	RE-LY, 2009	ROCKET AF, 2011	ARISTOTLE, 2011	ENGAGE AF-TIMI 48, 2013
Trial renal inclusion criteria	CrCl ≥30 mL/min	CrCl ≥30 mL/min	CrCl ≥25 mL/min and SCr ≤2.5 mg/dL	CrCl ≥30 mL/min
Number of trial participants with renal impairment	19% with CrCl <50 mL/min	21% with CrCl <50 mL/min	15% with CrCl 31–50 mL/min, 1.5% with CrCl ≤30 mL/min	19% with CrCl ≤50 mL/min
Trial dose for renal impairment	110 mg or 150 mg twice daily (standard dose for all participants)	15 mg daily for CrCl 30–49 mL/min	2.5 mg twice daily if ≥2 criteria met: age ≥80 years, weight ≤60 kg, SCr ≥1.5 mg/dL	15 mg or 30 mg daily if CrCl 30–50 mL/min
FDA approved dose for renal impairment	75 mg twice daily for CrCl 15–30 mL/min	15 mg daily for CrCl 15–50 mL/min	2.5 mg twice daily if ≥2 criteria met: age ≥80 years, weight ≤60 kg, SCr ≥1.5 mg/dL	30 mg daily for CrCl 15–50 mL/min

CKD chronic kidney disease, *CrCl* creatinine clearance, *DOAC* direct oral anticoagulant, *FDA* U.S. Food and Drug Administration, *min* minute, *mL* milliliter, *SCr* serum creatinine

Additional considerations for using DOACs in patients with CKD, including cost, monitoring, and drug interactions, are discussed in Chapter 8. See Table 9.2 for a summary of trial information and FDA approved renal dosing for the DOACs.

What Are Considerations When Using Warfarin in CKD?

General considerations for warfarin use are presented in Chapter 8. When determining a plan specifically for patients with moderate to severe renal dysfunction, consider that the majority of studies that have examined the use of warfarin in patients with atrial fibrillation and CKD have been observational studies in patients with end-stage renal disease. These studies have found conflicting results regarding bleeding and stroke risk [2]. Recently a large Danish observational cohort study was published that found a net clinical benefit with warfarin in non-dialysis dependent patients with CKD who have a CHA_2DS_2-VASc score >2 [19]. A meta-analysis that included this study also concluded that use of warfarin in this patient population is associated with a decrease in stroke, although the authors noted high heterogeneity [3].

There are some potential concerns when choosing warfarin for patients with CKD. Some studies have noted a possible relationship between warfarin use and vascular calcification [20]. Others note the potential for supratherapeutic INRs to contribute to faster progression of CKD. Warfarin use in CKD has also been associated with low bone density [2]. When dosing warfarin, consider that average dose requirements are typically lower in patients with CKD [21].

What Is the Best Anticoagulation Plan for this Patient?

Based on landmark DOAC study criteria, this patient would have been included in all of the above studies with her stable CrCl of 30 mL/min. Also, according to the FDA, dabigatran, rivaroxaban, and edoxaban are acceptable options with her current renal function. However, her CrCl is only one point away from meeting exclusion criteria for all trials except ARISTOTLE, and considering that DOAC data is limited for patients with moderate to severe renal dysfunction, these medications should be used with caution in this patient. Although less convenient in terms of monitoring, there is more data and experience supporting the safety of warfarin in severe CKD.

Key Points

- The risks of both stroke and bleeding are increased in patients with CKD.
- Patients were excluded from landmark DOAC trials if their CrCl was <25–30 mL/min. However, the FDA has approved the use of dabigatran, rivaroxaban, and edoxaban in patients with a CrCl as low as 15 mL/min based on extrapolated data.
- Limited data suggests benefit from warfarin in patients with non-dialysis dependent CKD and atrial fibrillation.

Self-Assessment Questions

1. The landmark trial involving which of the following anticoagulants included patients with CrCl as low as 25 mL/min?

    (a) Dabigatran
    (b) Rivaroxaban
    (c) Apixaban
    (d) Edoxaban

    C. Apixaban is the correct answer (ARISTOTLE trial). All other landmark trials (RE-LY, ROCKET AF, ENGAGE AF-TIMI 48) excluded patients with a CrCl <30 mL/min. However, the FDA has approved reduced dabigatran, rivaroxaban, and edoxaban dosing for patients with CrCl <25–30 mL/min based on pharmacokinetic modeling and extrapolation of study results.

2. What is a potential limitation of the HAS-BLED score when used to assess bleeding risk in patients with moderate to severe CKD?

Answer: The score does not account for bleeding risk in patients with less severe CKD.

Explanation: Abnormal renal function is only counted as a point in the HAS-BLED score if the patient is on long-term dialysis, has a history of kidney transplantation, or their SCr is ≥2.26 mg/dL. However, studies have shown that patients with less severe CKD still have an increased bleeding risk. When using this scoring system for patients with CKD who have a SCr <2.26, it may underestimate their risk of bleeding.

References

1. You JJ, Singer DE, Howard PA, et al. Antithrombotic therapy for atrial fibrillation: antithrombotic therapy and prevention of thrombosis, 9th ed: American College of Chest Physicians evidence-based clinical practice guidelines. Chest. 2012;141(2 Suppl):e531S–75S.
2. Ng KP, Edwards NC, Lip GY, et al. Atrial fibrillation in CKD: balancing the risks and benefits of anticoagulation. Am J Kidney Dis. 2013;62(3):615–32.
3. Providencia R, Marijon E, Boveda S, et al. Meta-analysis of the influence of chronic kidney disease on the risk of thromboembolism among patients with nonvalvular atrial fibrillation. Am J Cardiol. 2014;114(4):646–53.
4. Inker LA, Astor BC, Fox CH, et al. KDOQI US commentary on the 2012 KDIGO clinical practice guideline for the evaluation and management of CKD. Am J Kidney Dis. 2014;63(5):713–35.
5. Morrill AM, Ge D, Willett KC. Dosing of target-specific oral anticoagulants in special populations. Ann Pharmacother. 2015;49(9):1031–45.
6. Giugliano RP, Ruff CT, Braunwald E, et al. Edoxaban versus warfarin in patients with atrial fibrillation. N Engl J Med. 2013;369(22):2093–104.
7. Wilhelm SM, Kale-Pradhan PB. Estimating creatinine clearance: a meta-analysis. Pharmacotherapy. 2011;31(7):658–64.
8. Winter MA, Guhr KN, Berg GM. Impact of various body weights and serum creatinine concentrations on the bias and accuracy of the Cockcroft-Gault equation. Pharmacotherapy. 2012;32(7):604–12.
9. Connolly SJ, Ezekowitz MD, Yusuf S, et al. Dabigatran versus warfarin in patients with atrial fibrillation. N Engl J Med. 2009;361(12):1139–51.
10. Lehr T, Haertter S, Liesenfeld KH, et al. Dabigatran etexilate in atrial fibrillation patients with severe renal impairment: dose identification using pharmacokinetic modeling and simulation. J Clin Pharmacol. 2012;52(9):1373–8.
11. Fox KA, Piccini JP, Wojdyla D, et al. Prevention of stroke and systemic embolism with rivaroxaban compared with warfarin in patients with non-valvular atrial fibrillation and moderate renal impairment. Eur Heart J. 2011;32(19):2387–94.
12. Granger CB, Alexander JH, McMurray JJ, et al. Apixaban versus warfarin in patients with atrial fibrillation. N Engl J Med. 2011;365(11):981–92.
13. Hohnloser SH, Hijazi Z, Thomas L, et al. Efficacy of apixaban when compared with warfarin in relation to renal function in patients with atrial fibrillation: insights from the ARISTOTLE trial. Eur Heart J. 2012;33(22):2821–30.

14. Savaysa® [package insert], Parsippany, NJ: Daiichi Sankyo, Inc.; 2015
15. Eliquis® [package insert], Princeton, NJ: Bristol-Myers Squibb Company; 2015
16. Pradaxa® [package insert], Ridgefield, CT: Boehringer Ingelheim Pharmaceuticals, Inc.; 2015
17. Xarelto® [package insert], Titusville, NJ: Janssen Pharmaceuticals, Inc.; 2016
18. Patel MR, Mahaffey KW, Garg J, et al. Rivaroxaban versus warfarin in nonvalvular atrial fibrillation. N Engl J Med. 2011;365(10):883–91.
19. Bonde AN, Lip GY, Kamper AL, et al. Net clinical benefit of antithrombotic therapy in patients with atrial fibrillation and chronic kidney disease: a nationwide observational cohort study. J Am Coll Cardiol. 2014;64(23):2471–82.
20. Nimmo C, Wright M, Goldsmith D. Management of atrial fibrillation in chronic kidney disease: double trouble. Am Heart J. 2013;166(2):230–9.
21. Sakaan SA, Hudson JQ, Oliphant CS, et al. Evaluation of warfarin dose requirements in patients with chronic kidney disease and end-stage renal disease. Pharmacotherapy. 2014;34(7):695–702.

Chapter 10
Oral Anticoagulants in Patients with Variable Renal Function

James C. Lee

Abstract The ongoing use of direct oral anticoagulant therapy versus warfarin in individuals with varying renal function is challenging. The degree of renal function variability, the context in which renal function changes occur, and other patient and provider-specific factors must be carefully evaluated when assessing the benefits and risks of ongoing direct oral anticoagulant therapy.

Keywords Variable renal function • Direct oral anticoagulants • Atrial fibrillation Transitions of care • Acute kidney injury • Rivaroxaban • Overanticoagulation Renal dosing • Coagulation assays • Monitoring

Case Introduction

LJ is a generally healthy and independent 70-year-old African-American female with a prior medical history significant for atrial fibrillation, hypertension, congestive heart failure, dyslipidemia, recurrent urinary tract infections (UTI), baseline creatinine clearance (CrCl) of 55 mL/min, and weighs 82 kg. Previously, LJ took warfarin for 15 years, with a time in therapeutic range (TTR) of 90%. Her cardiologist started rivaroxaban 20 mg daily 1 year ago when she inquired about the "new blood thinners that are on TV." Her niece helps her obtain medications (all with reasonable Medicaid copays) and reliably drives her to clinic appointments.

LJ was hospitalized with worsening dyspnea, significant bruising on both arms, and edema and found to have acutely decompensated heart failure, and acute kidney injury. Serum creatinine was markedly elevated, with reduced CrCl of 13 mL/min. A CBC with differential was unremarkable.

J.C. Lee, PharmD, BCACP
University of Illinois Hospital & Health Sciences System, University of Illinois at Chicago College of Pharmacy, 833 S Wood St, MC 886, Chicago, IL 60612, USA
e-mail: jamlee1@uic.edu

Case Discussion

Background

Despite the various factors influencing effective warfarin therapy, the therapeutic intensity of warfarin is independent of renal function due to its extensive hepatic metabolism into inactive metabolites prior to renal elimination. In contrast, the therapeutic activity of non-warfarin anticoagulants such as low-molecular weight heparins (LMWH) and direct oral anticoagulants (DOACs) involve significant renal elimination unchanged, and are thus significantly affected by chronically or acutely impaired renal elimination [1].

Although recommendations for the use and monitoring of LMWH in renal insufficiency are more established, guidance for DOAC management is still emerging [2–5]. In the setting of normal renal function, DOACs do not require routine monitoring of therapeutic activity due to their predictable pharmacokinetic and pharmacodynamic profiles. Renal dosing for DOACs is recommended in atrial fibrillation, but not venous thromboembolism treatment or prophylaxis (except edoxaban) [6–9]. DOAC agent and dose selection should take into account both reduced (e.g. dabigatran, rivaroxaban, apixaban) and normal renal function (e.g. edoxaban).

Support for DOAC use in varying renal insufficiency is limited, and warfarin remains the preferred oral anticoagulant with established insufficiency [10, 11]. Compared to individuals with stable chronic kidney disease, acute clinical changes such as acute kidney injury may transiently increase the risk for DOAC accumulation and potentially lead to increased bleeding risk as a result of supratherapeutic DOAC drug concentrations. Varying renal function further complicates the selection of an appropriate maintenance DOAC dose in those with borderline renal insufficiency where the use of renally-adjusted DOAC doses would be potentially more appropriate.

As DOACs continue to be increasingly prescribed, routine renal function and complete blood count (CBC) monitoring are recommended at least annually and should be assessed more frequently in those with variable or reduced renal function [4, 11]. Measurement of DOAC therapeutic activity may be useful in those with varying renal function, but limited availability of useful coagulation assays to measure DOAC activity and limited recommendations for monitoring and coagulation assay interpretation represent significant barriers.

Considerations for DOAC Management in Variable Renal Function

Upon Admission

- **Assess renal function change**: Assess immediately upon admission and repeat frequently to assess trends and improvement. Compare current function with pre-admission function. Close attention should be paid to the DOAC used and anticoagulation indication, as the criteria for DOAC contraindication or DOAC dose reduction is agent and indication-specific. For LJ, rivaroxaban should initially be held given her markedly decreased function. Reducing rivaroxaban to 15 mg/day would have been an appropriate alternative if the decline was not as severe (e.g. CrCl was 15–50 mL/min) or if she had not been exhibiting clinical signs or consequences of potential drug accumulation.

- **Assess for bleeding**: Has declining renal function been accompanied by symptoms associated with drug accumulation and supratherapeutic activity (e.g. significantly increased bruising without clear cause, any bleeding, abnormal CBC)? Additionally, assess for recent falls or head trauma to determine if more extensive rule out screening is warranted (e.g. suspicion of intracranial processes). Consider DOAC therapeutic activity monitoring if reliable and appropriately sensitive coagulation assays are available (Table 10.1). DOAC reversal may be pursued if DOAC-specific reversal agents are available, in addition to alternative supportive measures. Given the concern for rivaroxaban accumulation in LJ, a CBC should be drawn to rule out any bleeding.

- **Assess medications adherence**: Assess DOAC adherence and for the presence of any significant drug-drug interactions (e.g. p-gp, CYP3A4, CYP2C9 inhibitors) known to increase DOAC drug concentrations. Evidence of poor DOAC adherence may decrease immediate concern for DOAC accumulation with accompanying worsened renal function, while excellent DOAC adherence may be cause for increased vigilance for bleeding. Investigate medication history directly from the patient, patient's caregiver, and patient's pharmacy. If an interacting medication is discovered and cannot be discontinued or substituted with an alternative agent, the DOAC should be discontinued.

Table 10.1 Coagulation assay utility for direct oral anticoagulants [5, 12]

PT/INR	Widely available, but sensitivity is agent-specific and limited to detecting DOAC presence. Possibly useful for apixaban and rivaroxaban. Least utility with dabigatran and edoxaban
aPTT	Widely available, but with utility limited to detecting dabigatran presence. No utility with apixaban, rivaroxaban, or edoxaban
Chromogenic anti-Factor Xa	Mixed utility with Factor X inhibitors due to lack of FDA-approved calibrations available. No utility with dabigatran
TT	Limited utility with dabigatran due to high sensitivity even at low drug concentrations
dTT	Not widely available. Limited utility and less sensitive to dabigatran at lower drug concentrations
ECT	Not widely available. Sensitive to dabigatran at all drug concentrations

aPTT active partial thromboplastin time, *dTT* diluted thrombin time, *ECT* ecarin clotting time, *TT* thrombin time

Case Continuation

Given LJ's increased bruising and concern for possible rivaroxaban accumulation with her worsened renal function, rivaroxaban was held for the duration of admission. Her hemoglobin and hematocrit were unchanged from her pre-hospitalization baseline and were within normal limits. Renally-adjusted rivaroxaban dosing was not considered as it was unclear if her renal function would continue to deteriorate. She was treated and prepared for discharge home as her primary symptoms resolved and renal function improved (CrCl 47 mL/min). Worsening of existing bruising was not noted.

Prior to Discharge

- **Consider dose reduction or alternative agent**: Does the patient have a history of frequent AKI, evidence of worsening renal insufficiency, or is taking medications known to be nephrotoxic or produce significant drug-drug interactions? Overall decline or acutely changing renal function may complicate the selection of an appropriate maintenance DOAC dose. The concurrent use of non-steroidal anti-inflammatory agents or antiplatelet agents could also increase the additive bleeding risk. Factors such as these complicate the selection of a standard versus renally-adjusted DOAC dose, especially in those with borderline renal function. Short-term or long-term use of P-gp and strong CYP3A4 inhibitors may not be able to be avoided, and if so, DOACs should be avoided. Appropriate rivaroxaban dosing for LJ is challenging since her baseline CrCl borders above the recommended CrCl cutoff (50 mL/min) for rivaroxaban dose reduction while her renal function on discharge indicates the need, at least temporarily, for the renally-adjusted dose. Apixaban could be considered depending on her serum creatinine. Dabigatran is inappropriate due to its more extensive renal elimination compared to the other DOACs. Warfarin is likely the best alternative if considering switching agents.
- **Recommend close outpatient follow-up of clinical status and renal function** especially if continuing a DOAC. More frequent phone follow-up to monitor for worsening bleeding or bruising during the transition of care period should be considered if any medications are modified. If LJ redevelops significant bruising and reduced renal function compared to baseline, consider continuing to hold rivaroxaban until post-hospitalization outpatient follow-up. Consider a temporary dose reduction in LJ to 15 mg daily if resuming anticoagulation is clinically appropriate based on her renal function status.
- **Assess the benefits and risks of continued anticoagulation**: If bleeding risk appears to outweigh the benefit of continued anticoagulation in the short-term, consider holding anticoagulation until outpatient follow-up, especially if thrombotic risk if low. LJ has a moderate stroke risk score, so rivaroxaban could be continued upon discharge as there is no evidence of additional or active bleeding.

- **Inform the anticoagulation provider** of any medication/anticoagulant changes, dose changes, or anticoagulant discontinuation. All changes should be reviewed upon discharge with the patient or patient's caregiver to avoid duplicate therapy with old prescriptions still located in the patient's home. Inform the patient's pharmacy to discontinue old anticoagulant prescriptions to avoid unintended refills.

Case Continuation

LJ's rivaroxaban was resumed upon discharge at her original dose. Two weeks following discharge during anticoagulation clinic follow-up, LJ was assessed for additional medication changes and adherence, and did not exhibit any signs or symptoms concerning for overanticoagulation (bleeding, bruising, etc). Repeat renal function testing was performed, with CrCl improving to 52 mL/min. Repeat CBC was unremarkable. LJ's anticoagulation provider discussed the major benefits (e.g. no need for regular therapeutic monitoring, improved bleeding risk profile with rivaroxaban vs warfarin, lack of dietary restrictions) and risks (e.g. concern for inappropriate dosing based with renal function decline/variable function, lack of reversal agent) of continuing rivaroxaban or transitioning to an alternative DOAC or warfarin.

During Hospitalization Follow-up

- **Reassess renal function** to assess recovery towards baseline function. More frequent monitoring of renal function, CBC, and resolution of clinical symptoms within 1–2 weeks should be considered until return to baseline function is confirmed. Consider repeating a CBC if concerns or evidence of new bleeding persist.
- **Reassess appropriateness of current dosing**: Has renal function and the patient's overall clinical picture returned to the pre-hospitalization baseline? Assess if the original DOAC dose should be resumed or if a modified dose or discontinuation is warranted. If renal function does not recover completely or a pattern of increasingly frequent events associated with variable and acutely worsened renal function becomes apparent, warfarin should be considered in place of continued DOAC therapy. If considering alternative DOACs, consider the differences in dosing frequency and differences in renal function criteria guiding dose adjustments. For LJ, it is reasonable to continue her current dose of rivaroxaban.
- **Reassess the benefits and risks of long-term anticoagulation**: Does the patient remain a good candidate for anticoagulation? If the patient is deemed to be at increased risk of poor anticoagulation safety outcomes (e.g. worsening renal function, increasing fall frequency) compared to the benefits, anticoagulation should be discontinued. LJ appears to be otherwise healthy, has good social support at home, and a history of adherence to her previous and current anticoagulation regimens.

The Outcome

Rivaroxaban 20 mg daily was continued. Given LJ's borderline renal function and concern for variation downwards, repeat labs were to be redrawn in 1 month. LJ would be contacted by telephone for clinical assessment again in 2 weeks and in 6 weeks to discuss lab results, as well as a decision on whether to continue or modify rivaroxaban therapy.

Key Points

- DOAC use in the setting of variable renal function should be scrutinized carefully or even avoided, especially if renal function severely fluctuates and borders cutoff criteria for dose adjustments. DOACs should be discontinued if it appears that renal insufficiency is worsening. Warfarin should be considered as the anticoagulant of choice in variable and severe renal insufficiency (e.g. approaching CrCl 30 mL/min) since its therapeutic intensity is not significantly altered by renal dysfunction.
- More frequent assessment of renal function and CBC should be performed in those with variable renal insufficiency. If available, drawing coagulation assays sensitive to the specific DOAC may be useful to determine the extent of accumulation if significant concern exists for severe DOAC accumulation. These coagulation assays are not currently widely available and/or standardized. Consider regular patient communication by phone or electronic messaging if in-clinic assessments are less frequent to ensure continued medication adherence and anticoagulation efficacy and safety.
- Consider all patient factors in addition to patient and provider convenience when considering continued DOAC use in those with variable renal insufficiency that borders criteria for DOAC dose adjustments. If renal function remains unstable and complicates the selection of a maintenance DOAC dose, warfarin may be a more manageable alternative.

Self-Assessment Questions

Please also reference Chap. 8 figures and tables.

1. Which of the following patients on direct oral anticoagulant therapy for atrial fibrillation should more frequent renal function monitoring be considered?
    (a) A 32-year-old 92 kg male patient on apixaban with a serum creatinine of 0.6 mg/dL being treated with oral vancomycin for Clostridium difficile.

(b) A 42-year-old male on rivaroxaban with no additional prior medical history other than hypertension.
(c) A 51-year-old male on dabigatran with stage III chronic kidney disease.
(d) A 76-year-old female on warfarin status-post renal transplantation and recently started on a 14-day course of sulfamethoxazole-trimethoprim DS for urinary tract infection.

Rationale for question #1

(a) Incorrect. Apixaban requires dose adjustment in those being treated for atrial fibrillation who possess two of the three following factors: Age of 80 years or older, body weight of 60 kg or less, or serum creatinine 1.5 mg/dL or greater. Patients on concomitant strong dual inhibitors of CYP 3A4 and P-gp should also use a reduced apixaban dose. Oral vancomycin is largely confined to the GI tract when taken orally.
(b) Incorrect. This patient likely does not require any closer monitoring than usual as he does not appear to have a complicated medical history that includes renal insufficiency.
(c) Correct. Stage III CKD is defined as GFR between 30 and 44 mL/min. Dabigatran requires dose adjustment in those being treated for atrial fibrillation with a CrCl 15–30 mL/min and is contraindicated in those with CrCl <15 mL/min. The CrCl cutoff for contraindication to dabigatran differs with anticoagulation indication.
(d) Incorrect. Although there is a clinically significant drug-drug interaction with warfarin, renal function is not expected to have a clinically relevant effect on warfarin elimination or INR.

2. Which of the following direct oral anticoagulants is correctly matched with the CrCl cutoff requiring a renally-adjusted dose when anticoagulating for atrial fibrillation?

(a) Apixaban—CrCl <30 mL/min
(b) Dabigatran—CrCl <30 mL/min
(c) Edoxaban—CrCl >50mL/min
(d) Rivaroxaban—CrCl >50 mL/min

Rationale

(a) Incorrect. Apixaban dose adjustments are considered based on serum creatinine, not creatinine clearance. Caution, however, should be heeded if renal insufficiency worsens.
(b) Correct. Dabigatran dose should be decreased starting at CrCl 30 mL/min.
(c) Incorrect. Edoxaban does not require dose adjustment at this level of function, but should be avoided if CrCl exceeds 95 mL/min.
(d) Incorrect. Rivaroxaban dose should be adjusted if CrCl is between 15 and 50 mL/min.

References

1. Nutescu EA, Burnett A, Fanikos J, et al. Pharmacology of anticoagulants used in the treatment of venous thromboembolism. J Thromb Thrombolysis. 2016;41(1):15–31.
2. Garcia DA, Baglin TP, Weitz JI, et al. Parenteral anticoagulants: antithrombotic therapy and prevention of thrombosis, 9th ed: American College of Chest Physicians evidence-based clinical practice guidelines. Chest. 2012;141(2 Suppl):e24S–43S.
3. Smythe MA, Priziola J, Dobesh PP, et al. Guidance for the practical management of the heparin anticoagulants in the treatment of venous thromboembolism. J Thromb Thrombolysis. 2016;41(1):165–86.
4. Burnett AE, Mahan CE, Vazquez SR, et al. Guidance for the practical management of the direct oral anticoagulants (DOACs) in VTE treatment. J Thromb Thrombolysis. 2016;41(1): 206–32.
5. Cuker A, Siegal DM, Crowther MA, et al. Laboratory measurement of the anticoagulant activity of the non-vitamin K oral anticoagulants. J Am Coll Cardiol. 2014;64(11):1128–39.
6. Pradaxa (dabigatran) package insert. Ridgefield, CT: Boehringer Ingelheim Pharmaceuticals, Inc; 2015.
7. Xarelto (rivaroxaban) package insert. Titusville, NJ: Janssen Pharmaceuticals, Inc; 2016.
8. Eliquis package insert. Princeton, NJ: Bristol-Myers Squibb Company; 2016.
9. Savaysa (edoxaban) package insert. Parsippany, NJ: Daiichi Sankyo, Inc; 2016.
10. Ageno W, Gallus AS, Wittkowsky A, et al. Oral anticoagulant therapy: antithrombotic therapy and prevention of thrombosis, 9th ed: American College of Chest Physicians evidence-based clinical practice guidelines. Chest. 2012;141(2 Suppl):e44S–88S.
11. January CT, Wann SL, Alpert JS, et al. 2014 AHA/ACC/HRS guideline for the management of patients with atrial fibrillation: executive summary. J Am Coll Cardiol. 2014;64(21): 2246–80.
12. Dager W, Hellwig T. Current knowledge on assessing the effects of and managing bleeding and urgent procedures with direct oral anticoagulants. Am J Health Syst Pharm. 2016;73(10 Suppl 2): S14–26.

Chapter 11
Patient with Concomitant Stable Coronary Artery Disease

Michael Brenner and Augustus Hough

Abstract There are no randomized controlled trials published for the use of either vitamin k antagonist or direct oral anticoagulants (DOACs) monotherapy in secondary heart prevention. There have been some pre-specified analyses from landmark trials studied for atrial fibrillation that have demonstrated a similar incidence of myocardial infarction between DOACs and warfarin.

Keywords Atrial fibrillation • Stable coronary artery disease (CAD) • Warfarin Direct oral anticoagulants • DOACs • Aspirin • Antiplatelet therapy

A 76 year old male presents to the office for routine follow-up. He complains of intermittent nosebleeds over the past few weeks. His past medical history consists of coronary artery disease (s/p coronary artery bypass grafting × 3 in 2007 and s/p myocardial infarction with drug-eluting stent in 2004), atrial fibrillation, hypertension, type 2 diabetes, anemia, and stage 3 chronic kidney disease. An echocardiogram was done recently that revealed normal left ventricular and right ventricular size and function, as well as normal valvular function. Vital signs today include blood pressure 126/78, pulse 62, height 70 in., and weight 80 kg. Pertinent laboratory values include SCr 1.8 (Est CrCl 39.5 mL/min), BUN 31, Hg 10.1 g/dL, Hct 35.4%, POC INR 2.7 (TTR >80% over past year), LFT within normal limits. Medications include warfarin with goal INR 2–3, aspirin, atorvastatin, lisinopril,

---

M. Brenner, PharmD, BCPS
VA Ann Arbor Healthcare System, Ann Arbor, MI 48105, USA
e-mail: Michael.Brenner@va.gov

A. Hough, PharmD, BCPS (✉)
West Palm Beach VA Medical Center, 7305 N. Military Trial, West Palm Beach, FL 33410-6400, USA
e-mail: Augustus.Hough@va.gov

chlorthalidone, pantoprazole, and glipizide. The patient has a $CHA_2DS_2\text{-}VAS_C$ score of 5 and $CHADS_2$ score of 3, and a HAS-BLED score of 3. Denies alcohol or tobacco use.

What is the most appropriate antithrombotic treatment option for this patient?

Case Discussion

Using antiplatelet therapy with anticoagulation can increase the risk for major bleeding and hospitalization for bleeding more than anticoagulation alone [1]. Antiplatelet agents such as aspirin and clopidogrel (if intolerant to aspirin) are cornerstone therapies for secondary prevention in stable coronary artery disease (CAD). Anticoagulation is important for stroke prevention in atrial fibrillation, but precaution must be made when used in combination with antiplatelet agents to minimize the risk for bleeding. For patients with an acute coronary syndrome or recent stent placement within the last year, continuing concomitant antiplatelet and anticoagulation therapies are ideal up to 12 months, but for stable CAD the evidence is less clear. Based on this patient's $CHA_2DS_2\text{-}VASc/CHADS_2$ score, continuing anticoagulation is recommended over aspirin monotherapy. Based on the patient's HAS-BLED score indicating a high risk of bleeding, complaints of nosebleed and anemia, discontinuing aspirin should be considered to allow continuation of anticoagulation.

No randomized trials exist on optimal antithrombotic therapy for stable CAD with concomitant atrial fibrillation. The 2012 CHEST antithrombotic therapy guidelines recommend warfarin rather than the combination of warfarin and aspirin [2]. The 2011 AHA-ACCF Secondary prevention guidelines recommend the combination of warfarin and aspirin in stable CAD patients if there is a compelling indication for anticoagulation [3]. The 2015 update for practical management of non-valvular atrial fibrillation by the European Heart Rhythm Association recommend avoiding antiplatelet agents in stable CAD patients receiving oral anticoagulants. There are no randomized controlled trials published in stable CAD with concomitant atrial fibrillation between vitamin K antagonist (VKA) and direct oral anticoagulants (DOACs). See Table 11.1 for summary of guideline recommendations. Data from the

Table 11.1 Summary of guideline recommendations for antiplatelet therapy with antithrombotic therapy in stable CAD patients

Clinical practice guidelines	Recommendation on antiplatelet therapy in stable CAD receiving warfarin
2012 CHEST Antithrombosis [2]	Recommend warfarin over the combination of antiplatelet therapy and warfarin
2011 AHA-ACCF secondary prevention [3]	Recommend continuing antiplatelet therapy while on warfarin
2015 European Heart Rhythm Association [4]	Avoid the combination of the antiplatelet therapy and anticoagulants

landmark atrial fibrillation trials of the DOACs versus VKA did not suggest that there would be heterogeneity in effects on background coronary disease outcomes. Specifically in the RELY study which compared dabigatran and VKA, the initial trial publication suggested a higher rate of MI in the dabigatran 150 mg twice daily arm than VKA. However, this was later found to be nonsignificant after all data was reviewed [5, 6]. A pre-specified substudy of the RE-LY trial was done for patients with a history of CAD or a previous MI to determine the relationship with myocardial ischemic events. A nonsignificant trend for an increase in MIs was observed in the dabigatran group for both doses compared with warfarin. Other myocardial ischemic events (unstable angina, need for revascularization, cardiac arrest, or cardiac death) were the same between both doses of dabigatran and warfarin. There was no dose-dependent effect on MI observed [7]. The FDA completed a study in Medicare patients comparing both medications for ischemic or clot-related stroke, gastrointestinal bleeding, MI, and death. The incidence of MI was similar between dabigatran and VKA. In the evaluations of the rivaroxaban, apixaban, and edoxaban versus VKA therapy there was no significant difference in MI rates in the trial arms [8–10]. Due to the lack of prospective data for the DOACs in stable CAD, it would be reasonable to prefer VKA at this point based on the presence of historic data.

The recommendations for use of VKA in stable CAD without concomitant antiplatelet therapy are derived from both direct and indirect data sources. Direct data comes from a meta-analysis of historic evaluation as well as the ASPECT-2 and WARIS II studies [11–13]. These evaluations did not show a significant reduction in cardiovascular or thromboembolic events in patients with CAD and atrial fibrillation when aspirin was added to VKA therapy. Secondary data supporting VKA therapy without antiplatelet therapy in stable CAD and atrial fibrillation comes from a sub-study from the SPORTIF trial. This study, which was nonrandomized, compared warfarin monotherapy to low dose aspirin (<100 mg/day) with warfarin (INR goal 2–3). The incidence of stroke/systemic embolism or myocardial infarction (MI) was similar between both groups, but major bleeding was significantly higher by two-fold for combination therapy [14]. Finally, a Danish cohort study evaluated patients with atrial fibrillation and the combinations of VKA, aspirin, and/or clopidogrel compared to VKA monotherapy. Coronary events or thromboembolism were similar between all groups and all combination therapies had more serious bleeds compared to VKA monotherapy [15].

Based on this patient's CHA_2DS_2-VASc and $CHADS_2$ score, anticoagulation is recommended over aspirin alone. This approach appears to provide better balance for thrombotic event prevention. It should be noted that the data with VKA in stable CAD is limited by its age as patients in these historic evaluations were not treated with modern approaches (e.g., second/third generation drug eluting stents). However in patients with stable CAD and atrial fibrillation, the data would still be expected to be relevant. Based on the patient's HAS-BLED score and hemoglobin level in the presence of stable CAD, aspirin should be discontinued to allow for continuation of anticoagulation while minimizing the risk for bleeding. There are no contraindications or any reason that the patient must switch from warfarin to a DOAC. Based on the information provided and clinical evidence, continuation of warfarin alone is the best clinical option of those provided.

Key Points

- Vitamin K antagonist (VKA) monotherapy has similar rates of coronary events compared to VKA and antiplatelet therapy in stable CAD and atrial fibrillation.
- There are no randomized controlled trials published in stable coronary artery disease with concomitant atrial fibrillation between vitamin K antagonist and direct oral anticoagulants.
- Pre-specified analyses have demonstrated similar rates of myocardial infarction between direct oral anticoagulants and vitamin K antagonist.

Self-Assessment Questions

1. Which of the following direct oral anticoagulants has similar rates of myocardial infarction to warfarin for secondary heart prevention?

    (a) Apixaban 5 mg twice daily
    (b) Edoxaban 60 mg once daily
    (c) Rivaroxaban 20 mg once daily
    (d) All of the above

    Correct Answer: D (All of the above)
    Rationale: All three direct oral anticoagulants mentioned above have shown a similar rate of myocardial infarction when compared to warfarin in their respective trials. Pre-specified analyses have been done in the ARISTOTLE and ROCKET AF trials for patients with coronary artery disease with the same results. No pre-specified analysis has been published for edoxaban at this time.

2. Which of the following provides the best summary of the outcomes of combining warfarin and aspirin versus warfarin alone in patients with atrial fibrillation and stable coronary artery disease?

    (a) More bleeding and less major adverse cardiovascular events
    (b) More bleeding and more major adverse cardiovascular events
    (c) More bleeding and similar major adverse cardiovascular events
    (d) Similar bleeding and less major adverse cardiovascular events

    Correct Answer: C (More bleeding and similar major adverse cardiovascular effects)
    Rationale: Based on direct and indirect data sources, such as the ASPECT II and WARIS II trials, and the sub-study of the SPORTIF trial, combining aspirin and warfarin showed higher bleeding rates and similar rates of cardiovascular events.

Disclaimer The views expressed in this chapter reflect those of the authors, and not necessarily those of the Department of Veterans Affairs.

References

1. Steinberg BA, Kim S, Piccini JP, et al. Use and associated risks of concomitant aspirin therapy with oral anticoagulation in patients with atrial fibrillation. Circulation. 2013;128:721–8.
2. You JJ, Singer DE, Howard PA, et al. Antithrombotic therapy for atrial fibrillation antithrombotic therapy and prevention of thrombosis, 9th ed: American College of Chest Physicians evidence-based clinical practice guidelines. Chest. 2012;141:e531S–75S.
3. Smith SC Jr., Benjamin EJ, Bonow RO, Braun LT, Creager MA, Franklin BA, Gibbons RJ, Grundy SM, Hiratzka LF, Jones DW, Lloyd-Jones DM, Minissian M, Mosca L, Peterson ED, Sacco RL, Spertus J, Stein JH, Taubert KA. AHA/ACCF secondary prevention and risk reduction therapy for patients with coronary and other atherosclerotic vascular disease: 2011 update: a guideline from the American Heart Association and American College of Cardiology Foundation. Circulation. 2011: published online before print November 3, 2011, doi:10.1161/CIR.0b013e318235eb4d
4. Heidbuchel H, et al. Updated European Heart Rhythm Association practical guide on the use of non-vitamin K antagonist anticoagulants in patients with non-valvular atrial fibrillation. Europace. 2015;17(10):1467–507. doi:10.1093/europace/euv309. Epub 2015 Aug 31.
5. Connelly SJ, et al. Newly identified events in the RE-LY trial. N Engl J Med. 2010;363(19):1875–6.
6. Connelly SJ, Ezekowitz MD, Yusuf S, et al. For the RE-LY Steering Committee and Investigators. Dabigatran versus warfarin in patients with atrial fibrillation. N Engl J Med. 2009;361:1139–51.
7. Hohnloser SH, Oldgren J, Yang S, et al. Myocardial ischemic events in patients with atrial fibrillation treated with dabigatran or warfarin in the RE-LY trial. Circulation. 2012;125:669–76.
8. Patel MR, Mahaffey KW, Garg J, et al. Rivaroxaban versus warfarin in nonvalvular atrial fibrillation (ROCKET AF). N Engl J Med. 2011;365(10):883–91.
9. Giugliano RP, Ruff CT, Braunwald E, et al. Edoxaban versus warfarin in patients with atrial fibrillation. N Engl J Med. 2013;369(22):2093–104.
10. Granger CB, Alexander JH, McMurray JJV, et al. Apixaban versus warfarin in patients with atrial fibrillation (ARISTOTLE). N Engl J Med. 2011;365:981–92.
11. Dentali F, Douketis JD, Lim W, Crowther M. Combined aspirin-oral anticoagulant therapy compared with oral anticoagulant therapy alone among patients at risk for cardiovascular disease. Arch Intern Med. 2007;167:117–1241.
12. Hurlen M, Abdelnoor M, Smith P, Erikssen J, Arnesen H. Warfarin, aspirin, or both after myocardial infarction. N Engl J Med. 2002;347:969–74.
13. Van Es RF, Jonker JJC, Verheugt FWA, Deckers JW, Grobbee DE. Aspirin and coumadin after acute coronary syndromes (the ASPECT-2 study): a randomized controlled trial. Lancet. 2002;360:109–13.
14. Flaker GC, Gruber M, Connolly SJ, et al. Risk and benefits of combining aspirin with anticoagulant therapy in patients with atrial fibrillation: an exploratory analysis of stroke prevention using an oral thrombin inhibitor in atrial fibrillation (SPORTIF) trials. Am Heart J. 2006;152:967–73.
15. Lamberts M, Gislason GH, Lip GY, et al. Antiplatelet therapy for stable coronary artery disease in atrial fibrillation patients taking an oral anticoagulant; a nationwide cohort study. Circulation. 2014;129:1577–85.

Chapter 12
Patient with Concomitant Acute Venous Thromboembolism

Lea E. dela Pena

Abstract In patients with atrial fibrillation who develop an acute venous thromboembolism, it is important to initiate anticoagulant dosing for the acute VTE, which may differ from dosing for atrial fibrillation depending on the particular agent. Parenteral anticoagulants are needed at the start of therapy if dabigatran, edoxaban, or warfarin is chosen, and should be prescribed at full treatment doses. The patient should be fully anticoagulated during the first 3 months of therapy after the VTE in order to prevent clot propagation and embolism.

Keywords Atrial fibrillation • Venous thromboembolism • Parenteral anticoagulant • Clot propagation

Case Introduction

A 55 year old male patient with past medical history significant for BPH, hypertension, and atrial fibrillation is in the hospital with a new diagnosis of deep vein thrombosis (DVT). He recently returned from an 8 hour international flight when he began complaining of leg swelling and tenderness. He travels internationally often for work. He currently takes tamsulosin, lisinopril, and aspirin. Vitals are stable, current height and weight is 70 in. and 85 kg, respectively, and hepatic/renal function is unremarkable. He has been started on a heparin drip, but physicians want to transition him to an oral medication in preparation for discharge.

L.E. dela Pena, PharmD, BCPS
Midwestern University Chicago College of Pharmacy,
555 W 31st St, Downers Grove, IL 60515, USA
e-mail: ldelap@midwestern.edu

Case Discussion

What oral anticoagulants can be utilized to treat this patient's atrial fibrillation and DVT?

- His oral options would be warfarin (bridged with a rapid acting agent, such as LMWH, until INR ≥2), dabigatran, rivaroxaban, apixaban, or edoxaban.

How would his provider choose among the various agents available to use?

- The provider should first make sure the patient does not have any contraindications to any of the medications; typically if a patient has a contraindication to a DOAC, he/she should be initiated on warfarin instead. Also, certain patient populations were not well studied in the clinical trials that led to approval of the DOACs, so these patients should be started on warfarin; these would include such populations as pediatric patients, patients with poor renal or hepatic function, patients with diagnosed thrombophilia, breastfeeding women, or patients with extremes of body weight [1]. Pregnant patients were also not adequately studied in the DOAC clinical trials; however, warfarin is not an option for these patients as it is considered teratogenic [2]. Our patient does not fall into any of the criteria for contraindications or populations that were not well-studied, so he is a candidate for warfarin or one of the DOACs.
- Drug interactions are also important to assess. Our patient does not have any clinically significant drug interactions with any of the anticoagulant medications up for consideration. His aspirin therapy will be stopped upon initiation of the anticoagulant.
- Patient adherence is important to assess as well. If a patient has issues with missing doses of medications, DOAC therapy may not be ideal as even missing just one dose can quickly put a patient at risk for a recurrent clot.
- The patient should also be brought into this conversation about choosing a particular anticoagulant. His preferences for once daily vs twice daily administration, dietary restrictions, frequent laboratory monitoring, and cost should be taken into consideration. Given his frequent travel for work, he may not be able to commit to the necessary laboratory monitoring needed for warfarin therapy, unless he is able to obtain a home INR monitor. Three of the medications (warfarin, dabigatran, and edoxaban) require a parenteral anticoagulant be administered prior to or at the beginning of therapy. The parenteral anticoagulant is usually a low molecular weight heparin (LMWH) such as enoxaparin or dalteparin, unfractionated heparin (UFH), or fondaparinux, given at treatment (not prophylactic) doses. If the patient is not agreeable to using an injectable medication, even for just a few days, these options may not be ideal for him.

What additional laboratory tests should be ordered prior to initiating therapy?

- A complete blood count, activated partial thromboplastin time, and prothrombin time should be ordered to ensure he does not have an underlying coagulopathy.

- A serum creatinine, as well as a calculated creatinine clearance, should be obtained to classify any underlying renal impairment which may affect dosing of certain agents.

Should the provider prescribe dosing for atrial fibrillation or DVT for this patient?

- The provider should prescribe anticoagulant dosing for the acute DVT (see Table 12.1). Some agents will have different dosing depending on the exact indication as discussed below.
- Warfarin dosing and target INR will be the same regardless if treating for atrial fibrillation or DVT.
- Rivaroxaban and apixaban have different initial dosing for DVT compared to atrial fibrillation as outlined in the Table 12.2, assuming no dosing adjustments needed based on patient characteristics such as reduced renal function [3–5].
- Dabigatran and edoxaban have the same dosing for atrial fibrillation as well as acute DVT: 150 mg BID and 60 mg daily, respectively. However, it is important to keep in mind that parenteral anticoagulant must be used for a few days prior to this initiation [1].

Table 12.1 Initial dosing for oral anticoagulants to treat acute DVT [2, 4–8]

Oral medication	Dosing	Dosing adjustments if applicable
Warfarin	Typically 2.5–10 mg po daily overlapped with parenteral anticoagulant for at least 5 days AND until two therapeutic INRs	N/A
Dabigatran	Parenteral anticoagulant × 5–10 days, followed by dabigatran 150 mg po BID	If CrCL ≤ 30 mL/min—no dosing recommendations provided by manufacturer
Rivaroxaban	15 mg po BID with food × 21 days, then change to 20 mg po daily with food	N/A
Apixaban	10 mg po BID × 7 days, then change to 5 mg po BID	N/A
Edoxaban	Parenteral anticoagulant × 5–10 days, followed by 60 mg po daily	If CrCL 15–50 mL/min, weight ≤ 60 kg or patient is on P-gp inhibitor, reduce edoxaban dose to 30 mg po daily

Table 12.2 Comparison of different dosing based on indication for rivaroxaban and apixaban

	Rivaroxaban	Apixaban
Atrial fibrillation dosing	20 mg daily with the evening meal	5 mg BID
VTE dosing	15 mg BID with food × 3 weeks then 20 mg once daily	10 mg BID × 7 days, then 5 mg BID

What is the expected duration of anticoagulation treatment for this patient?

- Since this is the patient's first DVT and likely due to a long international flight, he will only need anticoagulation for approximately 3 months for the DVT [9]. Patients need to be monitored closely during this time and must be fully anticoagulated in order to prevent further clot propagation and embolism.
- At the end of that time, therapy should be reassessed to see if further anticoagulation is needed for the DVT [9].

Which medication would be appropriate at the end of the first 3 months of anticoagulation therapy?

- Prior to the diagnosis of DVT, this patient's CHA_2DS_2-VASc score was one (hypertension) so aspirin therapy was selected and an appropriate choice for that indication although anticoagulation would also be an appropriate choice. The patient still has the same CHA_2DS_2-VASc score thus can continue the same antiplatelet therapy. This is an appropriate time to readdress the risk and benefit of antiplatelet versus anticoagulant therapy in stroke prevention to determine the patient's preference at this time.

Key Points

- Assess the patient for any contraindications or precautions to potential medications. Bring the patient into the conversation when discussing which medication to initiate.
- Initial dosing of rivaroxaban and apixaban is different for acute VTE compared to atrial fibrillation.
- Dabigatran, edoxaban, and warfarin require parenteral anticoagulation at the start of therapy. Parental therapy includes low molecular weight heparin, unfractionated heparin, or fondaparinux.
- Parenteral anticoagulation, if needed, should be prescribed at full treatment doses, instead of prophylactic doses.
- The patient needs to be fully anticoagulated during first 3 months of therapy in order to prevent clot propagation and embolism.

Self-Assessment Questions

1. A 50 year old female patient with history of atrial fibrillation, hypertension, dyslipidemia, and seasonal allergies has just been diagnosed with a new deep vein thrombosis. Her current medications include aspirin, hydrochlorothiazide, pravastatin, and loratadine. Her labwork is unremarkable. She prefers taking medications once a day, but she does have good prescription insurance through

her employer. If possible, she would like to avoid any injectable agents since she is afraid of needles. Which of the following medications would be best to initiate in this patient for her DVT?

(a) Warfarin with INR goal 2.0–3.0
(b) Rivaroxaban
(c) Apixaban
(d) Edoxaban

The correct answer is B. Cost does not seem to be an issue since she has good prescription coverage through her work. Rivaroxaban is taken once daily and does not require a parenteral agent prior to initiation. Her labwork is unremarkable which is important to assess for any coagulopathies or renal/hepatic dysfunction. Warfarin and edoxaban are not correct since both of these agents would require a parenteral anticoagulant be administered either prior to or concurrently with the oral agent. Apixaban is incorrect because this is dosed twice daily and the patient prefers a once daily regimen.

2. A 64 year old male patient with history of atrial fibrillation, hypertension, osteoarthritis, ESRD, and poor adherence is diagnosed with a pulmonary embolism. He is currently taking aspirin, lisinopril, and acetaminophen. He is retired and prefers generic medications whenever possible. Which of the following anticoagulants is the best choice to treat this patient's PE?

(a) Warfarin with INR goal 2.0–3.0
(b) Rivaroxaban
(c) Apixaban
(d) Edoxaban

The correct answer is A. Warfarin is generic, and thus less expensive than the DOACs. With this patient's history of poor adherence, missing even just one dose of a DOAC can put him at increased risk for a recurrent clot. Most DOACs were not studied in patients with ESRD. These reasons all make answers B, C, and D incorrect. Warfarin has been used in patients with ESRD. He will require overlap with a parenteral anticoagulant, likely unfractionated heparin, until his INR is in therapeutic range.

References

1. Burnett AE, Mahan CE, Vazquez SR, et al. Guidance for the practical management of the direct oral anticoagulants (DOACs) in VTE treatment. J Thromb Thrombolysis. 2016;41:206–32.
2. Coumadin [package insert]. Princeton, NJ: Bristol-Myers Squibb Company; 2015.
3. Mookadam M, Shamoun FE, Mookadam F. Novel anticoagulants in atrial fibrillation: a primer for the primary physician. J Am Board Fam Med. 2015;28:510–22.
4. Xarelto [package insert]. Titusville, NJ: Janssen Pharmaceuticals, Inc; 2016.
5. Eliquis [package insert]. Princeton, NJ and New York, NY: Bristol-Myers Squibb Company and Pfizer, Inc; 2016.

6. Ageno W, Gallus AS, Wittkowski A, et al. Oral anticoagulant therapy: antithrombotic therapy and prevention of thrombosis, 9th ed: American College of Chest Physicians evidence-based clinical practice guideline. Chest. 2012;141(2 Suppl):e44S–88S.
7. Pradaxa [package insert]. Ridgefield, CT: Boehringer-Ingelheim Pharmaceuticals, Inc; 2015.
8. Savaysa [package insert]. Parsippany, NJ: Daiichi Sankyo, Inc; 2015.
9. Kearon C, Akl EA, Ornelas J, et al. Antithrombotic therapy for VTE disease: CHEST guideline and expert panel report. Chest. 2016;149:315–52.

Chapter 13
Patient with Concomitant Mitral Valve Stenosis

Augustus Hough and Michael Brenner

Abstract Mitral stenosis is a significant risk factor for stroke in patients with atrial fibrillation and serves as an indication for anticoagulation regardless of the presence of other traditional stroke risk factors. The preferred oral anticoagulant in patients with atrial fibrillation and mitral stenosis is warfarin.

Keywords Mitral valve stenosis • Atrial fibrillation • Stoke risk factor Anticoagulation • Valvular atrial fibrillation

Case Introduction

A 63-year-old male presents to anticoagulation clinic for routine follow-up of warfarin therapy he takes for history of paroxysmal atrial fibrillation. He also has a PMH of moderate-severe mitral stenosis (class C), hypertension, BPH, and anxiety. Pertinent laboratory values include CrCl 74 mL/min, POC INR 2.2, CBC within normal limits. Patient's warfarin is generally very well controlled (time in therapeutic range 82%) but he is still employed and is having a difficult time leaving work to come to anticoagulation visits. He asks his provider whether continuing anticoagulation therapy is still necessary. He calculated his CHA_2DS_2-VASc score as 1 using an online calculator and would like to consider changing to aspirin alone to reduce bleeding risk and improved convenience of therapy. Alternatively, he asks about one of the direct oral anticoagulants and if he is a candidate because of lack of

---

A. Hough, PharmD, BCPS (AQ-Cardiology) (✉)
West Palm Beach VA Medical Center, 7305 N. Military Trial, West Palm Beach, FL 33410, USA
e-mail: Augustus.Hough@va.gov

M. Brenner, PharmD, BCPS (AQ-Cardiology)
VA Ann Arbor Healthcare System, Ann Arbor, MI 48105, USA
e-mail: Michael.Brenner@va.gov

monitoring. He has no other complaints at this time but would prefer to make things as simple as possible and reduce his risk of bleeding.

What is the most appropriate oral antithrombotic therapy for this patient?

Case Discussion

The decision regarding the use and selection of antithrombotic therapy (i.e., none, antiplatelet or anticoagulant) in patients with atrial fibrillation (AF) is generally made with consideration of thromboembolic risk as determined by the CHA_2DS_2-VASc score; however, patients with concomitant mitral stenosis (MS) are exceptions. Compared to normal sinus rhythm, AF increases the risk of stroke by approximately fivefold in the general population and up to 20-fold in patients with mitral stenosis [1]. Since there is a high risk of stroke in AF patients with mitral stenosis, anticoagulation is indicated regardless of other background risk factors for thromboembolism. The current 2014 AHA/ACC/HRS guidelines give a Class I (level of evidence B) recommendation for the use of anticoagulation (vitamin K antagonist (VKA) or heparin) in patients with MS and AF of any type [2]. Similarly, the 2012 CHEST guidelines on antithrombotic therapy in atrial fibrillation give a Grade IB recommendation for the use of anticoagulation with VKA therapy (INR target range 2–3) in AF patients with MS regardless of CHA_2DS_2-VASc risk score [3]. Therefore, barring any contraindications, anticoagulation should be recommended versus antiplatelet or no antithrombotic therapy.

The choice of anticoagulant is limited for patients with AF and MS as the only recommended oral anticoagulant to date is VKA therapy. The recommendation for use of VKA therapy is largely one of historic convention derived from positive observational findings rather than from a randomized evidence base [4]. Exclusion of direct oral anticoagulants (DOACs) from recommendations in this patient population is not based on an expectation of clinical failure versus VKA, but a lack of evaluation in this cohort. Patients with MS have consistently been excluded form major evaluations of antithrombotic therapies in AF (see Table 13.1 for detailed

Table 13.1 Exclusion criteria related to valvular disease in pivotal, modern anticoagulation trials

Trial	Selected exclusion criteria pertaining to valvular disease
RE-LY [5]	History of heart valve disorders (i.e., prosthetic valve or hemodynamically relevant valve disease)
ROCKET-AF [6]	Hemodynamically significant mitral stenosis or any valve prostheses (however, annuloplasty with or without prosthetic ring, commissurotomy and/or valvuloplasty were permitted)
ARISTOTLE [7]	Clinically significant (moderate or severe) mitral stenosis and conditions other than AF that require chronic anticoagulation (e.g., prosthetic mechanical heart valve)
ENGAGE AF-TIMI 48 [8]	Subjects with moderate or severe mitral stenosis or mechanical heart valve (however, subjects with bioprosthetic heart valves, mitral valve prolapse, mitral valve regurgitation, and aortic valve disease and/or valve repair were included)
ACTIVE W and A [9]	Requirement for oral anticoagulant for prosthetic mechanical heart valve) and mitral stenosis

exclusion criteria). This exclusion is based on several lines of reasoning. First, as noted earlier, MS significantly increases the thromboembolic risk beyond that seen in a typical AF cohort. Second, historical, non-controlled, findings have shown that while 91% of thrombi are isolated to the left atrial appendage (LAA) in non-rheumatic (non-MS) AF, only 57% of thrombi are localized to the LAA in rheumatic (MS) AF indicating that a different etiology of thrombi generation may be present, see Fig. 13.1 [10]. These findings provide both clinical and physiologic rationales to approach evaluations of MS and non-MS AF cohorts as separate entities.

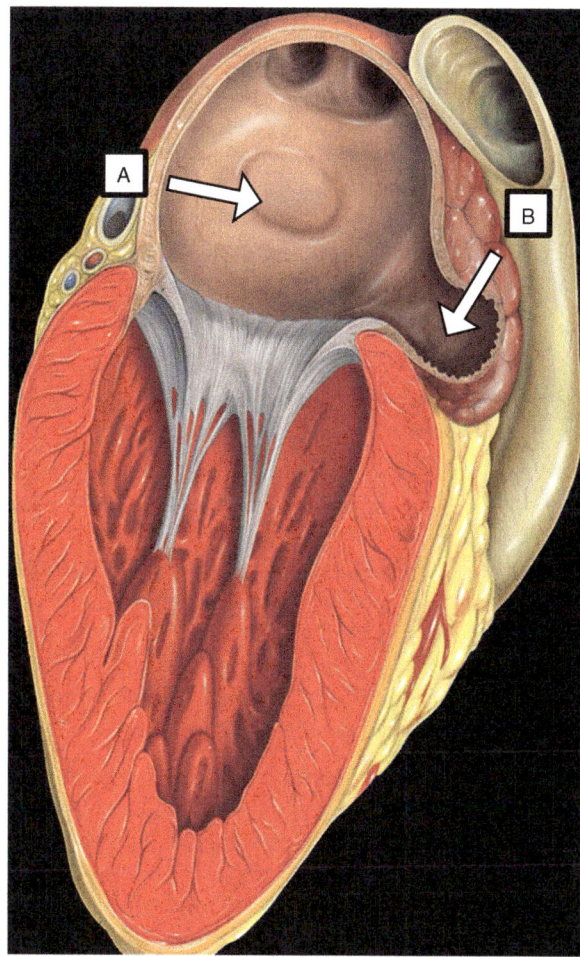

Fig. 13.1 (**a**) Left atrium, (**b**) left atrial appendage. The left atrial appendage (LAA) is site of 91% of thrombi isolation in non-rheumatic (non-mitral stenosis (non-MS)) atrial fibrillation (AF) while only 57% of thrombi are localized to the LAA in rheumatic (MS) AF. Illustration used with permission: By Patrick J. Lynch, medical illustrator (Patrick J. Lynch, medical illustrator) [CC BY 2.5 (http://creativecommons.org/licenses/by/2.5)], via Wikimedia Commons

A final consideration is that patients with MS may become candidates for valvular interventions (repair or replacement), a setting in which compiled evidence and clinical understanding supports VKA therapy (see Chap. 34). Thus, until data is available to support the efficacy and safety of DOACs in MS related AF, it is reasonable that warfarin should remain the therapy of choice for anticoagulation in these patients.

Our patient should be instructed to continue warfarin therapy at this time but perhaps considerations could be given to longer intervals between INR checks or patient self-testing of INR (see Chap. 16).

Key Points

- The development of atrial fibrillation in a patient with mitral stenosis is associated with a significant risk of stroke and is an indication for anticoagulation therapy regardless of background traditional risk factors for thromboembolism.
- The oral anticoagulant of choice in atrial fibrillation associated with mitral stenosis is warfarin.
- Mitral stenosis was a consistent exclusion criterion in evaluations of the direct oral anticoagulants (DOACs); thus, until more data is available the DOACs should not be pursued in patients with atrial fibrillation and mitral stenosis.

Self-Assessment Questions

1. What is the most appropriate antithrombotic therapy for a 58-year-old patient with the following medical history and no contraindications to any of the proposed therapies?
   Past Medical History: paroxysmal atrial fibrillation, depression, moderate-severe mitral stenosis, obesity, seizure history
   (a) No antithrombotic therapy
   (b) Aspirin 81 mg by month once daily
   (c) Aspirin 81 mg by mouth once daily along with clopidogrel 75 mg once daily
   (d) Warfarin by mouth dosed to INR target range of 2–3

   Correct answer: d (warfarin by mouth dosed to INR target range of 2–3)
   Rationale: In a patient with atrial fibrillation the presence of concomitant mitral stenosis is an indication for anticoagulation with vitamin K antagonist (VKA) therapy with target INR range 2–3 regardless of any other assessment of thromboembolic risk (i.e., regardless of CHA_2DS_2-VASc score). The CHEST AT9 guidelines on antithrombotic therapy in patients with atrial fibrillation and with mitral stenosis who are unable to take VKA therapy suggest aspirin and clopidogrel could be considered; but VKA is the preferred agent in patients without contraindications or intolerance.

2. In a 67-year-old male patient who has atrial fibrillation and asymptomatic moderate-severe mitral stenosis, which is the most appropriate recommendation for antithrombotic therapy? (Assuming CrCl >60 mL/min, SCr <1.5)
   (a) Warfarin by mouth dosed to INR target range of 2–3
   (b) Apixaban 5 mg by mouth twice daily
   (c) Rivaroxaban 20 mg by mouth once daily
   (d) All of the above are reasonable

   Correct answer: a (warfarin by mouth dosed to INR target range of 2–3)
   Rationale: Mitral stenosis was part of the exclusion criteria for the ARISTOTLE and ROCKET AF evaluations of apixaban and rivaroxaban respectively. Until data is available on the safety and efficacy of the direct oral anticoagulants in atrial fibrillation in patients with concomitant mitral stenosis warfarin remains the preferred anticoagulant.

Disclaimer The views expressed in this chapter reflect those of the authors, and not necessarily those of the Department of Veterans Affairs.

References

1. January CT, Wann LS, Alpert JS, et al. 2014 AHA/ACC/HRS guideline for the management of patients with atrial fibrillation: a report of the American College of Cardiology/American Heart Association task force on practice guidelines and the Heart Rhythm Society. J Am Coll Cardiol. 2014;64:e1–e76.
2. Nishimura RA, Otto CM, Bonow RO, et al. 2014 AHA/ACC guideline for the management of patients with valvular heart disease: a report of the American College of Cardiology/American Heart Association task force on practice guidelines. J Am Coll Cardiol. 2014;63:e57–185.
3. You JJ, Singer DE, Howard PA, et al. Antithrombotic therapy for atrial fibrillation antithrombotic therapy and prevention of thrombosis, 9th ed: American College of Chest Physicians evidence-based clinical practice guidelines. Chest. 2012;141:e531S–75S.
4. Whitlock RP, Sun JC, Fremes SE, Rubens FD, Teoh HK. Antithrombotic and thrombolytic therapy for valvular disease antithrombotic therapy and prevention of thrombosis, 9th ed: American College of Chest Physicians evidence-based clinical practice guidelines. Chest. 2012;141:e576S–600S.
5. Ezekowitz MD, Connolly S, Parekh A, et al. Rationale and design of RE-LY: randomized evaluation of long-term anticoagulant therapy, warfarin, compared with dabigatran. Am Heart J. 2009;157:805–10. e2
6. Patel MR, Mahaffey KW, Garg J, et al. Rivaroxaban versus warfarin in nonvalvular atrial fibrillation. N Engl J Med. 2011;365:883–91.
7. Lopes RD, Alexander JH, Al-Khatib SM, et al. Apixaban for reduction in stroke and other thromboembolic events in atrial fibrillation (ARISTOTLE) trial: design and rationale. Am Heart J. 2010;159:331–9.
8. Giugliano RP, Ruff CT, Braunwald E, et al. Edoxaban versus warfarin in patients with atrial fibrillation. N Engl J Med. 2013;369:2093–104.
9. Connelly S, Yusuf S, Budaj A, et al. Rationale and design of ACTIVE: the atrial fibrillation clopidogrel trial with irbesartan for prevention of vascular events. Am Heart J. 2006;151:1187–93.
10. Blackshear JL, Odell JA. Appendage obliteration to reduce stroke in cardiac surgical patients with atrial fibrillation. Ann Thoarc Surg. 1996;61:755–9.

Chapter 14
Patient with Concomitant Aortic Valve Stenosis

Augustus Hough and David Parra

Abstract Aortic valve stenosis, that does not require valvular surgery or intervention, does not impact decisions regarding the use of anticoagulation therapy in atrial fibrillation. If anticoagulation is indicated in a patient with atrial fibrillation based on presence of other traditional atrial fibrillation related stroke risk factors either warfarin or any of the nonwarfarin oral anticoagulants are reasonable choices.

Keywords Aortic valve stenosis • Atrial fibrillation • Anticoagulation • Nonvalvular atrial fibrillation

Case Introduction

A 73-year-old male with history of persistent atrial fibrillation, prior transient ischemic attack, heart failure with borderline left ventricular ejection fraction (LVEF) of 45–50% on past echocardiogram and moderate aortic stenosis is admitted for worsening heart failure. The patient complained on admission of worsening edema and dyspnea on exertion and 10 pound weight gain which he attributed to poor compliance with his low sodium diet and diuretic while on vacation. The hospital team repeats an echocardiogram during the admission finding an LVEF of 40–45% and unchanged moderate aortic valve stenosis. The patient is admitted for diuresis and

---

A. Hough, PharmD, BCPS (AQ-Cardiology) (✉)
West Palm Beach VA Medical Center, 7305 N. Military Trial, West Palm Beach,
FL 33410-6400, USA
e-mail: Augustus.Hough@va.gov

D. Parra, PharmD, FCCP, BCPS
Veterans Integrated Service Network 8 Pharmacy Benefits Management, Veterans Health Administration, Bay Pines, FL 33744, USA

Department of Experimental and Clinical Pharmacology, University of Minnesota
College of Pharmacy, Minneapolis, MN 55455, USA
e-mail: David.Parra@va.gov

© Springer International Publishing AG 2017
K. Kiser (ed.), *Oral Anticoagulation Therapy*,
DOI 10.1007/978-3-319-54643-8_14

prior to discharge a discussion takes place regarding appropriateness of his anticoagulation therapy given presence of aortic valve stenosis for which no valve surgery is indicated at this point. The patient was tolerating apixaban prior to admission, appreciates the convience of therapy, and wants to continue therapy with apixaban if appropriate. Pertinent laboratory values on discharge include SCr 1.5 mg/dL, CrCl 56 mL/min, weight 90 kg, CBC within normal limits. Medications prior to admission include apixaban, carvedilol, lisinopril, furosemide, and pravastatin.

Based on the above, what is the most appropriate regarding the discharge anticoagulation plan for this patient?

Case Discussion

The categorization of atrial fibrillation (AF) as either 'valvular' or 'non-valvular' has become a point of significant discussion regarding anticoagulation decisions in patients with AF. While the differentiation is necessary for patients with valvular heart disease (VHD) in whom embolic risk is sufficient that they warrant exclusion from standard cohorts of atrial fibrillation patients (see Chaps. 13 and 35 for discussions of mitral valve stenosis and mechanical valves) this does not capture all VHD patients. In fact, there were patients enrolled in the recent landmark trials of anticoagulants in AF that had some degree of VHD [1–4]. In light of this, several authors have suggested that the terms 'valvular' and 'non-valvular' AF may be misnomers as patients with non-critical VHD do not meet the spirit of the definition of 'valvular' AF [5, 6]. Unfortunately, the identification of critical 'valvular' AF patients is made more challenging in that the recent landmark trials of antithrombotic therapies in AF all differed on their definition of relevant VHD. A consensus reconciliation of these differences at the time of writing can be found in the American College of Cardiology/American Heart Association AF guidelines which define 'non-valvular' AF as AF "in the absence of rheumatic mitral stenosis, a mechanical or bioprosthetic heart valve, or mitral valve repair" [7].

With regard to the case at hand, patients with aortic valve stenosis (AVS) without pending valve intervention would not be labeled as having 'valvular' AF. As such, the decisions regarding use of anticoagulation should be made based on traditional risk factors rather than the presence of AVS alone. With regard to the choice of anticoagulant in the setting of non-critical AVS and AF with CHA_2DS_2-VASc ≥ 2 warfarin or any of the direct oral anticoagulants (DOACs) would be options as these patients were not excluded from the landmark trials involving these agents [1–4].

Post-hoc analyses of the ROCKET-AF and ARISTOTLE trials revealed that patients with VHD enrolled in the trials had similar efficacy outcomes compared to the non-VHD patients treated with rivaroxaban and apixaban respectively versus their warfarin based control arms (see Chap. 3 for discussion of these trials and outcomes) [5, 6]. Safety outcomes for apixaban versus warfarin were also consistent in the VHD and non-VHD arms in the ARISTOTLE trial [6]. In the ROCKET-AF trial VHD patients, but not the non-VHD patients, had higher rates of both major bleeding and combined major and clinically relevant non-major bleeding with rivaroxaban versus warfarin, a finding that was statistically significant but as post-hoc can only be hypothesis generating [5]. While these overall findings are promising and lend support to the use of DOACs in the setting of AF and non-critical VHD it should be noted that only 1.5 and 2% of the ROCKET-AF and ARISTOTLE trial cohorts respectively had AVS. In addition, no comparative data is available for patients in the landmark trials of dabigatran and edoxaban. As such, any conclusions need to be tempered based on the limited data pool from which they are drawn. However, at this point there does not appear to be any rationale to forgo the use DOACs for AF in the setting of non-critical AVS.

Given the finding that no intervention is planned for this patient's AVS and the present heart failure exacerbation can be attributed to factors outside of the AVS it is reasonable to label the patient as 'non-vavlular' AF. He can continue with apixaban as he has been tolerating it well and there is no contraindication to its use.

Key Points

- Patients with non-critical (i.e., not indicated for valvular surgery or intervention) aortic valve stenosis would generally not be labeled as having 'valvular' atrial fibrillation.
- At this point the presence of non-critical aortic valve stenosis does not impact the decision to pursue, or not purse, anticoagulation in patients with atrial fibrillation.
- Limited post-hoc analyses suggest generally similar effects of DOACs versus warfarin in patients with, and without, non-critical aortic valve stenois.
- If no aortic valve intervention pending or planned for a patients aortic valve stenosis the use of DOACs is reasonable with decisions regarding appropriateness made as would be done for any other atrial fibrillation patient.

Self Assessment Questions

1. Which of the following is the most appropriate antithrombotic therapy for a 77 year old patient with paroxysmal atrial fibrillation and moderate to severe aortic stenosis with a relevant drop in blood pressure with exercise who is being evaluated for aortic valve surgery?

    (a) Aspirin
    (b) Dabigatran
    (c) Apixaban
    (d) Warfarin
    (e) C or D

    Correct answer: D

Rationale: Based on presence of atrial fibrillation and age alone patient should be considered for anticoagulation, thus aspirin is not appropriate. In addition, because aortic valve intervention is imminent it would be reasonable to forgo direct oral anticoagulant therapy and give preference to warfarin.

2. Which clinical situation would be labeled as 'non-valavular' atrial fibrillation making it amenable to the use of a direct oral anticoagulant such as dabigatran?

   (a) AF in conjunction with moderate mitral valve stenosis with no planned intervention
   (b) AF in conjunction with moderate aortic valve stensosis with no planned intervention
   (c) AF in conjuction with severe aortic valve stenosis with possible intervention
   (d) A and B
   (e) None of the above

Correct answer: B

Rationale: Mitral stenosis of moderate to severe grading and aortic valve stensosis with possible intervention would be reasonable to categorize as critical types of valvular heart disease excluding the use of the direct oral anticoagulants. If aortic valve stenosis exists without planned intervention the use of direct oral anticoagulants would not be excluded and atrial fibrillation could be labeled as 'non-valvular'.

Disclaimer The views expressed in this chapter reflect those of the authors, and not necessarily those of the Department of Veterans Affairs.

References

1. Ezekowitz MD, Connolly S, Parekh A, et al. Rationale and design of RE-LY: randomized evaluation of long-term anticoagulant therapy, warfarin, compared with dabigatran. Am Heart J. 2009;157:805–10. e2
2. Patel MR, Mahaffey KW, Garg J, et al. Rivaroxaban versus warfarin in nonvalvular atrial fibrillation. N Engl J Med. 2011;365:883–91.
3. Lopes RD, Alexander JH, Al-Khatib SM, et al. Apixaban for reduction in stroke and other thromboembolic events in atrial fibrillation (ARISTOTLE) trial: design and rationale. Am Heart J. 2010;159:331–9.
4. Giugliano RP, Ruff CT, Braunwald E, et al. Edoxaban versus warfarin in patients with atrial fibrillation. N Engl J Med. 2013;369:2093–104.
5. Breithardt G, Baumgartner H, Berkowitz SD, et al. Clinical charateristics and outcomes with rivaroxaban vs. warfarin in patients with non-valvular atrial fibrillation but underlying native mitral and aortic valve disease participating in the ROCKET AF trial. Eur Heart J. 2014;35:3377–85.
6. Avezum A, Lopes RD, Schulte PJ, et al. Apixaban in comparison with warfarin in patients with atrial fibrillation and valvular heart disease: findings from the apixaban for reductgio in stroke and other thromboembolic events in atrial fibriallation (ARISTOTLE) trial. Circulation. 2015;132:624–32.
7. January CT, Wann LS, Alpert JS, et al. 2014 AHA/ACC/HRS guideline for the management of patients with atrial fibrillation: a report of the American College of Cardiology/American Heart Association task force on practice guidelines and the heart rhythm society. J Am Coll Cardiol. 2014;64:e1–e76.

Part III
Warfarin Management

Chapter 15
Best Practice for Switching Stable Warfarin Patients

Dave L. Dixon

Abstract While INR variability is frequently encountered in clinical practice, this is not true for all patients on warfarin. This case discusses pertinent factors to consider when considering direct oral anticoagulants (DOACs) in patients who are stable on warfarin.

Keywords Warfarin • Direct oral anticoagulants • Adherence • Monitoring

Case Introduction

A 66-year-old Caucasian male presents for his 8-week follow-up visit to check his INR. He has no new complaints. He has been taking warfarin for the past year after a diagnosis of atrial fibrillation. His INR has remained stable over the past 6 months. Other past medical history includes hypertension, GERD, hyperlipidemia, osteoarthritis (knees/hands) glaucoma, and depression. His current medications include metoprolol succinate, lisinopril, hydrochlorothiazide, esomeprazole, amlodipine, atorvastatin, timolol eye drops, acetaminophen, and sertraline. He smokes one pack of cigarettes daily, denies alcohol or illicit drug use. He lives in rural Appalachia and drives 150 mi round trip to come in for INR checks. He presents today and asks you about switching him to "one of the new blood thinners" as he is concerned about driving so far and the cost of gas for his car because he is on a fixed income. His most recent lab values indicate a serum creatinine of 1.0 mg/dL (CrCl = 86 mL/min) and normal hepatic function. An echocardiogram from 2 years ago found an ejection fraction of 55%, mild left ventricular hypertrophy, and no significant

---

D.L. Dixon, PharmD, BCACP, FCCP, FNLA, FACC
Department of Pharmacotherapy and Outcomes Science, VCU School of Pharmacy,
410 N. 12th St., PO Box 980533, Richmond, VA 23298-0533, USA
e-mail: dldixon@vcu.edu

valvulopathies. He reports no recent diet changes or signs/symptoms of any bleeding. His INR today is 2.7.

Case Discussion

What factors need to be considered before recommending a direct oral anticoagulants (DOACs)?

FDA-Approved Indications for Use

It is important to assess for an appropriate indication as the DOACs have limitations compared to warfarin. While each of the DOACs are approved for use in patients with atrial fibrillation, patients with valvular disease were not studied in the key clinical trials [1]. Furthermore, the RE-ALIGN trial evaluated the safety and efficacy of dabigatran in patients with mechanical prosthetic heart valves and observed a higher rate of thromboembolic events and excess of major bleeding in patients who received dabigatran, compared to warfarin [2]. This patient had a recent echocardiogram that showed no valvulopathies and he does not have a prosthetic heart valve. As such, he meets the current indications for a DOAC.

Comparison of DOACs with Warfarin

Overall, studies comparing DOACs with warfarin found similar efficacy and safety trends [1]. For the primary endpoint of stroke and venous thromboembolism, rivaroxaban, edoxaban, and dabigatran 110 mg twice daily were non-inferior to warfarin, while apixaban and dabigatran 150 mg twice daily were found to be superior to warfarin [1]. As for the safety comparison with warfarin, major bleeding rates were similar for rivaroxaban and dabigatran 150 mg twice daily, while apixaban, edoxaban, and dabigatran 110 mg twice daily were found to cause less major bleeding [1]. Table 15.1 summarizes the available safety and efficacy data. Additionally, a reduction in the incidence of intracranial haemorrhage was lower among all DOACs in comparison with warfarin [1]. Despite these data, differences in trial designs prevent us from comparing these agents to each other. Current guidelines do not necessarily favor one agent over another, but warfarin is the only oral anticoagulant given an A level of evidence rating [4]. In this patient case, shared-decision making and taking an individualized approach to anticoagulant selection would be appropriate [5].

Table 15.1 DOAC comparison of safety and efficacy [3]

Trial (DOAC dosing)	Stroke or systemic embolic event rate (%)				Major bleeding event rate (%)			
	DOAC	Warfarin	p-value	Clinical implication	DOAC	Warfarin	p-value	Clinical implication
RE-LY (Dabigatran 150 mg twice daily)	2.2	3.3	**0.001**	34% lower risk of stroke or embolic event with dabigatran compared to warfarin	6.2	6.6	0.34[a]	Dabigatran non-inferior to warfarin
ROCKET-AF (Rivaroxaban 20 mg daily)	3.8	4.3	0.12	Rivaroxaban non-inferior to warfarin	5.6	5.4	0.74	Rivaroxaban non-inferior to warfarin
ARISTOTLE (Apixaban 5 mg twice daily)	2.3	2.9	**0.012**	20% lower risk of stroke or embolic event with apixaban compared to warfarin	3.6	5.1	**<0.001**	29% lower risk of major bleeding with apixaban compared to warfarin
ENGAGE-AF (Edoxaban 60 mg once daily)	4.2	4.7	0.10	Edoxaban non-inferior to warfarin	6.3	7.9	**0.0002**	20% lower risk of major bleeding with edoxaban compared to warfarin

DOAC direct oral anticoagulant, *RR* risk ratio
[a]Dabigatran 110 mg twice daily was associated with a 20% relative risk reduction in major bleeding ($p = 0.003$)

Assessment of Renal Function

While it is well established that patients with renal impairment on warfarin have greater INR variability, warfarin is not renally cleared and has no "renal specific" dose adjustments [6]. However, each of the DOACs are eliminated by the kidneys. While renal dosing is provided for each of the agents, their use is limited in patients with advanced kidney disease. Apixaban is the only exception as dosing guidance for patients with end-stage renal disease is available in the package insert, but this has not yet been evaluated in clinical trials [7]. The patient in this case has normal renal function, and therefore, would be a reasonable candidate for a DOAC.

Adherence to Therapy

Adherence is especially important in patients receiving anticoagulant therapy. Warfarin is somewhat forgiving of the occasional missed dose and adherence can be measured indirectly using the INR. The short half-lives of DOACs requires an even greater emphasis on adherence as missed doses quickly diminishes the therapeutic effectiveness of these agents. Furthermore, the twice daily dosing of dabigatran and apixaban may present a problem for some patients if they do not take other medications at twice daily intervals.

Should self-monitoring be considered in light of this patient's transportation concerns?

Self-monitoring is a reasonable choice for patients who have difficulty getting to a clinic due to lack of transportation or living far from the nearest clinic. Furthermore, studies have shown self-monitoring to improve the quality of anticoagulation control, and even more importantly, a decrease in the number of thromboembolic events and mortality [8]. Despite this, patients must be able to execute self-testing correctly, which requires training and the physical (and mental) ability to perform the test. While this would be a reasonable choice for this patient who lives far from the nearest clinic, his arthritis and glaucoma may limit him physically to perform the testing accurately.

Which DOAC Would be Preferred in this Patient?

- Dabigatran is twice daily and strongly associated with dyspepsia, which is a concern given his history of GERD.
- Apixaban was superior to warfarin in preventing stroke and associated with a lower rate of major bleeding, but must be taken twice daily [1]. Patient preference should be considered here.

- Edoxaban is once daily, but is less effective in patients with normal renal function. The kidneys eliminate 50-60% of edoxaban, which may undertreat patients. As a result, edoxaban has a black box warning to avoid using edoxaban in patients with CrCl >95 mL/min. However, the ENGAGE-TIMI 48 trial found that a higher stroke risk was also observed in patients with CrCl ≥80 mL/min [9]. Thus, edoxaban may not be the most effective agent in this patient as his CrCl is 86 mL/min.
- Rivaroxaban is once daily and appears to be as safe and effective as warfarin [1]. It would be important to make sure the patient would take the rivaroxaban in the evening with a meal to maximize bioavailability and efficacy.
- Regardless of the DOAC selected, it is important to thoroughly educate the patient on the appropriate procedure for when to stop warfarin and begin the new agent. Table 15.2 summarizes the current conversion recommendations.

Table 15.2 DOAC and warfarin conversion [10–13]

DOAC	DOAC → Warfarin	Warfarin → DOAC
Apixaban	1. Stop apixaban 2. Begin warfarin + parenteral anticoagulant when the next apixaban dose would have been given 3. Stop parenteral anticoagulant when INR ≥ 2.0	1. Stop warfarin 2. Start apixaban when INR < 2.0
Dabigatran	Based on creatine clearance (mL/min): • If ≥50, start warfarin 3 days before stopping dabigatran • If 30–50, start warfarin 2 days before stopping dabigatran • If 15–30, start warfarin 1 day before stopping dabigatran • If <15, no recommendations can be made	1. Stop warfarin 2. Start dabigatran when INR < 2.0
Edoxaban	Option 1: • Reduce the patients dose by half and discontinue edoxaban when INR ≥ 2.0 Option 2: • Begin warfarin + parenteral anticoagulant when the next apixaban dose would have been given • Stop parenteral anticoagulant when INR ≥ 2.0	1. Stop warfarin 2. Start edoxaban when INR ≤ 2.5
Rivaroxaban	1. Stop apixaban 2. Begin warfarin + parenteral anticoagulant when the next apixaban dose would have been given 3. Stop parenteral anticoagulant when INR ≥ 2.0	1. Stop warfarin 2. Start rivaroxaban when INR <3.0

DOAC direct oral anticoagulant

Key Points

- The primary benefits of switching patients from warfarin to a DOAC include convenience for the patient and a reduced risk of intracranial haemorrhage.
- In most cases, patients on warfarin with stable INRs should remain on warfarin.
- Before switching from warfarin to a DOAC, special consideration should be given to ensure appropriate indication for use, renal function, and adherence considerations.
- Self-monitoring is a reasonable solution for select patients with transportation barriers to attending clinic visits for INR monitoring.

Self-Assessment Questions

1. Use the patient case scenario above (Case-13): The decision was made to switch the patient to rivaroxaban as he was willing to take it at night with his evening meal. Given today's INR (2.7) and that he took his last dose of warfarin the evening before, which of the following is the best plan for switching this patient from warfarin to rivaroxaban?

    (a) Discontinue warfarin and initiate rivaroxaban when the INR is <2.0
    (b) Discontinue warfarin and initiate rivaroxaban when the INR is <2.5
    (c) Since his INR is <3.0, switch to rivaroxaban beginning with tonight's dose
    (d) Although his INR is <3.0, he should wait 72 h before beginning rivaroxaban

    The correct answer is C. According to the package insert for rivaroxaban, it is appropriate to discontinue warfarin and start rivaroxaban as soon as the INR is below 3.0. Considering the patients last warfarin dose was the night before and his INR is <3.0 in clinic, it would be appropriate to start rivaroxaban in place of the next scheduled warfarin dose. Answer A is incorrect because this is the recommendation for converting patients to dabigatran or apixaban. Answer B is incorrect because this is the recommendation for converting patients to edoxaban. Answer D is incorrect because waiting 72 h would most likely lead to a subtherapeutic anticoagulation.

2. A 68-year-old female presents to the warfarin clinic for routine INR follow up. Her past medical history includes atrial fibrillation, hypertension, St. Jude mitral valve replacement (2 years ago), dyslipidemia, depression, type 2 diabetes, and stage 4 CKD (eGFR ~20 mL/min). She has been quite stable on warfarin 7.5 mg daily and comes to clinic monthly to have her INR checked. Her INR today is 2.8. She voices frustration with the monthly visits and asks if she could be switched to one of the "new drugs" instead. Which of the following reasons best supports why she is NOT a good candidate for a DOAC? (SELECT ALL THAT APPLY)

(a) Age > 65 years
(b) Severely reduced renal function
(c) Type 2 diabetes
(d) Valvular disease
(e) Stable on current regimen

The correct answer is B and D. There is little benefit for most patients in switching to a DOAC if they are stable on warfarin. Indication for use is a major consideration, especially in this case. This patient has a St. Jude mitral valve, thus she is not a candidate for any of the DOACs as they are ONLY approved for use in patients with non-valvular atrial fibrillation. Additionally, dabigatran was associated with significant adverse events when studied in patients with valvular disease. She also has stage 4 CKD and is nearing end-stage disease that will warrant dialysis in the near future. While renal dose adjustments are available for dabigatran and edoxaban, it would not be advisable given the potential for increased risk of bleeding. Apixaban may be considered but it's use in patients with end-stage renal disease has not been formally studied. Age > 65 years and the presence of type 2 diabetes would not prohibit the use of DOAC, but are merely risk factors for having an embolic event.

References

1. Savelieva I, Camm AJ. Practical considerations for using novel oral anticoagulants in patients with atrial fibrillation. Clin Cardiol. 2014;37(1):32–47.
2. Eikelboom JW, Connolly SJ, Brueckmann M, et al. Dabigatran versus warfarin in patients with mechanical heart valves. N Engl J Med. 2013;369:1206–14.
3. Ruff CT, Giugliano RP, Braunwald E, et al. Lancet. 2014;383(9921):15–21.
4. January CT, Wann LS, Alpert JS, et al. 2014 AHA/ACC/HRS guidelines for the management of patients with atrial fibrillation: executive summary. J Am Coll Cardiol. 2014;64(21):2246–80.
5. Seaburg L, Hess E, Coylewright M, et al. Shared decision making in atrial fibrillation. Circulation. 2014;129:704–10.
6. Limdi NA, Beasley TM, Baird MF, et al. Kidney function influences warfarin responsiveness and hemorrhagic complications. J Am Soc Nephrol. 2009;20(4):912–21.
7. Eliquis® [package insert]. New York, NY: Bristol-Myers Squibb Company and Pfizer Inc; 2012.
8. Nutescu EA, Bathija S, Sharp LK, et al. Anticoagulation patient self-monitoring in the United States: considerations for clinical practice adoption. Pharmacotherapy. 2011;31(12):1161–74.
9. Giugliano RP, Ruff CT, Braunwald E, et al. Edoxaban versus warfarin in patients with atrial fibrillation. N Engl J Med. 2013;369:2093–104.
10. Pradaxa [package insert]. Ridgefield, CT: Boehringer-Ingelheim Pharmaceuticals, Inc; 2015.
11. Xarelto [package insert]. Titusville, NJ: Janssen Pharmaceuticals, Inc; 2016.
12. Eliquis [package insert]. Princeton, NJ and New York, NY: Bristol-Myers Squibb Company and Pfizer, Inc; 2016.
13. Savaysa [package insert]. Parsippany, NJ: Daiichi Sankyo, Inc; 2015.

Chapter 16
Patient-Centered Strategies for Improving Warfarin Management

James C. Lee

Abstract The need for regular monitoring of warfarin therapeutic therapy is a commonly cited barrier to optimal patient adherence. Alternative warfarin monitoring and management strategies which involve significant patient participation should be considered in select patients and may improve patient adherence and satisfaction with ongoing warfarin therapy.

Keywords Patient self-testing • Patient self-management • Warfarin • Anticoagulation clinic • Distance-based management • Independent diagnostic testing facility • Extended interval monitoring • Patient education

Case Introduction

AM is a 55-year-old Hispanic male with a prior medical history significant for atrial fibrillation, prostate cancer (complete remission), type 2 diabetes, chronic kidney disease stage III, and obesity who has been anticoagulated on warfarin for the past 4 years. He is predominantly Spanish-speaking but is conversationally fluent in English. He is employed full-time as a custodian for the public school district and works Monday through Friday from 9:00 a.m. to 3:30 p.m. He was previously considered for direct oral anticoagulant (DOAC) but continued warfarin due to his chronic renal insufficiency. He has a history of good anticoagulation control with warfarin (85% time in therapeutic range), exhibits good medication adherence, and able to remember his weekly warfarin regimen when asked. He is usually 30–45 min late for afternoon INR follow-up appointments despite rushing from work, and would need to take vacation time for appointments during work hours. He occasionally misses appointments but always promptly calls the clinic to reschedule and is ultimately seen every 6–8 weeks.

J.C. Lee, PharmD, BCACP
University of Illinois Hospital and Health Sciences System, University of Illinois at Chicago College of Pharmacy, 833 S Wood St, MC 886, Chicago, IL 60612, USA
e-mail: jamlee1@uic.edu

At today's appointment, he asks about the availability of weekend clinic appointments, weekend laboratory draws, or even obtaining a point-of-care testing (POCT) coagulometer. The clinic is only open weekdays from 9:00 a.m. to 4:00 p.m. and the affiliated medical center's outpatient phlebotomy service is open Monday through Saturday.

Case Discussion

The complexity of anticoagulation treatment requires regular monitoring to ensure continued safety and efficacy [1, 2]. The positive impact of anticoagulation clinics on patient clinical and financial outcomes compared to usual care has been previously reported [3–5]. Telephone-based management provides patients with greater convenience in testing times and locations, and even potentially improved clinical outcomes compared to clinic-based care [6, 7]. DOACs do not require routine monitoring of therapeutic activity in most patients as with warfarin, but due to the significance of DOAC dependence on renal clearance, regular renal and hematologic assessment are still recommended.

Patient-centered warfarin management includes patient self-testing (PST) and patient self-management (PSM). PST and PSM are suggested for highly-motivated patients capable of demonstrating competency in self-management strategies [2, 8]. PST is defined as patients self-testing their international normalized ratio (INR) via a POCT device with an anticoagulation provider managing dosing and testing frequency. PSM incorporates patient self-testing INR and patient self-adjustment of dosing and testing frequency.

The clinical benefits of patient self-care are well documented in Europe and increasingly in the United States (US) [9–12] Although evidence points towards improved patient satisfaction, expanded utilization in the US has lagged in part due to cost of testing equipment and supplies, and provider apprehension [13, 14]. Patient self-care is inherently distance-based, and provider staffing and lack of reimbursement remain barriers to expansion. Other novel patient-provider communication (e.g. web-based) modalities continue to be developed.

Patient Considerations

- **Competing obligations and day-to-day responsibilities**: Consider work schedule flexibility and other time-sensitive life responsibilities that are barriers to timely anticoagulation monitoring. Are schedule changes made on short notice easily accommodated by the patient or is more advanced notice required? If arranging in-person care remains challenging, consider extended interval monitoring, distance-based laboratory draws, or PST if on warfarin. Clinicians may also consider extending follow-up INR monitoring to 12 weeks intervals if a patient demonstrates a reliable history of therapeutic anticoagulation control,

follow-up appointment adherence, and medication adherence. Transitioning to a DOAC may also be considered given decreased monitoring requirements. AM appears to have inflexible work hours, so more flexible means of testing outside of normal clinic hours needs to be considered.
- **History of treatment and appointment adherence**: Is there a persistent history of missed appointments and difficulty in rescheduling appointments? Consider barriers leading to poor adherence as well. Strategies such as consolidating appointments on a single day may be helpful. AM is seen regularly at acceptable intervals despite his limited availability and need for rescheduling appointments. Continuing clinic-based monitoring may be reasonable, but if more frequent testing is required, use of laboratory services outside normal clinic hours or PST, or PSM would also be reasonable.
- **Insurance**: DOACs are excellent alternatives to warfarin if clinically appropriate (e.g. adequate renal function) and if increased copays are acceptable to the patient. Small increases in copay may be significant barriers to medication acquisition and adherence for some patients.
- **Reliable communication**: Assess consistency of provider- and patient-initiated communication. Is the patient reliably reachable and do patients timely respond when contacted by providers? If communication is unreliable or lacking, PST and distance-based management may not be viable due to an impediment of communicating critical treatment instructions. AM's ability to be contacted at work during normal clinic hours should be assessed before proceeding with distance-based management.
- **Patient decision-making capacity**: Is the patient capable of reliably communicating health status changes with providers and pursuing care independently when necessary? Patients with poor cognition but with good social support may benefit from DOAC simplicity. AM appears aware of his limitations to care but also has a good history of patient-provider communication and anticoagulation stability, making distance-based management viable.
- **Patient motivation for self-management/self-testing competency**: Is the patient physically and cognitively capable of performing the steps required for self-testing? Is the patient agreeable and highly motivated to provide self-care and capable of seeking emergency care when indicated? If yes, PST and PSM are viable options. Highly motivated and physically competent patients capable of administering self-care are good candidates for PST, PSM, or telephone-based laboratory management. AM should be assessed on his comfort, willingness, and physical ability to self-test or self-manage warfarin therapy.

Provider/Clinic Considerations

- **Specialty anticoagulation clinic referral**: Directories of anticoagulation clinic locations are available online (e.g. Anticoagulation Forum: http://acforum.org/clinics.php), although patient referral requirements and clinic services offered may vary.

Patients managed by medical generalists may benefit from anticoagulation specialist management if alternative monitoring approaches (e.g. distance-based management, extended interval follow-up, PST/PSM etc.) and dedicated anticoagulation management services are not provided by the current clinician. Distance-based services incorporating local laboratory draws and PST/PSM may also be available.
- **Individualized patient training for PST/PSM**: Individualized training and initial trial periods to assure patient self-testing competency should be implemented for all patients initiated on PST/PSM. Consider weekly testing intervals followed by progressively longer intervals based on patient success. Regularly address physical and cognitive issues as part of the patient assessment. Patients not qualified for PST/PSM, but with otherwise good social support, may benefit from local laboratory testing with subsequent provider telephone follow-up. If long-term equipment and supply costs limit the ability for patients to self-test at clinically appropriate intervals, PST/PSM should be avoided.
- **Development of distance-based management protocols**: Clinician policies and procedures guiding effective and safe distance-based anticoagulation management should be in place prior to implementation of distance-based management. Issues such as patient-provider communication, patient qualification criteria, treatment non-adherence, and resolution of abnormal lab values and treatment complications should be addressed. PSM policy and procedures should additionally define treatment and communication protocols, eligibility criteria, and patient and provider responsibilities in the role of self-management.
- **Provider billing and time allocation of distance-based management**: Insurance reimbursement for non-clinic-based monitoring is inconsistent. Providers must ensure adequate time to address and resolve simple and complex clinical scenarios. AM appears to be a reliable and clinically stable patient who would likely self-test when instructed and not require a significant amount of time for provider phone-follow-up.

The Outcome

AM was able to successfully demonstrate self-testing competency with his primary care provider's office coagulometer. After completing a training session and meeting self-testing competencies, a prescription for a POCT coagulometer and test strips were written. AM's insurance company would not cover the cost of the meter or supplies. He was instead able to lease the same coagulometer model used by the clinic through an independent diagnostic testing facility (see Table 16.1 for additional resources) and is paying for test strips on his own. During the initial 3 week once-weekly home testing trial period, AM required multiple testing attempts to acquire a successful measurement, but improved by the second and third testing dates. He was then instructed to test his INR again in 4 weeks. Language barriers have not been an issue during telephone follow-up and he has agreed to present to clinic in person for assessment once every 6 months.

Table 16.1 Resources for Patients and Professionals

Alere home INR monitoring	**Frequently asked questions** Example of an Independent Diagnostic Testing Facility (IDTF) and its criteria for patient eligibility and testing supply reimbursement http://www.alerecoag.com/ww/pat/alere-home-inr-monitoring/frequently-asked-questions.html **Home testing candidates** Example of patient factors to evaluate when considering home INR monitoring http://www.alerecoag.com/ww/pat/alere-home-inr-monitoring/am-I-a-good-candidate.html
Anticoagulation Forum	**Anticoagulation clinic directory** Online directory of anticoagulation clinics in the United States and Canada http://acforum.org/clinics.php
Anticoagulation Forum Centers of Excellence	**Resource center** Comprehensive library for healthcare providers of anticoagulation and operational management resources http://excellence.acforum.org/?page=resource_center **Disease state management >> patient self testing** Includes example documentation, information guides, patient educational material, and guidelines http://excellence.acforum.org/?page=resource_list&resource_page=Disease%20State%20Management
ClotCare	**Patient self-testing** Patient-friendly information page on the state and benefits of patient self-testing http://www.clotcare.com/pst.aspx **Self-management of oral anticoagulation** Patient-friendly review of a study evaluating the utility of patient-self management of warfarin http://www.clotcare.com/oral_anticoagulation_self_management.aspx
Clot Connect	**INR self-testing** Comprehensive patient information sheet discussing patient suitability and descriptions of various point-of-care devices http://files.www.clotconnect.org/INR_Self_Testing.pdf
National Blood Clot Alliance	**INR self-testing** Comprehensive patient information sheet discussing patient suitability and descriptions of various point-of-care devices https://www.stoptheclot.org/article120.htm

Key Points

- Assess patient motivation and competency for patient self-care. If physical, cognitive, or social support barriers exist, PST or PSM with warfarin therapy may not be appropriate. If patients demonstrate high motivation and competency with self-testing technique, PST and PSM may be viable. PSM can be considered for a subset of highly-motivated and competent patients who possess reliable means of communication and predictably stable anticoagulation control.

- Assess existing factors that may be barriers to consistent medication and monitoring adherence. Determine if any issues can be improved or are essentially non-modifiable. Consistent and reliable patient-provider communication is critical to high quality distance-based anticoagulation management.
- Consider provider barriers to timely distance-based patient care prior to implementation. Is the provider or clinic resourced with appropriate time and staffing to manage distance-based patients in addition to existing clinic-based responsibilities? Are providers able to safely and adequately resolve questions and treatment-related complications in a timely manner? Consider if the effort expended on distance-based management is clinically safe and financially justifiable.

Self-Assessment Questions

1. Which of the following patients taking warfarin is best qualified for patient self-testing?

    (a) A 7 year old boy status-post Fontan procedure who relies on his parents to administer his warfarin. He has good TTR, but his parents regularly forget his appointments and are difficult to contact by clinic staff when attempting to reschedule the missed appointments.
    (b) A 32-year-old African American male with difficulty presenting to appointments during regular business hours due to significant overlap with his full-time work schedule. He is adherent with medications, reliably reschedules his appointments in a timely manner, and possess good anticoagulation control (90% time in therapeutic range).
    (c) A 55-year-old white female with previous stroke and left-sided unilateral weakness who is wheelchair-bound. She is highly adherent with appointments with the help of her children and possesses good anticoagulation control.
    (d) A 67-year-old Chinese female with elementary English proficiency and without health insurance. She requires an interpreter at clinic visits, regularly misses 1–2 doses of warfarin per week, and has difficulty recalling her dose when asked during appointments.

    Rationale for question #1

    (a) Incorrect. This patient is not a good candidate due to his reliance on his parents as his main caregivers. His parents' unreliability has negatively impacted the patient's appointment patient adherence. Additionally, it is difficult to communicate with his parents when rescheduling missed appointments.
    (b) Correct. This patient is likely missing his appointments due to his work schedule overlapping with the clinic's normal operating hours. He appears reliable based on his medication adherence and responsibility with rescheduling appointments.

(c) Incorrect. This patient's physical limitations are likely a physical barrier to good testing technique. If her children are willing to assist with testing, PST may become viable.

(d) Incorrect. Language barriers may impede effective patient-provider communication, particularly if language support services are unavailable. Additionally, inability of the patient to consistently adhere or remember her dose may also be of concern and should be further evaluated.

2. Which of the following patients is the best candidate for continued self-testing?

    (a) A patient self-testing for 12 months who is punctual with reporting INR results on scheduled testing days and adherent with annual clinic follow-up.
    (b) A patient self-testing for 9 months who was recently hospitalized for a stroke 2 months ago, but with improving physical function.
    (c) A patient self-testing for 6 months who requires occasional reminder calls from the clinic to test INR on scheduled testing days.
    (d) A patient self-testing for 2 months who reliably tests on scheduled days and calls in INR results to the clinic voicemail, but is difficult to contact when providers attempt to follow up results.

Rationale for question #2

(a) Correct. The patient demonstrates punctuality with appointments and is likely able to be consistently contactable by clinic staff.
(b) Incorrect. Physical ability to self-test should be reassessed based on the severity of the patient's physical deficits.
(c) Incorrect. Although patient reliability may not be poor, this patient is not the best candidate given the need for occasional reminder calls to ensure the patients tests at appropriate intervals.
(d) Incorrect. This patient is not reliably reachable by the clinic. The most significant concern is ensuring appropriate care if significantly abnormal INR or treatment-related complications are reported to the clinic.

References

1. The Joint Commission. Hospital National Patient Safety Goals. Available at: http://www.jointcommission.org/assets/1/6/2016_NPSG_HAP.pdf. Accessed April 20, 2016.
2. Holbrook A, Schulman S, Witt DM, et al. Evidence-based management of anticoagulant therapy: antithrombotic therapy and prevention of thrombosis, 9th ed: American College of Chest Physicians evidence-based clinical practice guidelines. Chest. 2012;141:e152S–84S.
3. Rudd KM, Dier JG. Comparison of two different models of anticoagulation management services with usual medical care. Pharmacotherapy. 2010;30(4):330–8.
4. Chiquette E, Amato MG, Bussey HI. Comparison of an anticoagulation clinic with usual medical care. Arch Intern Med. 1998;158:1641–7.
5. Ernst ME, Brandt KB. Evaluation of 4 years of clinical pharmacist anticoagulation case management in a rural, private physician office. J Am Pharm Assoc. 2003;43:630–6.

6. Staresinic AG, Sorkness CA, Goodman BM, et al. Comparison of outcomes using 2 delivery models of anticoagulation care. Arch Intern Med. 2006;166:997–1002.
7. Wittkowsky AK, Nutescu EA, Blackburn J, et al. Outcomes of oral anticoagulant therapy managed by telephone vs in-office visits in an anticoagulation clinic setting. Chest. 2006;130:1385–9.
8. Witt DM, Clark NP, Kaatz S, et al. Guidance for the practical management of warfarin therapy in the treatment of venous thromboembolism. J Thromb Thrombolysis. 2016 Jan;41(1):187–205.
9. Gadisseur APA, Breukink-Engbers WGM, van der Meer FJM, et al. Comparison of the quality of oral anticoagulant therapy through patient self-management and management by specialized anticoagulation clinics in the Netherlands. Arch Intern Med. 2003;163:2639–46.
10. Matchar DB, Jacobson A, Dolor R, et al. Effect of home testing of international normalized ratio on clinical events. N Engl J Med. 2010;363(17):1708–20.
11. Bloomfield HE, Krause A, Greer N, et al. Meta-analysis: effect of patient self-testing and self-management of long-term anticoagulation on major clinical outcomes. Ann Intern Med. 2011;154:472–82.
12. Bussey HI, Bussey M. Warfarin management; international normalized ratio self-testing and warfarin self-dosing. Circulation. 2012;126:e52–4.
13. Verret L, Couturier J, Rozon A, et al. Impact of a pharmacist-led warfarin self-management program on quality of life and anticoagulation control: a randomized trial. Pharmacotherapy. 2012;32(10):871–9.
14. Wittkowsky AK, Sekreta CM, Nutescu EA, et al. Barriers to patient self-testing of prothrombin time: national survey of anticoagulation practitioners. Pharmacotherapy. 2005;25(2):265–9.

Part IV
Venous Thromboembolism (VTE)

Chapter 17
Provoked Versus Unprovoked Venous Thromboembolism

Jasmine M. Pittman

Abstract Acute VTE anticoagulant treatment selection and duration is based on categorization of the VTE as provoked or unprovoked. Malignancy in particular as a provoking factor for VTE has different treatment strategies compared to other provoking factors. Dosing of LMWH can also be complicated by obesity, and additional monitoring of anti-factor Xa levels may be appropriate to ensure adequate anticoagulation in these patients.

Keywords VTE • Provoked • Unprovoked • Malignancy • LMWH and cancer Monitoring LMWH • Anti-factor Xa

Case Introduction

MS is a 37 y/o WF admitted to the hospital with a proximal deep vein thrombosis (DVT) in her left leg. Around 4 months ago, she was diagnosed with an unprovoked proximal DVT in her right leg. After her initial DVT diagnosis, MS was put on appropriately-dosed rivaroxaban (Xarelto®) for 3 months, but she stopped that medication 2 weeks ago as directed by her physician. Her PMH includes h/o proximal DVT in right leg, HTN, and seasonal allergies. Current medications include lisinopril, loratadine, and St. John's wort. She has NKDA. Vital signs: BP 132/78 mmHg, HR 67 BPM, RR 17, Ht 69″, Wt 122.3 kg, BMI 39.8 kg/m². SCr 0.77 mg/dL, Hgb 13.7 g/dL, Hct 41.1%, Plt 210, PT 13.0 s, and INR 1.05. Upon additional diagnostic evaluation during this hospitalization, MS was diagnosed with ovarian cancer, which is hypothesized to be a provoking factor for both of her DVTs. MS reports being able to afford the co-pays of all of her current medications.

What is the best treatment option for MS, including a drug, dose, and duration of therapy?

J.M. Pittman, PharmD, BCACP
Parkwest Medical Center, Knoxville, TN, USA
e-mail: jmckee@covhlth.com

Case Discussion

What are risk factors for venous thromboembolism (VTE) development?

There are many risk factors associated with VTE formation. Risk stratification of VTE risk is complicated by the fact that many of these risks have shown different degrees of association with VTE development [1–4]. Table 17.1 lists these risk factors.

In the situation of recurrent VTE, it is important to assess the patient's history for any risk factors that may contribute to VTE recurrence, such as antiphospholipid syndrome or cancer. Medications that may increase the risk of VTE formation should be assessed for appropriateness of therapy, and, if possible, switched to another agent without the same degree of risk of VTE occurrence [4].

For this patient, her history of a previous DVT and her recently-diagnosed cancer contribute to her risk of VTE formation. Her cancer diagnosis makes both of her recent DVTs considered "provoked" VTEs.

How is an active VTE treated? Is the treatment of cancer-associated VTE different from other types of VTE?

Active VTE is treated with an immediate-acting anticoagulant to decrease the odds of clot propagation and embolism [5]. Examples of immediate-acting anticoagulants are apixaban, argatroban, fondaparinux, low-molecular weight heparin (LMWH),

Table 17.1 Risk factors associated with VTE formation [1–4]

Risk factors for nonsurgical patients
Active malignancy
Acute infection (e.g., sepsis)
Acute ischemic stroke
Acute myocardial infarction
Acute rheumatologic disorder
Age $\geq$ 70 y/o
BMI $\geq$ 30
Chemotherapy[a]
Heart failure
Hormone therapy (i.e., estrogens)
Previous VTE
Reduced mobility (bedrest for $\geq$3 days)
Recent surgery (especially orthopedic and open-abdominal and pelvic surgeries)
Recent trauma
Respiratory failure
Thrombophilic conditions

[a]Only some chemotherapy agents are associated with increasing VTE risk

rivaroxaban, and unfractionated heparin (UFH). Active VTE, without additional complications, is recommended to be treated with a direct oral anticoagulant (DOAC) over a vitamin K antagonist (VKA), UFH, or a LMWH [4]. The DOACs are recommended over VKA for both initial and maintenance VTE treatment based upon evidence that the risk of VTE recurrence is similar between both groups, but the DOACs demonstrate less bleeding risk [4]. Additionally, DOACs offer greater convenience for patients and healthcare providers, with a lack of known dietary restrictions and no necessary monitoring [4].

MS's treatment is further complicated by her malignancy, as initial treatment (the first 10 days of treatment) of a cancer-associated VTE is recommended to be a LMWH [4]. LMWH is recommended over UFH for this indication because of a decrease in mortality rate, although there is no difference in VTE recurrence rate [6]. In comparison to fondaparinux for cancer-associated VTE, the rate of VTE recurrence was lower with a LMWH [6]. VKA is not appropriate to be used for the initial treatment phase due to its long onset to treatment effect, although it may be started with a LMWH or UFH to bridge therapy until the VKA is considered to be therapeutic (INR of 2.0–3.0) [4, 7].

In the early maintenance phase of cancer-associated VTE, defined as the time from the eleventh day to the third month of therapy, LMWH was associated with a decreased rate of recurrent VTE without any difference in bleeding or mortality rate when compared to VKA [6]. The LMWHs are all assumed to be equally as effective for cancer-associated thrombosis, as there have been no studies directly comparing them for this indication. Table 17.2 below shows dosing and duration for commercially-available LMWHs used in cancer-associated VTE.

DOACs seem promising in the treatment of VTE associated with cancer, as they are oral agents with a rapid onset of effect and reduced laboratory monitoring [10]. In a trial comparing dabigatran to VKA in cancer patients with active VTE, dabigatran was as effective in preventing recurrent VTE without a difference in bleeding risk; a recent meta-analysis showed similar results—that the DOACs are as effective and as safe as VKA in cancer-associated VTE [11, 12]. While this data seems promising for potential use of DOACs for cancer-associated VTE, they have not yet been compared to the gold standard of treatment in cancer-associated VTE—LMWH [10]. The results of various indirect comparisons are inconclusive, with some studies showing a potential benefit for DOACs and others showing that LMWHs are more effective [12–14]. In data presented at the American College of

Table 17.2 Dosing of commercially-available LMWHs for cancer-associated VTE [6, 8, 9, 21]

Drug	Dosage	Maximum dosage
Dalteparin	200 international units/kg/day × 1 month, **then** 150 international units/kg/day	18,000 international units/day
Enoxaparin	1.5 mg/kg/day **or** 1 mg/kg BID	None listed[a]

[a]In a study comparing warfarin to enoxaparin in patient with cancer, only 11.3% of patients on enoxaparin had a BMI > 30 kg/m^2, with a maximum weight in that study of 106 kg [23]. With obese patients using the 1.5 mg/kg once daily dose, the mean AUC is higher in obese patients than in non-obese patients, suggesting additional monitoring may be needed in obese patients to ensure efficacy and safety [9]

Cardiology 65th Annual Scientific Session and Expo, when rivaroxaban was compared to LMWH in cancer-associated VTE, there was no significant difference in VTE recurrence or mortality rates when participants were followed for around 6 months, but the study did have a small sample size of 135 patients [15]. In summary, the DOACs should not be used as first-line for cancer-associated VTE until they have been proven to be as effective and safe as LMWHs in a direct comparison that those results are reproducible. Select-d is a study that is currently underway that compares rivaroxaban (Xarelto®) to a LMWH in cancer-associated VTE [16]. As the evidence supporting the efficacy of DOACs continues to develop in this patient population, the recommendations for the first-line treatment may continue to evolve in future years.

What patient characteristics are important for making a decision regarding MS's VTE treatment?

Risk of bleeding: Cancer patients are at a 2–6 times higher risk of bleeding on anticoagulant therapy than other VTE patients [10]. While the risk of bleeding may influence the treatment duration of VTE in patients with non-provoked or VTE provoked by a reversible risk factor, patients with cancer-associated VTE are recommended to receive extended-duration anticoagulation regardless of their bleeding risk [4]. In patients who have a high bleeding risk on extended duration anticoagulation, consider using a therapy that has a reversal agent (like UFH, enoxaparin, VKA, or dabigatran) to ensure safety.

Insurance coverage: Selecting an item that is affordable for the patient will help to ensure adherence, especially in a patient population that is likely to experience a high financial healthcare burden [17]. Some of the financial burdens that cancer patients experience are an inability to afford co-payments and inadequate coverage of aspects of their treatment [18]. Choosing a therapy that is covered by the patient's insurance or is considered affordable by the patient should be a priority for this patient population to help ensure adherence. It is still important to ensure that patients are receiving the guideline-recommended therapy, as those therapies have been shown to have additional benefits in comparison to other anticoagulant options [4, 6]. Patient assistance programs may be helpful in aiding patients' obtaining their medications. NeedyMeds (available at Needymeds.org) is a reliable resource to help find coupon cards and patient assistance programs for patients. The website can be searched by medication name or by disease state to see what assistance programs are available for patients who need financial assistance for their treatments and disease states [19].

Patient preference: Patient participation in therapeutic decision making should influence therapy selection. In a study reviewing the experiences of patients with cancer and VTE, many patients reported preferring LMWH injections to VKA therapy because of less frequent monitoring and the lack of dietary restrictions [20]. For patients with an aversion to injections that would influence adherence to therapy, oral medications may be appropriate. While VKA was shown to be less effective than LMWH in VTE recurrence in clinical trials of cancer-associated VTE, it is still considered to be an appropriate treatment option, especially if the patient refuses to give self-injections [6]. There are a variety of factors that may influence the efficacy of VKA therapy, including drug interactions, dietary restrictions, and a variable dose-response relationship [7, 10]. These factors may be especially influential in a cancer patient, where various chemotherapy agents and inconsistent dietary intake due to nausea or anorexia can influence maintaining a therapeutic INR [10].

How long is VTE treated in patients with cancer?

Table 17.3 reviews the duration of anticoagulation based on indication, bleeding risk, and what strength of evidence that recommendation holds. Active, non-provoked VTE is typically treated for 3 months. In patients with cancer-associated thrombosis, like MS, there should be no scheduled stop date. The use of treatment should be reassessed at least annually and upon remission of the malignancy [4].

Table 17.3 Duration of anticoagulation based on indication [4]

Indication for anticoagulation	Bleeding risk	Duration of therapy	Strength of recommendation & grade of evidence
Unprovoked isolated distal DVT	All	3 months	1B and 2C
Unprovoked proximal DVT or PE	Low—moderate	Extended	2B
	High	3 months	1B
DVT or PE provoked by surgery	All	3 months	1B
DVT or PE provoked by transient nonsurgical risk factor	All	3 months	1B
Cancer-associated VTE	Low—moderate	Extended	1B
	High	Extended	2B
Recurrent unprovoked DVT or PE	Low	Extended	1B
	Moderate	Extended	2B
	High	3 months	2B

Recommendation strength: 1 = strong, 2 = weak/conditional. Evidence strength: A = high, B = moderate, C = low/very low. Extended = no scheduled stop date

Case Outcome

MS is put on enoxaparin (Lovenox®) 120 mg SubQ BID, but she develops another DVT a month later. What considerations should be kept in mind? How should her treatment change?

The first step in this situation is to assess the patient's adherence to her anticoagulant. If the patient is non-adherent, addressing the cause of her non-adherence would be the recommended intervention. If the non-adherence is related to cost, finding a cheaper alternative for the patient may be necessary. Education regarding the importance of adherence for this medication may also help adherence.

If the patient was adherent to the treatment regimen, a change in the regimen is required. For a patient who is maintained on VKA, change the patient to a LMWH. If the patient was maintained on a LMWH, the dose should be increased by 20–30%. This dose of enoxaparin 120 mg SubQ BID is appropriately dosed for the patient's weight and renal function. If a dose adjustment is needed, increasing the dose by 20% would be a dose of 144 mg SubQ BID; increasing the dose by 30% would be a dose of 156 mg SubQ BID. For ease of administration, choosing a 150 mg SubQ BID dose is an appropriate option, since syringes are commercially available in that strength.

Of note, because the patient is obese and still developed a VTE on full anticoagulation, it may be appropriate to monitor her anti-factor Xa concentrations in order to ensure therapeutic efficacy of the medication [9, 21]. Peak anti-factor Xa concentrations are reached around 4 h after a subcutaneous dose; peak levels are most closely associated with therapeutic efficacy [22]. Table 17.4 shows recommended dose adjustments for treatment doses of LMWH based on anti-factor Xa concentrations.

Table 17.4 Dose adjustments of treatment-dosing of LMWH based off of anti-factor Xa concentrations[a] [4, 22]

Drug	When to check anti-factor Xa concentration (U/mL)	Target anti-factor Xa concentration (U/mL)	Dose adjustment if anti-factor Xa concentration < target	When to repeat anti-factor Xa concentration
Dalteparin once daily	4–6 h after dose	Around 1.05	Increase by 25–30%	4–6 h after next dose
Enoxaparin BID	4 h after dose	0.5–1.0	Increase by 25–30%	4 h after dose

[a]Of note, monitoring anti-factor Xa concentrations is not typically performed in practice for otherwise healthy patients. In some patients, anti-factor Xa monitoring may be performed to ensure adequate dosing for therapeutic efficacy

Key Points

- LMWH is the preferred treatment for VTE associated with malignancy.
- Use extended anticoagulant therapy for patients with a VTE associated with malignancy.
- Patient-specific factors may influence the selection of the therapy that is chosen.
- Dosing of LMWH is complex in obese patients because of pharmacokinetic changes associated with obesity. Use weight-based dosing and consider additional monitoring with anti-factor Xa levels.

Self-Assessment Questions

1. TL is a 62 y/o male who was admitted to the hospital with a diagnosis of a new PE, provoked by his hepatic cancer. He has no known drug allergies. His PMH includes CKD (unknown stage) and he is currently on lisinopril 20 mg PO daily. He is expected to undergo chemotherapy soon. His vital signs today are BP 128/82 mmHg, HR 72 BPM, RR 20, Temp 97.6°F, Ht 72″, Wt 210 lbs. Pertinent labs include SCr 3.2 mg/dL. Which of the following medications would be the best anticoagulation option for this patient?

    (a) Dalteparin (Fragmin®) 18,000 units SubQ Q24H + warfarin 5 mg PO daily
    (b) enoxaparin (Lovenox®) 100 mg SubQ Q24H
    (c) rivaroxaban (Xarelto®) 15 mg PO BID
    (d) rivaroxaban (Xarelto®) 20 mg PO daily

    ANS: B

    B is the best answer choice because LMWH is first-line therapy for initial and extended duration treatment of cancer-associated VTE; this patient would require a renally-adjusted dose of Lovenox, as his calculated CrCl <30 mL/min. A is not an appropriate answer choice because VKA was shown to have a higher VTE recurrence rate in comparison to LMWH in patients with cancer-associated VTE. C would have been a correct answer choice for this patient if his VTE was not associated with a malignancy. D is the non-valvular AFib dosing of rivaroxaban.

2. How long should TL receive anticoagulation for his cancer-associated VTE?

    (a) 10 days
    (b) 3 months
    (c) 6 months
    (d) 1 year
    (e) No scheduled stop date

    ANS: E

E is the best answer choice because anticoagulation should be continued with no scheduled stop date in patients with cancer-associated VTE and in those with a second unprovoked VTE with low to moderate bleeding risk. A is considered the initial treatment period, and anticoagulation is recommended to go beyond the initial treatment period for all types of VTE. B would have been the correct answer if the patient had an unprovoked VTE or a VTE provoked by surgery or a transient risk factor. C and D are not timeframes specifically mentioned in the CHEST 2016 guidelines, but may be appropriate in certain clinical situations, such as a provoked VTE with a transient risk factor that has not yet resolved.

References

1. Falck-Ytter Y, Francis CW, Johanson NA, et al. Prevention of VTE in orthopedic surgery patients: Antithrombotic therapy and prevention of thrombosis, 9th ed.: American College of Chest Physicians evidence-based clinical practice guidelines. Chest. 2012;141(2 Suppl):e278S–325S.
2. Gould MK, Garcia DA, Wren SM, et al. Prevention of VTE in nonorthopedic surgical patients: antithrombotic therapy and prevention of thrombosis, 9th ed: American College of Chest Physicians evidence-based clinical practice guidelines. Chest. 2012;141(2 Suppl):e227S–77S.
3. Kahn SR, Lim W, Dunn AS, et al. Prevention of VTE in nonsurgical patients: antithrombotic therapy and prevention of thrombosis, 9th ed: American College of Chest Physicians evidence-based clinical practice guidelines. Chest. 2012;141(2 Suppl):e195S–226S.
4. Kearon C, Akl EA, Ornelas J, et al. Antithrombotic therapy for VTE disease: CHEST guideline and expert panel report. Chest. 2016;149(2):315–52.
5. Claxton R, Arnold RM. Pharmacologic treatment of acute venous thromboembolism in patients in advanced cancer #236. J Palliat Med. 2012;15(7):828–9.
6. Farge D, Debourdeau P, Beckers M, et al. International clinical practice guidelines for the treatment and prophylaxis of venous thromboembolism in patients with cancer. J Thromb Haemost. 2013;11(1):56–70.
7. Coumadin®—warfarin sodium tablet [package insert]. New York, NY: Bristol-Myers Squibb Pharma Company; 2015.
8. Fragmin®—dalteparin sodium injection [package insert]. New York, NY: Pfizer Laboratories Div Pfizer Inc.; 2015.
9. Lovenox®—enoxaparin sodium injection [package insert]. Bridgewater, NJ: Sanofi-Aventis U.S. LLC; 2013.
10. Short NJ, Connors JM. New oral anticoagulants and the cancer patient. Oncologist. 2014;19(1):82–93.
11. Schulman S, Goldhaber SZ, Kearon C, et al. Treatment with dabigatran or warfarin in patients with venous thromboembolism and cancer. Thromb Haemost. 2015;114(1):150–7.
12. Vedovati MC, Germini F, Agnelli G, et al. Direct oral anticoagulants in patients with VTE and cancer: a systematic review and meta-analysis. Chest. 2015;147(2):475–83.
13. Posch F, Königsbrügge O, Zielinski C, et al. Treatment of venous thromboembolism in patients with cancer: a network meta-analysis comparing efficacy and safety of anticoagulants. Thromb Res. 2015;136(3):582–9.
14. Carrier M, Cameron C, Delluc A, et al. Efficacy and safety of anticoagulant therapy for the treatment of acute cancer-associated thrombosis: a systemic review and meta-analysis. Thromb Res. 2014;134(6):1214–9.

15. McBane RD, Simmons B, Saadiq R, et al. Rivaroxaban compared to low molecular weight heparin in treatment of malignancy associated venous thromboembolism. J Am Coll Cardiol. 2016;67(13):2257.
16. Young A, Phillips J, Hancocks H, et al. OC-11—anticoagulation therapy in selected cancer patients at risk of recurrence of venous thromboembolism. Thromb Res. 2016;140(Suppl 1):S172–3.
17. Bernard DSM, Farr SL, Fang Z. National estimates of out-of-pocket health care expenditure burdens among nonelderly adults with cancer: 2001 to 2008. J Clin Oncol. 2011 Jul;29(20): 2821–6.
18. Sharpe K, Shaw B, Seiler MB. Practical solutions when facing cost sharing: the American Cancer Society's health insurance assistance service. Am J Manag Care. 2016;22(4 Suppl): S92–4.
19. NeedyMeds, Inc. NeedyMeds: find help with the cost of medicine [Internet]. 2016. http://www.needymeds.org
20. Mockler A, O'Brien B, Emed J, et al. The experience of patients with cancer who develop venous thromboembolism: an exploratory study. Oncol Nurs Forum. 2012;39(3):E233–40.
21. Patel JP, Roberts LN, Arya R. Anticoagulating obese patients in the modern era. Br J Haematol. 2011;155(2):137–49.
22. Nutescu EA, Spinler SA, Wittkowsky A, et al. Low-molecular-weight heparins in renal impairment and obesity: available evidence and clinical practice recommendations across medical and surgical settings. Ann Pharmacother. 2009;43(6):1064–83.
23. Meyer G, Marjanovic Z, Valcke J, et al. Comparison of low-molecular-weight heparin and warfarin for the secondary prevention of venous thromboembolism in patients with cancer: a randomized controlled study. Arch Intern Med. 2002;162:1729–35.

Chapter 18
Venous Thromboembolism (VTE) Prophylaxis in Hip and Knee Replacement Surgery

Mary G. Amato and Danielle Carter

Abstract This case presentation describes an elderly patient with osteoarthritis undergoing hip replacement and reviews risks and benefits of the various options for venous thromboembolism (VTE) prophylaxis. Evidence-based guidelines are reviewed as well as patient-specific and institution-specific factors that influence selection of therapy for VTE prophylaxis for this type of surgery.

Keywords Orthopedic surgery • Total hip arthroplasty • Total knee arthroplasty • Post-operative venous thromboembolism prophylaxis • Perioperative anticoagulation

Case Introduction

A 74-year-old male with hip osteoarthritis will be having a right total hip arthroplasty next month. He has had disabling pain over the past year despite treatment with acetaminophen and naproxen, limiting his walking distance, and use of a cane. He has a history of well controlled hypertension and BPH and he has no history of VTE or bleeding disorder. His current medications are lisinopril, naproxen extended release and doxazosin. His weight is 81 kg, blood pressure 140/72, pulse 76, and labs show normal CBC, renal and liver function. The medical team asks what regimen

---

M.G. Amato, PharmD, MPH, BCPS, FCCP (✉)
MCPHS University, 179 Longwood Ave, Boston, MA 02115, USA

Brigham and Women's Hospital, 75 Francis St, Boston, MA 02115, USA
e-mail: mary.amato@mcphs.edu

D. Carter, PharmD, BCPS, CACP
Brigham and Women's Hospital, 75 Francis St, Boston, MA 02115, USA
e-mail: dcarter8@bwh.harvard.edu

© Springer International Publishing AG 2017
K. Kiser (ed.), *Oral Anticoagulation Therapy*,
DOI 10.1007/978-3-319-54643-8_18

would be recommended post-operatively for this patient to prevent VTE. The patient has no specific concerns about bleeding or objections to receiving subcutaneous injections.

Case Discussion

What factors should be considered when developing a plan for VTE prophylaxis after total hip (THA) or knee (TKA) replacement surgery?

Risk of Postoperative VTE

Recent studies have shown a decline in postoperative VTE risk with improved surgical techniques and early ambulation. However, risk without any prophylactic treatment remains substantial with a rate of symptomatic VTE in the first 35 days postop estimated at 4.3% based on recent studies [1, 2]. Pharmacologic VTE prophylaxis reduces the risk of VTE by about 50%, although the benefit is partially offset by increased risk of bleeding for several agents [2]. Use of graded compression stockings has been shown to reduce asymptomatic, but not symptomatic DVT (RR 0.92, CI 0.77–1.09). Low quality data support over 50% reduction in DVT and PE with intermittent pneumatic compression devices (IPC) for up to 14 days postoperatively compared to no thromboprophylaxis, with no increased risk of bleeding. There are issues, however, with compliance with devices that require external power sources and logistical issues with use of these devices in the hospital [1].

Risk for Bleeding

Baseline risk for major bleeding events associated with hip and knee replacement surgeries without VTE prophylactic agents is estimated to be 1–2%. General risk factors for bleeding after these procedures include previous major bleeding, severe renal failure, concomitant antiplatelet agent and individual surgical factors. Compared to no treatment, significant increases in minor bleeding were seen with pharmacologic treatment (RR 1.67, CI 1.18–2.38). Non-significant trends were seen for increased major bleeding for Vitamin K antagonists (VKAs, such as warfarin), and fondaparinux, compared to no prophylaxis. A significant increase in major bleeds was seen for warfarin compared to low molecular weight heparins (LMWH) (RR 3.9, CI 1.9–8.1) and non-significant trends for increased major bleed for fondaparinux and rivaroxaban compared to LMWHs. [1, 3, 4].

Choice of Agent for VTE Prophylaxis

The 2012 American College of Chest Physician (ACCP) guidelines recommend VTE prophylaxis for at least 10–14 days with pharmacologic therapy or IPC in all patients undergoing THA or TKA [1]. Pharmacologic therapy is recommended unless there is particular concern about bleeding complications. See Table 18.1 for agent dosing recommendations for prophylaxis after total hip or total knee arthroplasty. IPC or no prophylaxis can be used in patients with high risk for bleeding. IPC as dual therapy with pharmacologic therapy should be considered if there is availability of battery powered IPC devices in the hospital and patients are willing to comply with wearing the devices.

ACCP recommends that LMWH be used first line starting 12 h preoperatively or 12 h postoperatively, and continued for at least 10–14 days. Extended therapy up to 35 days for an additional reduction in symptomatic VTE should also be considered [1]. Fondaparinux, apixaban, dabigatran, rivaroxaban, low-dose unfractionated heparin, adjusted-dose VKA, aspirin, or IPC are also acceptable choices.

Table 18.1 Dosing of agents recommended for VTE prophylaxis after total hip (THA) or knee arthroplasty (TKA)

Pharmacologic agent	Dose	Duration	Adjustment for renal insufficiency
Enoxaparin	30 mg SC q12 h or 40 mg SC 24 h (THA) 30 mg SC q12 h (TKA)	10–14 days; consider an additional 3wk after initial phase for THA	30 mg q24 h if CrCl <30 mL/min
Dalteparin	5000 IU SC once daily (THA)	5–14 days	Not defined; may not need adjustment
Fondaparinux	2.5 mg SC q24 h	10–14 days; up to 35 days	Avoid if CrCl <30 mL/min
Apixaban	2.5 mg PO BID	12 days (TKA); 35 days (THA)	No adjustment
Dabigatran	110 mg PO × 1 dose (THA), then 220 mg PO daily	28–35 days	Avoid if CrCl <30 mL/min
Rivaroxaban	10 mg PO once daily	12 days (TKA); 35 days (THA)	Avoid if CrCl <30 mL/min
Unfractionated heparin	5000 units SC q8–12 h	at least 10–14 days	None
Vitamin K antagonist warfarin	Adjusted to INR (1.8–2.3 or 2–3)	at least 10–14 days	None
Aspirin	81 mg BID; 325 mg daily-BID	10–14 days, up to 4 weeks	None

Limitations of LMWH include inconvenience of daily injections and risk of heparin induced thrombocytopenia. Potential limitations based on published studies for fondaparinux, rivaroxaban and VKAs include the possibility of increased bleeding compared to LMWH. Potential limitations for low dose unfractionated heparin, VKA, aspirin, and IPC alone include potential decreased efficacy compared to LMWH [1, 5, 6]. Given the similar efficacy and similar rates of bleeding with apixaban and dabigatran, these agents have been recommended by ACCP as next choices after LMWH. The American Academy of Orthopaedic Surgeons (AAOS) guidelines do not recommend one choice of pharmacologic agent over another [7].

Despite the publication of evidence-based guidelines by ACCP and AAOS, the treatments used for VTE prophylaxis are highly variable among orthopedic practices [8]. Experience with various hospitals and informal discussions with practitioners and patients has revealed that warfarin for two (TKA) to four (THA) weeks, and aspirin are commonly used in practice in addition to rivaroxaban, LMWH, and other agents. At some institutions, centralized anticoagulation clinics or monitoring programs are able to achieve better results for time in therapeutic range than was reported in clinical trials for patients receiving VKAs such as warfarin, increasing provider confidence in using VKAs over other agents at those locations. A lower INR target (1.8-2.3) is used at some institutions, despite lack of sufficient evidence for efficacy. Some practitioners use individual patient risk factors for VTE such as prior VTE to guide duration of treatment. Although the evidence to support efficacy of aspirin is not as strong as other agents, it continues to be frequently used by surgeons for VTE prophylaxis. There have been concerns about lack of long-term safety data and unavailability of reversal agents with the newer oral agents apixaban, dabigatran and rivaroxaban. These concerns may be decreasing with the availability of longer term safety data and development of reversal agents such as idarucizumab (for dabigatran reversal), and andexanet alfa (for factor Xa inhibitors). Idarucizumab has been approved by the FDA for use currently, while andexanet alfa has yet to be approved for use in the US.

Dosing recommendations for pharmacologic agents are listed in Table 18.1. FDA-approved prescribing information includes recommendations for achievement of hemostasis, then administering the first dose of dabigatran 1–4 h after surgery, fondaparinux 6–8 h after surgery, rivaroxaban 6-10 hr after surgery, and enoxaparin or apixaban 12–24 h after surgery, with options for preoperative and postoperative starts for dalteparin.

As this patient has no objection or contraindication to receiving LMWH, it is recommended he receive prophylaxis with a low molecular weight heparin beginning at least 12 h before or after surgery, for example, enoxaparin 40 mg SC q24 h, continued at least 10–14 days, and up to 35 days. The patient should discontinue his naproxen 3–7 days before surgery. It is recommended that patients discontinue use of aspirin 7–10 days prior to surgery and any other antiplatelet agents as recommended prior to elective THA or TKA (those with history of recent acute coronary syndrome/coronary interventions would generally not be candidates for this surgery as stopping antiplatelet agents would significantly increase thrombotic risk). Patients should also undergo early mobilization after surgery [7].

Additional Considerations

1. Screening asymptomatic patients for VTE with Doppler/Duplex ultrasound is not recommended [1].
2. IVC filter placement is not recommended in patients with contraindications to other treatments [1].
3. Increasing the VTE prophylaxis dose of LMWH by 30% may be appropriate in morbidly obese patients (BMI >40 kg/m^2) [9].
4. Decreasing VTE prophylaxis dose of enoxaparin may also be appropriate in patients with low body weight (<45 kg for women and <57 kg for men).

Key Points

- Total hip replacement and total knee replacement surgery are significant risk factors for post-operative VTE.
- Pharmacotherapy for prophylaxis is recommended over IPC or no prophylaxis in patients without an unacceptably high risk of bleeding.
- Antiplatelet agents should be discontinued prior to elective THA and TKA as appropriate for the patient's indication.
- VTE prophylaxis with low molecular weight heparin, fondaparinux, apixaban, dabigatran, rivaroxaban, low dose unfractionated heparin, vitamin K antagonist, or aspirin may be used.
- The 2012 ACCP Antithrombotic guidelines recommend LMWH over other agents unless contraindicated or refused by patient.
- Prophylaxis should be continued at least 10–14 days, and considered for up to 35 days postoperatively.

Self-Assessment Questions

1. A 55-year-old woman undergoing hip replacement surgery does not wish to receive SC injections. Which of the following regimens would be most acceptable for VTE prophylaxis?

    (a) Intermittent pneumatic compression
    (b) No thromboprophylaxis
    (c) Fondaparinux
    (d) Apixaban

    The best answer is D. Intermittent pneumatic compression or no thromboprophylaxis are likely not as effective as pharmacologic therapies. Patient does not wish to receive subcutaneous injections so that would make C. fondaparinux not an appropriate choice. An oral agent such as apixaban is an appropriate second choice. Warfarin, dabigatran, rivaroxaban or aspirin therapy would also be appropriate.

2. A 65-year-old man with renal insufficiency (CrCl 23 mL/min) will be having a total knee arthroplasty (TKA). He is willing to take SC injections and has no history of prior bleeding events. If LMWH is used for VTE prophylaxis, what dosing should be used?

   (a) He should not be treated with LMWH.
   (b) Dalteparin 5000 IU SC once daily
   (c) Enoxaparin 30 mg SC q24 h
   (d) Enoxaparin 40 mg SC q24 h

   The best answer is C. Enoxaparin dose adjustment recommendation is 30 mg SC q24 h for patients with CrCl <30 mL/min. The standard doses may increase risk of bleeding. Dosing of dalteparin in renal insufficiency is less defined and may need to be dosed according to anti-Xa levels.

References

1. Falck-Ytter Y, Francis CW, Johanson NA et al. Prevention of VTE in orthopedic surgery patients. Antithrombotic therapy and prevention of thrombosis, 9th ed: American College of Chest Physicians. Chest 2012;141(2)(Suppl):e278s–e325s.
2. Adam SS, McDuffie JR, Lachiewicz PF, Ortel TL, Williams JW. Comparative effectiveness of new oral anticoagulants and standard thromboprophylaxis in patients having total hip or knee replacement: a systematic review. Ann Intern Med. 2013;159:275–84.
3. Chan NC, Siegal D, Lauw MN, et al. A systematic review of contemporary trials of anticoagulants in orthopaedic thromborophylaxis: suggestions for a radical reappraisal. J Throm Thrombolysis. 2015;40:231–9.
4. Soberaj DM, Coleman CE, Tongbram V et al. Venous thromboembolism in orthopedic surgery. Comparative Effectiveness Review no 49. AHRQ Publication no. 12-EHC020-EF. Rockville, MD: Agency for Healthcare Research and Quality: March 2012. www.effectivehealthcare.ahrq.gov/reports/final.cfm. Accessed 12 Aug 2016.
5. Drescher F, Sirovich BE, Lee A, et al. Aspirin versus anticoagulation for prevention of venous thromboembolism major lower extremity orthopedic surgery: a systematic review and meta-analysis. J Hosp Med. 2014;9:579–85.
6. Stewart DW, Frshour FE. Aspirin for the prophylaxis of venous thromboembolic events in orthopedic surgery patients: a comparison of the AAOS and ACCP guidelines with review of the evidence. Ann Pharmacother. 2013;47:63–74.
7. Mont MA, Jacobs JJ. AAOS clinical practice guideline summary: preventing venous thromboembolic disease in patients undergoing elective hip and knee arthroplasty. J Am Acad Orthop Surg. 2011;19:768–76.
8. Flierl MA, Messina MJ, Mitchell JJ, et al. Venous thromboembolism prophylaxis after total joint arthroplasty. Orthopedics. 2015;38:252–63.
9. Nutescu EA, Spinler SA, Wittkowsky A, Dager WE. Low-molecular-weight heparins in renal impairment and obesity: available evidence and clinical practice recommendations across medical and surgical settings. Ann Pharmacother. 2009;43:1064–83.

Chapter 19
Venous Thromboembolism (VTE) Prophylaxis in the Intensive Care Unit (ICU)

Dillon Elliott

Abstract Critical illness puts patients at an increased risk for developing venous thromboembolism (VTE). Contraindications to pharmacologic VTE prophylaxis and/or organ dysfunction can be common in critical illness and can complicate the decision of VTE prophylaxis method or agent being used.

Keywords Critical care • Venous thromboembolism (VTE) • Prophylaxis • Trauma Renal impairment • Intermittent pneumatic compression (IPC)

Case Introduction

A 74-year-old male (Ht: 69″, Wt: 75 kg) is admitted to the medical intensive care unit for sepsis. His wife states that he received a course of oral antibiotics 2 weeks ago for pneumonia, but never seemed to get better. His blood pressure is 89/53 mm Hg, pulse 95 bpm, and O_2 saturation is 92% on mechanical ventilation after undergoing endotracheal intubation in the ER. He has received 2.5 L of fluid resuscitation and is now requiring a norepinephrine infusion at 4 µg/min to maintain his blood pressure. His past medical history includes type 2 diabetes, stage III chronic kidney disease, and COPD. Home medications include: insulin lispro via sliding scale, insulin glargine, lisinopril, and fluticasone/salmeterol. Current labs are as follows: BUN 31 mg/dL, SCr 1.6 mg/dL, WBC count 18,000/mm^3, Hemoglobin 12 g/dL, Hematocrit 36%, Platelets 150,000/mm^3, Liver panel within normal limits including INR of 1.02. The medical team has started the patient on empiric antibiotics and famotidine for stress ulcer prophylaxis. What would you recommend as appropriate venous thromboembolism (VTE) prophylaxis for this patient?

D. Elliott, PharmD, BCPS, BCCCP
South College School of Pharmacy, 400 Goody's Lane, Knoxville, TN 37922, USA
e-mail: delliott@southcollegetn.edu

Case Discussion

What Factors Should Be Considered When Evaluating Options for VTE Prophylaxis in This Critically Ill Patient?

In order to properly assess the need for VTE prophylaxis in this patient, risk factors for the development of VTE must be considered. See Table 19.1 for a summary of risk factors in critically ill patients. Unfortunately, no widely validated stratification tool exists for use in critically ill patients. VTE can occur in critically ill patients despite the administration of prophylaxis and lead to poor outcomes. It is generally safe to assume that critically ill patients carry high risk of developing VTE and pharmacologic prophylaxis, mechanical prophylaxis, or both should be administered unless contraindications exist [4]. Our patient is acutely ill, elderly, and currently receiving mechanical ventilation warranting the need for some form of VTE prophylaxis.

Risk of bleeding must be assessed in combination with risk of VTE. Many critically ill patients are at high risk of bleeding due to their various disease states, invasive interventions, and concomitant medications. Bleeding risk varies depending on the patient and must be individually assessed when considering pharmacologic prophylaxis [4]. See Table 19.2 for bleeding risk factors and contraindications to pharmacologic VTE prophylaxis. When bleeding risk is considered a contraindication to pharmacologic prophylaxis, mechanical prophylaxis with graduated compression stockings (GCS) or intermittent pneumatic compression (IPC) should be initiated and continued until risk has resolved and pharmacologic prophylaxis can be initiated [1, 6]. Our patient has not received any anticoagulants and does not have active bleeding or increased bleeding risk based on laboratory values.

Table 19.1 Risk factors for VTE [1–3]

VTE risk factors in critically ill patients
Previous VTE or stroke
Active or history of cancer
Prolonged immobilization
Age > 60
Sepsis
Surgery (higher risk with orthopedic)
Mechanical ventilation
Sedative use
Trauma
Spinal cord injury
Obesity
Pregnancy
Vasopressors
Central venous catheterization

Table 19.2 Risk of bleeding [4, 5]

Contraindications to pharmacologic VTE prophylaxis
Active bleeding
Use of thrombolytics (alteplase etc.) in the last 24 h
Risk factors for bleeding with pharmacologic VTE prophylaxis
Active gastroduodenal ulcer
Bleeding in the past 3 months
Platelet count <50,000/μL
Hepatic failure (INR >1.5)
Renal failure
ICU admission
Concomitant anticoagulant or antiplatelet use
Invasive procedures
Acute stroke

Table 19.3 Dosing of pharmacologic agents [10]

Pharmacologic agent	CrCl ≥30 mL/min	CrCl 20–30 mL/min	CrCl ≤20 mL/min
Enoxaparin	40 mg SQ q24 h[a]	30 mg SQ q24 h	Not recommended
Dalteparin	5000 units SQ daily		No accumulation observed in critically ill patients with severe renal impairment
Unfractionated Heparin	5000 units SQ Q8 h or q12 h[b]		

[a]In trauma patients, enoxaparin 30 mg SQ BID
[b]Preferred in patients with CrCl <20 mL/min

Choice of Pharmacologic Agent

Without contraindication to anticoagulants or high bleeding risk, the use of subcutaneous low molecular weight heparin (LMWH) or unfractionated heparin (UFH) for VTE prophylaxis in critically ill patients are recommended over no prophylaxis [1, 6]. See Table 19.3 for dosing of anticoagulants for VTE prophylaxis. The possibility of one of these two available choices for pharmacologic VTE prophylaxis being superior has been evaluated in clinical trials. While several trials have found no difference in the occurrence of deep vein thrombosis (DVT) with the two agents, one study found dalteparin to have a significantly lower incidence of pulmonary embolism (PE) over UFH as a secondary endpoint with no difference in DVT occurrence [7]. Based on current literature, both LMWH and UFH are preferred options for pharmacologic VTE prophylaxis in medical/surgical critically ill patients with UFH being the agent of choice in patients with severe renal impairment (estimated CrCl <20 mL/min). Most trials evaluating subcutaneous unfractionated heparin for VTE prophylaxis used q12 h dosing intervals and no head to head trials exist evaluating q8 h vs. q12 h dosing. Warfarin is not recommended for VTE prophylaxis due to increased absolute risk of bleeding [6]. Direct oral anticoagulants have been studied in critically ill patients and are not recommended [4]. In trauma patients, enoxaparin administered at a dose of 30 mg SQ BID is preferred in patients with estimated creatinine clearance >30 mL/min due to a statistically significant reduction of DVT over subcutaneous unfractionated heparin [8, 9].

Obesity

An increase in dosage of prophylactic enoxaparin to 0.5 mg/kg SQ daily or 40 mg SQ Q12 h and UFH to 7500 units SQ q8 h may be considered in morbidly obese patients with BMI ≥ 40 [11, 12].

Monitoring

Platelets

Patients receiving VTE prophylaxis with LMWH or UFH should have a baseline platelet level drawn prior to initiation of therapy. Heparin-induced thrombocytopenia (HIT) is generally defined as a decrease in platelet level by 50% from baseline and below an absolute value of <150,000/mm^3 (though HIT can rarely occur with a platelet level above 150,000/mm^3). Onset of HIT most often occurs within 5–10 days from initiation of therapy. The 4 T's score can be used to evaluate probability of HIT in patients with suspected clinical criteria using a summative point score of thrombocytopenia, timing of platelet fall, thrombosis, and whether the patient has a therapeutic cause for thrombocytopenia. If the clinical suspicion of HIT is likely, heparin products should be stopped immediately, alternate anticoagulation should be initiated, and further laboratory investigation is warranted [13].

Serum Creatinine

Serum creatinine should be monitored at baseline and intermittently throughout therapy for patients receiving LWMH in order to appropriately adjust dosing of these medications or switch to UFH should the patient's renal function deteriorate.

Hemoglobin and Hematocrit

Hemoglobin and hematocrit should be monitored at baseline and in patients with suspicion of bleeding or who have multiple risk factors for bleeding.

Anti-Factor Xa Assay

Though monitoring of anti-Factor Xa levels with UFH and LMWH therapy for VTE prophylaxis has not correlated well in general patient populations, there may be utility in patients with BMI > 40 using a reference range of 0.2–0.5 IU/mL for enoxaparin and 0.1–0.4 IU/mL for UFH [11].

How Should This Patient Be Managed?

This patient is at high risk of developing a VTE based on his age and acute illness requiring mechanical intubation. He does not have active bleeding and is not at high risk of bleeding based on stable hemoglobin/haematocrit, platelets, and an INR within normal limits. It would be reasonable for this patient to receive pharmacologic prophylaxis with enoxaparin 40 mg SQ q24 h, heparin 5000 units SQ q8 h or q12 h, or dalteparin 5000 units SQ q24 h. While he does have an elevated creatinine (estimated CrCl of 40 mL/min) and chronic kidney disease, he is not considered to have severe renal impairment. Subcutaneous heparin would be preferred if this patients renal function worsens, which should be closely monitored given the potential for organ failure with sepsis. This patient could also receive mechanical prophylaxis with GCS or IPC, as the combination is generally considered acceptable in high-risk patients with multiple risk factors for developing VTE.

Key Points

- Critically ill patients are at increased risk for developing VTE
- No VTE risk stratification tools are available for critically ill patients
- In patients at high risk of bleeding or with active bleeding mechanical VTE prophylaxis is preferred until bleeding or bleeding risk has resolved
- UFH and LMWH are the preferred agents to be used for pharmacologic VTE prophylaxis.
- Pharmacologic agents should be dosed appropriately for renal function with UFH being the preferred agent in patients with severe renal impairment.
- Trauma patients should receive VTE prophylaxis with enoxaparin at a dose of 30 mg SQ q12 h as a preferred agent in the absence of severe renal impairment.

Self-Assessment Questions

1. A 54-year-old woman is admitted to the neurological intensive care unit from the emergency room. She was brought to the hospital early this morning roughly 1 h after onset of right-sided weakness. After a CT scan showed an occlusion of the

right middle cerebral artery with no evident hemorrhage, the neurologist ordered the patient to receive alteplase 0.9 mg/kg with 10% given as a bolus and the remaining amount administered over 1 h for ischemic stroke. Current labs are within normal limits. Vitals include a blood pressure of 140/86 mm Hg, heart rate of 85 bpm, and respiratory rate of 18 bpm. The attending physician has not addressed VTE prophylaxis. What would be an appropriate recommendation for VTE prophylaxis in this patient?

(a) Enoxaparin 40 mg subcutaneously daily
(b) Heparin 5000 units subcutaneously every 12 h + intermittent pneumatic compression devices
(c) Intermittent pneumatic compression devices with no pharmacologic prophylaxis
(d) This patient has a contraindication to both pharmacologic and mechanical VTE prophylaxis

The correct answer is C. The appropriate VTE prophylaxis recommendation for this patient would be to initiate intermittent pneumatic compression devices upon admission to the unit and after 24 h bleeding risk should be assessed again. This patient's risk of bleeding is extremely high immediately after receiving alteplase for an ischemic stroke. It is recommended to wait at least 24 h after alteplase administration before initiating any anticoagulants or antiplatelet agents, therefore Answers A and B are incorrect. The patient is still at risk of VTE and does not have contraindications to mechanical prophylaxis, therefore Answer D would be insufficient. Pharmacologic prophylaxis should be initiated with or without mechanical prophylaxis when contraindications to pharmacologic prophylaxis no longer exist.

2. A 73-year-old man has been in the medical intensive care unit for 5 days after admission from his nursing home for shock secondary to urosepsis. He is receiving enoxaparin 40 mg subcutaneously q24 h for VTE prophylaxis. He has developed acute kidney injury over the last 5 days and his current creatinine clearance is estimated to be 15 mL/min. What recommendation can be made regarding his VTE prophylaxis?

(a) Continue his current regimen of enoxaparin 40 mg subcutaneously q24 h
(b) Decrease his dose of enoxaparin to 30 mg subcutaneously q24 h
(c) Discontinue enoxaparin and begin heparin 5000 units subcutaneously every 12 h
(d) Discontinue enoxaparin and begin intermittent pneumatic compression devices

This patient's estimated creatinine clearance has worsened to below 20 mL/min due to acute kidney injury and enoxaparin has not been studied in patients with extreme renal impairment. Therefore, Answers A and B would not be appropriate choices for pharmacologic prophylaxis due to concern for drug accumulation. The correct answer is C. Unfractionated heparin does not rely on renal elimination and is preferred in severe renal impairment. Answer D would be insufficient for this patient as they do not have contraindications to pharmacologic therapy and are at high risk for developing VTE due to critical illness.

References

1. Kahn SR, Lim W, Dunn AS, et al. Prevention of VTE in nonsurgical patients: antithrombotic therapy and prevention of thrombosis, 9th ed: American College of Chest Physicians evidence-based clinical practice guidelines. Chest. 2012;141(2 Suppl):195S–226S.
2. Minet C, Potton L, Bonadona A, et al. Venous thromboembolism in the ICU: main characteristics, diagnosis and thromboprophylaxis. Crit Care. 2015;19(1):287.
3. Spyropoulos AC, Anderson Jr FA, Fitzgerald G, Decousus H, Pini M, Chong BH, et al. Predictive and associative models to identify hospitalized medical patients at risk for VTE. Chest. 2011;140(3):706–14.
4. Boonyawat K, Crowther MA. Venous thromboembolism prophylaxis in critically ill patients. Semin Thromb Hemost. 2015;41:68–74.
5. Jobin S, Kalliainen L, Adebayo L, Agarwal Z, Card R, Christie B, Haland T, Hartmark M, Johnson P, Kang M, Lindvall B, Mohsin S, Morton C. Venous thromboembolism prophylaxis. Bloomington, MN: Institute for Clinical Systems Improvement (ICSI); 2012. p. 51.
6. Gould MK, Garcia DA, Wren SM, et al. Prevention of VTE in nonorthopedic surgical patients: antithrombotic therapy and prevention of thrombosis, 9th ed: American College of Chest Physicians evidence-based clinical practice guidelines. Chest. 2012;141(2 Suppl):227S–77S.
7. Cook D, Meade M, Guyatt G, et al. PROTECT investigators for the Canadian critical care trials group and the Australian and New Zealand Intensive Care Society Clinical Trials Group. Dalteparin versus unfractionated heparin in critically ill patients. N Engl J Med. 2011;364(14):1305–14.
8. Geerts WH, Jay RM, Code KI, et al. A comparison of low-dose heparin with low-molecular weight heparin as prophylaxis against venous thromboembolism after major trauma. N Engl J Med. 1996;335:701–7.
9. Toker S, Hak DJ, Morgan SJ. Deep vein thrombosis prophylaxis in trauma patients. Thrombosis. 2011;2011:505373.
10. Douketis J, Cook D, Meade M, et al. Prophylaxis against deep vein thrombosis in critically ill patients with severe renal insufficiency with the low molecular weight heparin dalteparin: an assessment of safety and pharmacodynamics: the DIRECT study. Arch Intern Med. 2008;168(16):1805–12.
11. Freeman A, Homer T, Pendleton RC, Rondina MT. Prospective comparison of three enoxaparin dosing regimens to achieve target anti-factor Xa levels in hospitalized, medically ill patients with extreme obesity. Am J Hematol. 2012;87(7):740–3.
12. Wang TF, Milligan PE, Wong CA, Deal EN, Thoelke MS, Gage BF. Efficacy and safety of high-dose thromboprophylaxis in morbidly obese patients. Thromb Haemost. 2014;111(1):88–93.
13. Linkins LA, Dans AL, Moores LK, et al. Treatment and prevention of heparin-induced thrombocytopenia: antithrombotic therapy and prevention of thrombosis, 9th ed: American College of Chest Physicians evidence-based clinical practice guidelines. Chest. 2012;141(2 Suppl):e495S–530S.

Chapter 20
VTE and Recent Drug Eluting Stent (DES) Placement

Wendy M. Gabriel

Abstract If a patient with recent stent placement develops a VTE, triple oral antithrombotic therapy may be indicated if the stent was placed within the past 6 months. The most evidence based regimen is a combination of clopidogrel, aspirin, and warfarin.

Keywords Triple oral antithrombotic therapy • Dual antiplatelet therapy • Venous thromboembolism • Anticoagulation • P2Y12 inhibitor • New oral anticoagulant • Warfarin • Aspirin

Case Introduction

A 72 year old male presents to the emergency room with complaints of right leg swelling and pain. The symptoms began at 12 PM yesterday and have not gotten better with rest overnight. He is from a different state and has been in the car driving across the country to help his granddaughter move into college. He has spent the past 2 days in the car for 12 h each day. He has a past medical history of hypertension, dyslipidemia, tobacco use (1/2 pack per day for 55 years), and coronary artery disease. He had one drug eluting stent placed emergently 8 months ago due to non-ST segment elevation myocardial infarction (NSTEMI). His home medications include aspirin, prasugrel, atorvastatin, lisinopril, metoprolol tartrate, SL nitroglycerin PRN, and albuterol PRN. Physical exam reveals that the right leg is swollen and is warm and tender to touch. An ultrasound of the right leg shows evidence of acute DVT. His serum creatinine is 1.2 mg/dL, current blood pressure is 142/88 mmHg, and weight is 76 kg. The emergency room physician starts the patient on enoxaparin 80 mg subcutaneously q12 h.

W.M. Gabriel, PharmD, BCPS
South College School of Pharmacy, 400 Goody's Lane, Knoxville, TN 37922, USA
e-mail: wgabriel@southcollegetn.edu

What factors should be considered when developing a plan for acute VTE in a patient with CAD?

Case Discussion

In patients with acute venous thromboembolism (VTE), treatment with anticoagulation is necessary to prevent complications and further thrombosis [1]. Complications may include clot extension, pulmonary embolus, and death. For patients with provoked VTE due to transient causes, 3 months of anticoagulation is indicated provided there are no contraindications to anticoagulation therapy [2]. This patient's VTE is most likely caused by immobility after several days of driving in the car across the country. If this was not a provoked VTE, would the duration change? The CHEST guidelines recommend at least 3 months of anticoagulation if it is a first unprovoked VTE, however extended therapy with no stop date can be considered if the patient is a low or moderate bleeding risk [2]. This recommendation does not change if the patient experiences a second unprovoked VTE.

Choosing an Anticoagulant

Dabigatran, rivaroxaban, apixaban, and edoxaban are recommended over warfarin, and warfarin is recommended over low-molecular weight heparins for treatment of VTE [2]. All four new oral anticoagulants (DOACs) were found to be non-inferior to standard therapy warfarin and unfractionated heparin/low-molecular weight heparin in treatment of VTE [3–6]. Further, DOACs have been associated with similar rates of recurrent VTE and major bleeding [7], and decreased all-cause mortality [8]. This data suggests that DOACs have similar efficacy and a similar if not better safety profile when used to treat VTE. The DOACs also offer benefits for patients such as no monitoring, no dietary restrictions, and fewer drug interactions. Because none of the DOACs have been studied head-to-head, one drug cannot be conclusively considered superior to another. However, a 2015 network meta-analysis compared the DOACs indirectly and reported the relative risks of major bleeding between each agent. The analysis reported similar risks with the exception that apixaban had a lower relative risk of major bleeding when compared to dabigatran (RR: 0.42; 95% CI: 0.21–0.87) and edoxaban (RR: 0.37; 95% CI: 0.19–0.73) [9].

Due to lack of data directly comparing the DOACs to one another, choice of anticoagulant is often based on patient specific factors and affordability of the medication. For this patient, any of the DOACs would be appropriate because he has no cytochrome P-450 or p-glycoprotein interactions with the DOACs, good renal function, no hepatic dysfunction, no contraindications to DOACs, and no history of bleeding. Selection for this patient would largely rest on patient preference and affordability. Using the HAS-BLED scoring system, he has a score of 1, which indicates he is low risk for bleeding [10]. Even though bleeding risk assessments are not as well validated, the HAS-BLED model has the best predictive value to predict bleeding events in the first 3 months of therapy [11].

Considering Antiplatelet Therapy

When determining anticoagulation needs of a patient who is also requiring dual-antiplatelet therapy (DAPT), evidence-based recommendations come from trials that often do not have the power to make conclusions on both safety and efficacy. Most of the literature on triple oral antithrombotic therapy (TOAT) references patients with acute coronary syndromes requiring stent placement who were previously on oral anticoagulants for atrial fibrillation. If this data is extrapolated to treatment with VTE, the recommendation would be to complete TOAT for 6 months post drug-eluting stent (DES) placement and then de-escalate to dual treatment with an anticoagulant and a single antiplatelet [12, 13]. See Fig. 20.1 for treatment algorithm. The WOEST trial results suggest that clopidogrel, and not aspirin, would be the antiplatelet of choice in this situation [14]. By de-escalating therapy, bleeding risks and mortality are minimized. This evidence would suggest that because the patient's stent was placed 8 months ago, his aspirin could be discontinued to minimize bleeding risk now that an oral anticoagulant (OAC) is being started. Would it

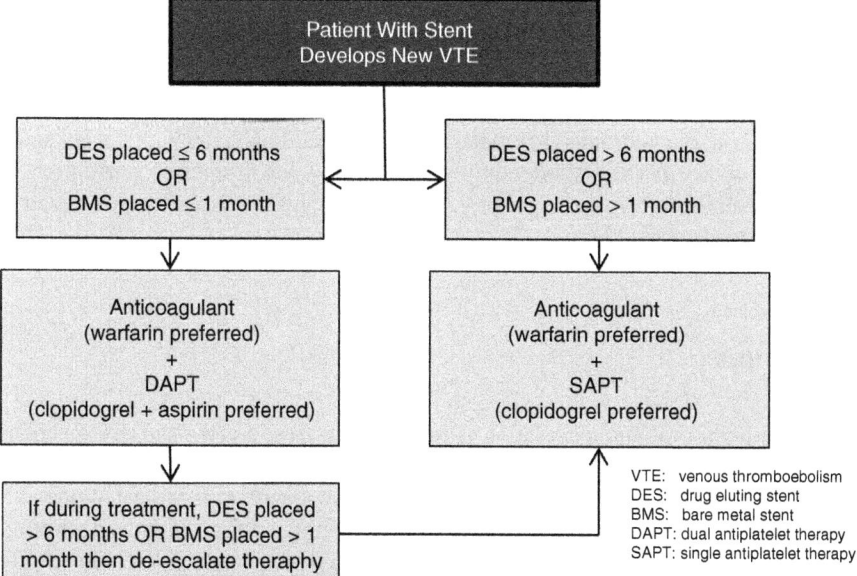

Fig. 20.1 Treatment algorithm for new VTE in patient with a stent

be wise to keep prasugrel as the antiplatelet agent or should the patient be switched to clopidogrel?

All of the studies on TOAT therapy were conducted using clopidogrel, warfarin, and aspirin. Little data exists on regimens with any of the DOACs or newer P2Y12 agents. This presents a challenge when trying to use the DOACs for treatment of acute VTE as the CHEST guidelines recommend. A prospective cohort analysis found an increased risk in major and minor bleeding in patients receiving TOAT with prasugrel when compared to TOAT with clopidogrel ($p < 0.001$) after placement of DES [15]. Both agents had similar risk of individual components and composite endpoint of death, myocardial infarction, ischemic stroke, and stent thrombosis ($p = 0.61$). This study only had a small number of patients on prasugrel ($n = 21$), however included patients with indications other than atrial fibrillation for OAC. The results of this study are not surprising, because prasugrel has been shown to have increased risk of bleeding when compared to clopidogrel. At this time, there are no studies evaluating the safety and efficacy of ticagrelor used in TOAT.

There is a small amount of evidence in using newer DOAC in TOAT therapy. A sub-group analysis from the RE-LY trial compared dabigatran to warfarin in patients on DAPT. Data was presented at the 2011 European Society of Cardiology Congress and suggests that dabigatran was associated with less major bleeding when compared to warfarin. [16]. Rivaroxaban has been evaluated in post-ACS medication regimens, but doses used in that study were much lower than those used for atrial fibrillation or acute treatment of VTE. No data evaluating apixaban or edoxaban safety and efficacy as a part of TOAT therapy has been published at this time.

Antiplatelet in Coronary Artery Disease

DAPT is indicated 12 months after stent placement, bare metal or drug eluting, due to acute coronary syndrome [17]. After this time period, patients with CAD should be treated with life-long single-antiplatelet therapy for secondary prevention of coronary events. Aspirin is the preferred antiplatelet and clopidogrel may be used in those with an aspirin allergy.

Key Points

- 3 months of oral anticoagulation is necessary to treat a provoked acute venous thromboembolism.
- If therapy with aspirin, P2Y12 inhibitor and anticoagulant is indicated, the evidence suggests that TOAT therapy should be continued for 6 months post drug-eluting stent (DES) placement. Clopidogrel would be the best P2Y12 inhibitor to use because it has more evidence when used in TOAT regimens.

- After 6 months, TOAT therapy should be de-escalated to dual treatment with an anticoagulant and a single antiplatelet to minimize bleeding risks associated with TOAT therapy. Literature suggests that clopidogrel, and not aspirin, would be the best antiplatelet to continue at this time. Clopidogrel showed less bleeding than aspirin when used with an anticoagulant in the WOEST trial.
- Anticoagulant choice will depend on patient specific factors because warfarin is the only anticoagulant with robust data describing risk and benefit when used concomitantly with dual-antiplatelet therapy. DOACs might be appropriate to use so long as a patient is not high risk of gastrointestinal bleeding. Apixaban is the only DOAC that did not show increased GI bleeding when compared to warfarin.

Self-Assessment Questions

1. AC is a 67 year old male (82 kg) with new acute proximal DVT that is unprovoked. He has a past medical history of coronary artery disease, CABG × 2 four years ago, dyslipidemia, hypertension, gastrointestinal bleed (6 months ago), and depression. The patient is taking aspirin 81 mg PO once daily and no other medications that pre-dispose him to bleeding. His serum creatinine is 0.8 mg/dL and his blood pressure is controlled at 122/76 mmHg. Which of the following would be the best treatment plan for AC's VTE?

    (a) Enoxaparin 80 mg subcutaneously Q12H and warfarin 5 mg daily. Titrate to INR 2–3 and discontinue enoxaparin when INR is therapeutic for 24 h or for 5 days. Total duration of treatment should be 3 months.
    (b) Enoxaparin 80 mg subcutaneously Q12H for 10 days followed by dabigatran 150 mg PO BID for indefinite duration.
    (c) Apixaban 10 mg PO BID for 7 days, followed by apixaban 5 mg PO BID. Total duration of treatment should be 3 months.
    (d) Rivaroxaban 15 mg PO BID for 21 days followed by rivaroxaban 20 mg PO once daily for indefinite duration.

    ANSWER: The correct response is C. The patient has three risk factors for bleeding: Age ≥ 65 years, GI bleed, and aspirin use. The CHEST guidelines recommend that if a patients has three or more risk factors, treatment for unprovoked DVT should be 3 months. After treatment, consideration can be made for further treatment at patient and physician discretion. Because of his coronary artery disease, he cannot discontinue the aspirin, and thus eliminate one of his risk factors. All DOACs are recommended over warfarin for treatment of VTE and thus consideration should be made to pick the best anticoagulant given patient specific factors. Apixaban has the lowest bleeding rates when compared to warfarin and is the only DOAC that does not have increased GI bleeds when compared to warfarin. Due to this patient's history of a GI bleed, apixaban would be the best option.

2. MG is a 40 year old male who is admitted for acute DVT 2 days after receiving an elective catheterization secondary to progressive angina pains. His past medical history includes STEMI 3 months ago with three DES placed, dyslipidemia, hypertension, depression, anxiety, and seasonal allergies. His current medications include aspirin 81 mg daily, ticagrelor 90 mg BID, atenolol 50 mg once daily, ramipril 2.5 mg once daily, citalopram 20 mg once daily, and alprazolam 1 mg TID prn anxiety. Which of the following would be the best recommendation for his antithrombotic regimen?
    (a) Triple therapy with clopidogrel, aspirin, and dabigatran.
    (b) Triple therapy with ticagrelor, aspirin, and warfarin.
    (c) Dual therapy with clopidogrel and dabigatran.
    (d) Dual therapy with aspirin and warfarin.

ANSWER: The correct response is A. The patient should be triple therapy because his stents were placed only 3 months ago. After 6 months, it would be appropriate to discontinue the aspirin and only treat with a P2Y12 inhibitor and oral anticoagulant. Because there is no data with ticagrelor, the P2Y12 inhibitor of choice would be clopidogrel. Although the literature is not robust, there is a small amount of evidence that shows dabigatran has lower bleeding in TOAT when compared to warfarin. Dabigatran is also recommended over warfarin for treatment of VTE.

References

1. Ramzi DW, Leeper KV. DVT and pulmonary embolism: part II. Treatment and prevention. Am Fam Phys. 2004;69(12):2841–8.
2. Kearon C, Aki EA, Ornelas J, et al. Antithrombotic therapy for VTE disease: CHEST guidelines. Chest. 2016; doi:10.1016/j.chest. 2015.11.026.
3. Schulman S, Kearon C, Kakkar AK, et al. RE-COVER Study Group. Dabigatran versus warfarin in the treatment of acute venous thromboembolism. N Engl J Med. 2009;361:2342–52.
4. Investigators EINSTEIN. Oral rivaroxaban for symptomatic venous thromboembolism. N Engl J Med. 2010;363:2499–510.
5. Agnelli G, Buller HR, Cohen A, et al. AMPLIFY Investigators. Oral apixaban for the treatment of acute venous thromboembolism. N Engl J Med. 2013;369:799–808.
6. Hokusai-VTE Investigators. Edoxaban versus warfarin for the treatment of symptomatic venous thromboembolism. N Engl J Med. 2013;369:1406–15.
7. Gomez-Outes A, Lecumberri R, Suarez-Gea ML, et al. Case fatality rates of recurrent thromboembolism and bleeding in patients receiving direct oral anticoagulants for the initial and extended treatment of venous thromboembolism: a systematic review. J Cardiovasc Pharmacol Ther. 2015;20:490–500.
8. Kakkos SK, Kirkilesis G, Tsolakis IA. Editors' choice-efficacy and safety of the new oral anticoagulants dabigatran, rivaroxaban, apixaban, and edoxaban in the treatment and secondary prevention of venous thromboembolism: a systematic review and meta-analysis of phase III trials. Eur J Vasc Endovasc Surg. 2014;48:565–75.
9. Mantha S, Ansell J. Indirect comparison of dabigatran, rivaroxaban, apixaban and edoxaban for the treatment of acute venous thromboembolism. J Thromb Thrombolysis. 2015;39:155–65.

10. Lip GY, Frison L, Halperin JL, Lane DA. Comparative validation of a novel risk score for predicting bleeding risk in anticoagulated patients with atrial fibrillation: the HAS-BLED (Hypertension, abnormal renal/liver function, stroke, bleeding history or predisposition, labile INR, elderly, drugs/alcohol concomitantly) score. J Am Coll Cardiol. 2011;57(2):173–80.
11. Riva N, Bellesini M, Di Minno MN, et al. Poor predictive value of contemporary bleeding risk scores during long-term treatment of venous thromboembolism. A multicentre retrospective cohort study. Thromb Haemost. 2014;112:511–21.
12. Fiedler KA, Maeng M, Mehilli J, et al. Duration of triple therapy in patients requiring oral anticoagulation after drug-eluting stent implantation: the ISAR-TRIPLE trial. J Am Coll Cardiol. 2015;65:1619–29.
13. You JJ, Singer DE, Howard PA, et al. Antithrombotic therapy for atrial fibrillation; antithrombotic therapy and prevention of thrombosis, 9th ed. American College of Chest Physicians evidence-base clinical practice guidelines. Chest. 2012;141(2 Suppl):e531S–75S.
14. Dewilde W, Oirbans T, Verheugt F, et al. Use of clopidogrel with or without aspirin in patients taking oral anticoagulant therapy and undergoing percutaneous coronary intervention: an open-label, randomized, controlled trial. Lancet. 2013;381:1107–15.
15. Sarafoff N, Martischnig A, Wealer J, et al. Triple therapy with aspirin, prasugrel and vitamin k antagonists in patients with drug-eluting stent implantation and an indication for oral anticoagulation. J Am Coll Cardiol. 2013;61(20):2060–6.
16. Dans AL. Concomitant use of antiplatelet therapy with dabigatran or warfarin: a sub-analysis from RE-LY. Paris, France: European Society of Cardiology Congress. Accessed 28 Aug 2011.
17. Levin GN, Bates ER, Bittl JA, et al. 2016 ACC/AHA guideline focused update on duration of dual antiplatelet therapy in patients with coronary artery disease. Circulation. 2016;134(10):e123–55.

Chapter 21
Acute VTE in a Patient with Moderate Chronic Kidney Disease

Brenda Pahl and Douglas Anderson

Abstract This case discusses therapeutic options for treating an acute VTE in a patient with moderate chronic kidney disease. The focus of the treatment is patient specific considerations when selecting an oral anticoagulant for outpatient treatment.

Keywords Moderate chronic kidney disease • Acute VTE • Direct oral anticoagulants • Oral anticoagulant considerations

Case Introduction

AF is a 78 year old female who has presented to the emergency department with complaints of lower left leg pain and swelling. She recently returned home from travel abroad by airplane on an 8 hour flight. She was diagnosed with an acute DVT in the proximal popliteal vein after confirmation by an abnormal D dimer and duplex ultrasound. As the emergency room provider, you have been asked to manage therapy for this patient. She has a medical history of hypertension, congestive heart failure (CHF), type 2 diabetes, obesity (BMI of 30) and moderate renal insufficiency (Wt. 125 lb, SCr 1.0 mg/dL, CrCL of 41.2 mL/min). Her risks of bleeding include age and type 2 diabetes as well as being on aspirin therapy. She has no prior history of a VTE. Her risk factors for VTE include CHF and recent travel, her current medications include lisinopril, amlodipine, furosemide, potassium chloride, aspirin, Lantus, and Humalog as per a sliding scale prior to meals. She is compliant with taking her medications, however due to the fact that she does not drive, she has difficulty making her medical appointments. She does not qualify for home health care, therefore home laboratory monitoring cannot be considered.

B. Pahl, RPh, PharmD (✉) • D. Anderson, PharmD, DPh
Cedarville University School of Pharmacy, 251 N. Main Street, Cedarville, OH 45314, USA
e-mail: bpahl@cedarville.edu; andersond@cedarville.edu

Case Discussion

Chronic kidney disease (CKD) has become a common health problem. The increase in CKD in the United States is the result of an aging population and a high prevalence of type 2 diabetes as is the patient described in the case presented above. The CDC estimates that more than 10% of adults in the United States, more than 20 million people, may have some degree of CKD [1]. Several studies have also shown that patients with any stage of CKD are at an increased risk for venous thromboembolic (VTE) events [2]. Therefore, the incidence of treating a patient with some degree of renal impairment for an acute VTE event will be high.

In January of 2016, the American College of Chest Physicians (CHEST) released revised guidelines for VTE management [3]. At the same time, the Anticoagulation Forum published guidelines on VTE treatment in the January, 2016 edition of the Journal of Thrombosis and Thrombolysis [4]. Both of these guidelines for anticoagulation management address the use of the direct oral anticoagulants (DOACs), warfarin, and low molecular weight heparins (LMWH) for the treatment of VTE. It is recommended that most patients with DVTs and some with PEs can be managed on an outpatient basis. The guidelines also recommend therapy should be customized according to clinical circumstances of each individual patient. Patients with renal dysfunction require special considerations when selecting an anticoagulant therapy.

What Is the Preferred Anticoagulant for VTE Treatment in Patients with Mild Renal Dysfunction?

Warfarin has long been the mainstay of treatment for VTE and can be safely prescribed for patients with severe renal function with no specific dose adjustments based on renal clearance. However, recent studies have shown that patients on warfarin that have CKD require lower maintenance doses and need to be seen more often due to decreased stability in dosing [5, 6]. Since warfarin doses are adjusted based on the INR, the INR must be monitored on a regular basis. If a patient is unable to adhere to the need for frequent lab draws, e.g. patients with transportation issues, other options should be considered. Treatment with warfarin must be overlapped with either unfractionated heparin, requiring an inpatient stay, or LMWH which can be used on an outpatient basis. The LMWHs enoxaparin and dalteparin have recommended dose reductions when CrCl is <30 mL/min. One must also consider if the patient is able to self-administer the LMWH or is in need of assistance. Home monitoring of the INR during warfarin therapy is a possibility, however the patient's ability to perform the point of care test and insurance coverage would need to be considered.

For patients with VTE, who do not have cancer, the 2016 CHEST guidelines recommend the use of a direct oral anticoagulant agent over warfarin. DOACs have

Table 21.1 DOACs dosing for VTE according to renal function [8–10, 14]

DOAC	DVT/PE treatment	CrCL 30–50 mL/min	CrCL <30 mL/min	Other considerations
Dabigatran	150 mg twice daily after 5–10 days of parenteral anticoagulation	CrCl <50 mL/min with any P-gp inhibitor- avoid use	No recommendation. Patients were excluded from clinical trials	
Edoxaban	60 mg daily after 5–10 days of parenteral anticoagulant	30 mg daily	For CrCl 15–30 mL/min, dose is 30 mg daily	Weight < 60 kg or use with specific P-gp inhibitors dose is 30 mg daily
Rivaroxaban	15 mg twice daily for 10 days, followed by 20 mg daily	No dose adjustment	Avoid use in CrCl <30 mL/min	
Apixaban	10 mg twice daily for 7 days, then 5 mg twice daily	No dose adjustment	No recommendation or evidence in CrCl <25 mL/min	

been proven to be at least as effective and safe as the combination of heparin and warfarin in treating acute VTE [7]. Evidence from clinical trials demonstrated that DOACs have a lower risk of bleeding, especially intracranial bleeding. Due to the fact that DOACs have fixed dosing, they do not require close monitoring to measure anticoagulant effect thus offering a convenient alternative for those patients who have difficulty maintaining lab appointments. DOACs would be an excellent option for AF who has transportation issues. The drawback of these agents is that they all possess some degree of renal elimination leading to an increased risk of bleeding due to drug accumulation in patients with decreased renal function. Therefore, dosing needs to be adjusted according to the patient's estimated CrCl (see Table 21.1) using the Cockcroft-Gault equation [7].

Which of the DOACs Is the Best Option for Treating the DVT in AF?

The new CHEST guidelines as well as the guidance document from the Anticoagulation Forum, do not recommend one DOAC over another. The clinical scenario of the patient should be the deciding factor in the selection of a DOAC. (See Table 21.2).

Dabigatran (Pradaxa®), a direct thrombin inhibitor, was the first oral, non-vitamin k antagonist approved for prevention of stroke in patients with atrial fibrillation October 19, 2010. It was approved for treatment of VTE on April 7, 2014. Elimination

Table 21.2 Patient specific considerations when considering oral anticoagulant for VTE [3]

Patient concern	Suggested anticoagulant
Need for once daily dosing	Edoxaban, rivaroxaban, warfarin
Poor compliance (missed doses)	Warfarin (INR monitoring would detect)
Avoidance of laboratory monitoring	Apixaban, dabigatran, edoxaban, rivaroxaban
Avoidance of parenteral therapy	Apixaban, rivaroxaban
CrCL <30 mL/min	Warfarin
History or high risk of bleeding	Apixaban, warfarin
Coronary artery disease	Apixaban, edoxaban, rivaroxaban
Need for a reversal agent	Dabigatrin, warfarin
Pregnancy	No oral options. Use LMWH
Financial concerns	Varies by patient insurance. Warfarin least expensive

of dabigatran is primarily renal with 80% of an intravenous dose excreted in this manner [8]. Dosing for the treatment of venous thromboembolism is 150 mg twice daily to begin after 5–10 days of parenteral anticoagulation based on RE-COVER and RE-COVER II trials. This would require a hospital admission if using unfractionated heparin or the ability to inject a LMWH. For patients ≥75 years, the risk of bleeding increases with dabigatran. Therefore elderly patients should be monitored for signs of bleeding or consider other treatment options. Dosing adjustments for renal dysfunction include only those patients who are currently receiving a P-gp inhibitor. For these patients, if the CrCl is <50 mL/min while on these medications, co-administration should be avoided. There are no dosing recommendations for CrCl ≤30 mL/min [8].

Rivaroxaban (Xarelto®) is an oral, reversible, direct Factor Xa inhibitor. Rivaroxaban has a dual mode of elimination. Following oral administration, approximately two thirds of the dose undergoes hepatic metabolism where the metabolized drug is eliminated partly via renal excretion and the other half eliminated via a hepatobiliary route. The remaining one-third of the absorbed dose is excreted unchanged through the kidneys. The dose of rivaroxaban approved for acute VTE is 15 mg twice daily with food for 21 days, followed by 20 mg daily. If the CrCl is less than 30 mL/min, rivaroxaban should be avoided [9]. Rivaroxaban does not require a 5–10 day treatment of a parenteral agent prior to initiation. This fact, along with a once daily dosing option, makes rivaroxaban a good choice for a patient who does not want to use a parenteral therapy.

Apixaban (Eliquis®) is another oral direct Factor Xa inhibitor. It is eliminated in both urine and feces with renal excretion accounting for about 27% of total clearance, the least of all the DOACs. The recommended dose for VTE treatment is 10 mg twice daily for 7 days followed by 5 mg twice daily. While there is no dose adjustment specifically based on renal function suggested by the manufacturer, it should be noted that patients with a serum creatinine >2.5 mg/dL or CrCl <25 mL/min were excluded from clinical trials [10]. In clinical trials, apixaban was associated with a significantly lower risk of bleeding compared to warfarin [11]. It would be the recommended DOAC if the risk of bleeding was a concern.

Edoxaban (Savaysa®) is the newest oral direct Factor Xa inhibitor. The renal clearance for edoxaban is 50%. Edoxaban is unique in that it is not recommended for use in atrial fibrillation patients with a CrCl >95 mL/min. In the ENGAGE AF-TIMI 48 study non-valvular atrial fibrillation patients with CrCL >95 mL/min had an increased rate of ischemic stroke with edoxaban 60 mg once daily compared to patients treated with warfarin [12]. In these patients another anticoagulant should be used. In the Hokusi-VTE trial, this was not a finding [13]. The recommended dose for DVT and PE treatment is 60 mg once daily after 5–10 days of initial therapy with a parenteral agent. It is recommended to reduce the dose to 30 mg once daily if CrCl is 15–50 mL/min. For CrCl ≤15 mL/min, it is not recommended to use edoxaban [14].

To address the patient case presented earlier, warfarin dose adjusted based on INR with overlapping parenteral anticoagulation, would be an acceptable treatment. However, the patient may have difficulty adhering with the required monitoring. A DOAC, which does not require frequent lab visits, should be considered. Rivaroxaban and apixaban do not require initial parenteral anticoagulant therapy and can be used as initial therapy for patients with acute VTE. Because of the patient's CrCl of 41.2 mL/min, the dose of either apixaban or rivaroxaban would be the normal dose for DVT treatment. Edoxaban 30 mg daily after 5–10 days of parenteral anticoagulation therapy could also be an option. This patient is a diabetic who self-administers insulin therapy so co-therapy with a short-course of an LMWH would not be a barrier, however the patient may want to avoid additional injections. Dabigatran 150 mg twice daily could also be given after 5–10 days of parenteral therapy but should be used with caution as the patient is over 75 years of age. The patient's insurance coverage should also be considered when selecting between these agents.

Key Points

- Warfarin has been the main treatment for acute VTE and is recommended in patients with severe renal impairment.
- The new, oral anticoagulants offer a safe and effective treatment option for the treatment of VTE without intense laboratory monitoring.
- All of the new oral anticoagulants have some degree of renal elimination, therefore renal function must be considered when determining appropriate doses.
- Warfarin, dabigatran and edoxaban all require initial treatment of a parenteral anticoagulant agent when treating an acute VTE.
- Apixaban and rivaroxaban offer a single agent therapy option for treatment of acute VTE.

- Rivaroxaban and dabigatran should be avoided if CrCl is ≤30 mL/min, while edoxaban should be avoided when CrCl ≤15 mL/min.
- The clinical scenario of the patient should be considered when selecting an anticoagulant for treating VTE.

Self-Assessment Questions

1. If AF's renal function worsened and her CrCl is now 25 mL/min, which of the following anticoagulants could be used to treat her VTE? (Select all that apply).

   (a) Dabigatran 75 mg twice daily
   (b) Rivaroxaban 20 mg daily
   (c) Apixaban 5 mg twice daily
   (d) Edoxaban 30 mg once daily
   (e) Warfarin dose adjusted based on INR

   Correct answer(s): C, D, E

   (a) Dabigatran 75 mg twice daily would not be a correct choice as there are no dosing recommendations for a CrCl ≤30 mL/min for dabigatran.
   (b) Rivaroxaban 20 mg daily would not be an option as it should be avoided if the CrCl is less than 30 mL/min.
   (c) Apixaban 5 mg twice daily would be an anticoagulant that could be used to treat the patient as no dose adjustments are recommended for treating acute DVT/PE.
   (d) Edoxaban 30 mg once daily would be an anticoagulant that could be used as this is the recommended dose for CrCl 15–50 mL/min.
   (e) Warfarin dose adjusted based on INR would also be an option as this is the suggested therapy in patients with severe renal dysfunction.

2. Which of the following anticoagulants require 5–10 days of parenteral anticoagulant therapy either prior to or during treatment when initiating therapy for a DVT. (choose all that apply)

   (a) Warfarin
   (b) Edoxaban
   (c) Apixaban
   (d) Rivaroxaban
   (e) Dabigatran

   Correct Answer(s): A, B, E

   (a) Warfarin requires the use of low molecular weight heparin or unfractionated heparin until the INR is therapeutic.
   (b) Edoxaban requires 5–10 days of parenteral anticoagulant therapy prior to initiation per the manufacturer.
   (c) Apixaban does not require the use of a parenteral anticoagulant.
   (d) Rivaroxaban does not require the use of a parenteral anticoagulant.
   (e) Dagibatran requires 5–10 days of parenteral anticoagulation therapy prior to initiation per the manufacturer.

References

1. Citation Centers for Disease Control and Prevention (CDC). National chronic kidney disease fact sheet: general information and national estimates on chronic kidney disease in the United States, 2014. Atlanta, GA: US Department of Health and Human Services, Centers for Disease Control and Prevention; 2014.
2. Wattanakit K, Cushman M, Stehman-Breen C, Heckbert S, Folsom A. Chronic kidney disease increases risk for venous thromboembolism. J Am Soc Nephrol. 2008;1:135–40.
3. Kearon C, Akl EA, Ornelas J, et al. Antithrombotic therapy for VTE disease: chest guideline and expert panel report. Chest. 2016;149(2):315–52.
4. Burnett AE, Mahan CE, Vazquez SR, Oertel LB, Garcia DA, Ansell J. Guidance for the practical management of the direct oral anticoagulants (DOACs) in VTE treatment. Journal of Thrombosis and Thrombolysis. 2016;41:206–232. doi:10.1007/s11239-015-1310-7.
5. Kleinow ME, Garwood CL, Clemente JL, Whittaker P. Effect of chronic kidney disease on warfarin management in a pharmacist-managed anticoagulation clinic. J Manag Care Pharm. 2011;17(7):523–30.
6. Hughes S, Szerki I, Nash MJ, Thachil J. Anticoagulation in chronic kidney disease patients—the practical aspects. Clin Kidney J. 2014;7:442–9.
7. Becattini C, Agnelli G. Treatment of venous thromboembolism with new anticoagulant agents. J Am Coll Cardiol. 2016;67:1941–55.
8. Pradaxa (dabigatran) package insert. Ridgefield, CT: Boehringer Ingelheim Pharmaceuticals, Inc.; 2015 Nov.
9. Xarelto (rivaroxaban) package insert. Titusville, NJ: Janssen Pharmaceuticals, Inc; 2016 May.
10. Eliquis (apixaban) package insert. Princeton, NJ: Bristol-Myers Squibb Company; 2015 Sept.
11. Granger CB, Alexander JH, McMurray JJ, Lopes RD, Hylek EM, Hanna M, et al. Apixaban versus warfarin in patients with atrial fibrillation. N Engl J Med. 2011;365(11):981–92.
12. Giugliano RP, Ruff CT, Braunwald E, Murphy SA, Wiviott SD, Halperin JL, et al. Edoxaban versus warfarin in patients with atrial fibrillation. N Engl J Med. 2013;369(22):2093–104.
13. Investigators Hokusai-VTE, Buller HR, Decousus H, Grosso MA, Mercuri M, Middeldorp S, et al. Edoxaban versus warfarin for the treatment of symptomatic venous thromboembolism. N Engl J Med. 2013;369:1406–15.
14. Savaysa (edoxaban) package insert. Parisppany, NJ: Daiichi Sankyo, Inc; 2015 Sept.

Chapter 22
Oral Anticoagulation and Duration in Recurrent Venous Thromboembolism (VTE)

Regina Arellano

Abstract Long-term anticoagulant therapy for recurrent venous thromboembolism (VTE) is determined based on a patient's underlying thromboembolic risk and bleeding risk. Patient characteristics and preferences should be considered when selecting appropriate anticoagulant therapy.

Keywords Recurrent deep vein thrombosis • Pulmonary embolism • Venous thromboembolism • Duration • Selecting oral anticoagulation therapy • Thromboembolic risk • Bleeding risk

Case Introduction

A 68-year-old male presents to clinic complaining of pain and swelling in his left lower extremity (LLE). His past medical history is significant for unprovoked pulmonary embolism (PE) one year ago for which he completed approximately 5 months of oral anticoagulation therapy with warfarin targeted to an INR range of 2–3. Patient has a family history of VTE. His current weight and height is 148 kg and 77 in., respectively. His most recent vital signs and labs are within normal limits, except for most notably serum creatinine of 1.2 mg/dL. His primary care physician ordered a LLE venous duplex ultrasound, which revealed a non-occlusive deep vein thrombus (DVT) confined to the left popliteal vein. Today this patient presents to discuss oral anticoagulant options and he does not want injections. Patient reports a history of non-adherence to INR monitoring and inconsistency with vitamin K intake. Upon further discussion, he admits he does not like to take medications and he was uncomfortable with taking more than one tablet at a time which often resulted in less than optimal time in therapeutic range (TTR). He also did not like

---

R. Arellano, PharmD, BCPS
Midwestern University Chicago College of Pharmacy,
555 31st Street, Downers Grove, IL 60515, USA
e-mail: rarell@midwestern.edu

having restrictions to his diet because he frequently travels (note: travel was ruled out as a possible etiology for previous and current VTE).

Case Discussion

What should be considered in developing a plan to manage this patient's recurrent VTE?

Duration of Therapy

Venous thromboembolism (VTE) includes (DVT) and (PE). Recurrent VTE is particularly common in patients who present with unprovoked (idiopathic) VTE. One study found the risk of recurrence at 2 years to be 4.8% in patients with a provoked event versus 12.1% in patients with an unprovoked event [1]. After a second unprovoked VTE, long-term anticoagulant therapy is recommended for patients who do not have risk factors for bleeding [1]. Long-term anticoagulant therapy is highly recommended if unprovoked event was a PE or if a second unprovoked VTE occurs [2]. This patient presents with a history of unprovoked PE and second unprovoked VTE. Long-term therapy should have been considered for his first VTE, however it is common in clinical practice to discontinue therapy after approximately 6–12 months, especially if patient is having difficulty with adherence to oral anticoagulant and/or appropriate monitoring parameters such as INR monitoring.

Risk of Thrombosis Versus Risk of Major Bleeding

History of VTE is the main risk factor (see Table 22.1) for a second VTE [1]. The risk of recurrence is categorized according to underlying etiology (see Table 22.2). The risk is considered high if thrombosis was unprovoked or is associated with an irreversible risk factor such as underlying hypercoagulable disorder. The risk is deemed intermediate if thrombosis was provoked by a minor transient risk factor such as prolonged travel and immobility [2]. The incidence of VTE varies by the type and duration of travel and by individual risk factors, but the association between air travel and VTE is strongest for flights >8–10 h [4]. This patient presents with history of unprovoked VTE and a recurrent, acute unprovoked VTE, both factors place him at high risk for recurrence. It is also important to recognize that this patient reports a lifestyle involving frequent travel which may also increase patient's risk depending on type and duration of travel. Also important to note, in patients who discontinue anticoagulation therapy after 3–6 months following an incident VTE, the risk of a recurrent event is approximately 10% in the first year, 5% in the

Table 22.1 Risk factors for VTE [3]

Risk factor	Example
Age	Risk doubles with each decade after age 50
Prior history of VTE	Strongest known risk factor for DVT and PE
Venous stasis	Major medical illness, major surgery, paralysis, obesity, varicose veins, immobility
Vascular injury	Major orthopedic surgery (e.g., knee and hip replacement), trauma (especially fractures of the pelvis, hip, or leg), indwelling venous catheters
Hypercoagulable states	Malignancy (diagnosed or occult), activated protein C resistance/factor V Leiden, prothrombin gene mutation, protein C/S deficiency, antithrombin deficiency, antiphospholipid antibodies, pregnancy/postpartum
Drug therapy	Estrogen-containing oral contraceptives, estrogen replacement therapy, selective estrogen receptor modulators, heparin induced thrombocytopenia, chemotherapy, testosterone

Table 22.2 Risk for recurrent VTE [2]

	Clinical presentation of VTE	Example
High	Unprovoked Associated with an irreversible risk factor	Incurable malignancy >1 occurrence of unprovoked VTE
Intermediate	Provoked by a reversible factor	Leg trauma (immobilization) Within 6 weeks of estrogen therapy Prolonged air travel (>10 h)
Low	Provoked by a major reversible factor	Surgery

second year, and 2–4% for each subsequent year [5]. Risk factors that increase the risk of recurrent VTE in patients with an unprovoked VTE include male sex, increasing age and obesity [6]. This patient discontinued therapy within 3–6 months following his first VTE and is an obese male. While this patient would be deemed at high risk for recurrent VTE suggesting long-term anticoagulant therapy, risk factors for bleeding are important to consider. Risk factors for bleeding include age 65 years or older, previous stroke, previous bleeding (e.g., gastrointestinal), active peptic ulcer disease, renal impairment, anemia, thrombocytopenia, liver disease, diabetes mellitus, use of antiplatelet therapy, poor patient compliance, and decreased TTR. One or two risk factors suggests moderate risk of bleeding and ≥3 risk factors suggest high risk of bleeding [7]. This patient is >65 years old and presents with a history of poor compliance to appropriate INR monitoring and decreased TTR. While evaluating a patient's risk for both thrombosis and bleeding, it is also important to assess whether there is an alternative therapy option which can reduce the risk of thrombosis without increasing the risk of bleeding.

Therapeutic Options Available

Treatment options for the initial phase of an acute VTE include rapid-onset anticoagulant agents to achieve therapeutic anticoagulation allowing stabilization of the thrombus and reducing risk of embolism. This patient presents with an acute VTE which requires rapid-onset anticoagulant therapy. Available options include (1) an oral anticoagulant bridged with low molecular weight heparin (LMWH) or (2) unmonitored subcutaneous unfractionated heparin [9] for a minimum of 5 days, or (3) a single-drug approach with an oral anticoagulant without the need for bridging with a parenteral agent. For VTE in patients without active malignancy, dabigatran, rivaroxaban, apixaban, or edoxaban is suggested over vitamin K antagonists (VKA) therapy as long-term anticoagulant therapy, while VKA therapy is suggested over LMWH [7]. Drug characteristics are an important factor to consider when selecting an appropriate anticoagulant therapy (see Table 22.3). Major differences that are important to patients include differences in the need for bridging with a parenteral agent and dosing frequency. Variation in drug characteristics that are important to providers include efficacy profiles, pharmacokinetic differences such as renal elimination (see Fig. 22.1),

Table 22.3 Recommended dosing for DOACs in treatment and secondary prevention of VTE

	Treatment	Secondary prevention	Renal adjustments	Potential for adverse effects	Considerations
Rivaroxaban	15 mg BID × 21 days then 20 mg daily	20 mg daily	CrCl < 30: Avoid	GIB, dyspepsia	No parenteral lead-in Acute VTE: BID dosing × 3 weeks F ↑ with food
Dabigatran	LMWH × 5 days 150 mg BID	150 mg BID	CrCl < 30: Avoid	GIB	Parenteral lead-in for acute VTE BID dosing
Apixaban	10 mg BID × 7 days then 5 mg BID × 6 months	2.5 mg BID	CrCl < 25 or Scr > 2.5: not included trials	N/A	No parenteral lead-in BID dosing Strong dual inhibitors of CYP 3A4 and Pg-P: reduce dose of 10 or 5 mg bid by 50% OR AVOID if already taking 2.5 mg bid
Edoxaban	LMWH × 5–10 days 60 mg daily	60 mg daily	CrCl > 95: Avoid CrCl 30–50/≤60 kg/ Pg-P inhibitor: 30 mg daily CrCl < 30: Avoid	N/A	Parenteral lead-in for acute VTE FDA approval ONLY for treatment

BID twice daily, *GIB* gastrointestinal bleed, *F* bioavailability

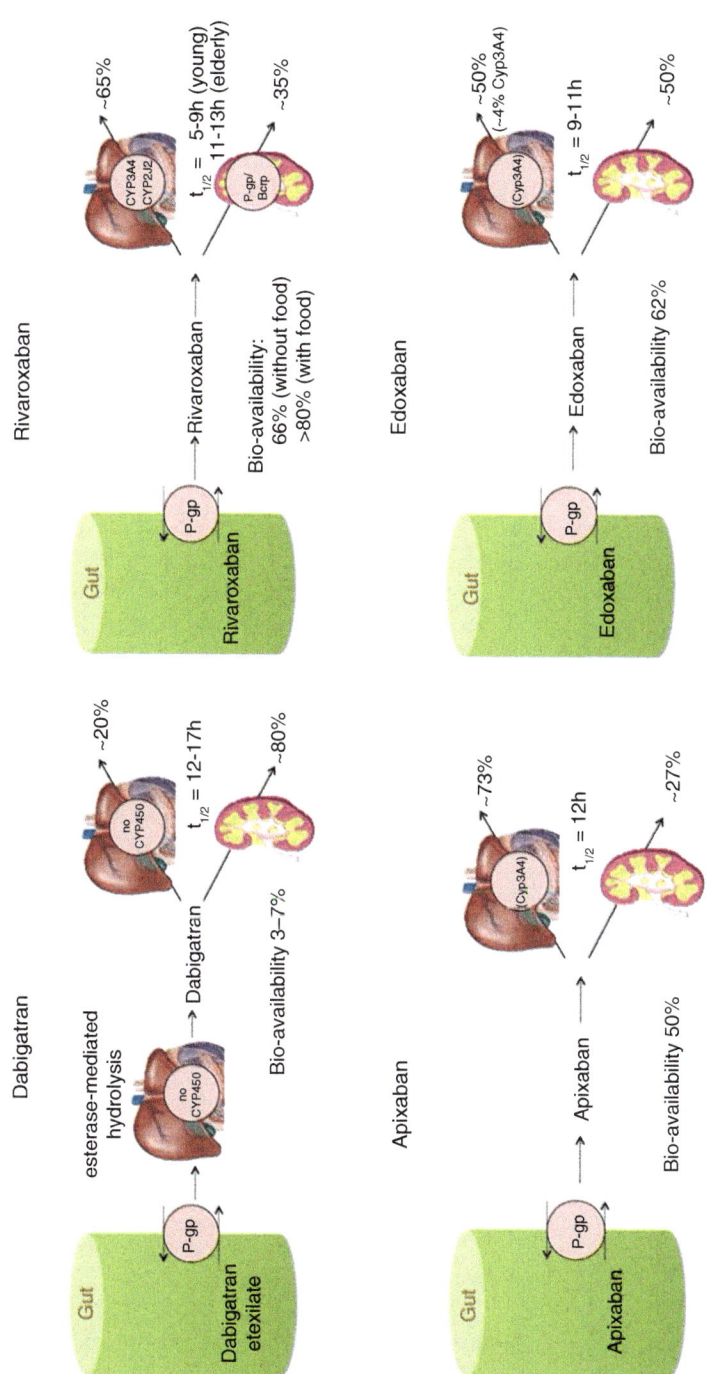

Fig. 22.1 Absorption and metabolism of the different direct oral anticoagulants [8]

potential for drug interactions and safety profile. The risk reduction for recurrent VTE with direct oral anticoagulants (DOACs) appears to be similar to the risk reduction with VKA, however, the risk of intracranial bleeding is less with DOACs [7]. In trials including patients with atrial fibrillation, gastrointestinal bleeding may be higher with dabigatran, rivaroxaban, and edoxaban compared to VKA, but has not been seen in trials including patients with VTE [7]. Another important consideration is that the exclusion criteria varied slightly among the trials including patients with VTE. In general, important exclusion criteria to consider include need for thrombolytic therapy, clinically significant liver disease (acute or chronic hepatitis or cirrhosis), creatinine clearance (CrCl) <30 mL/min (<25 mL/min for apixaban), aspirin use >100 mg/day, and other interacting medications. The updated CHEST guideline suggests VKA as the preferred agent in renal disease and CrCl <30 mL/min and in patients with poor compliance unless compliance is not expected to be an issue with a DOAC [10].

Patient Characteristics/Preferences

Based on differences in drug characteristics and to assess potential for adverse effects, baseline labs should be performed including serum creatinine for appropriate dosing, liver function tests for potential underlying liver disease, and complete blood count for potential underlying anemia or thrombocytopenia when selecting an appropriate anticoagulant therapy. In addition, concomitant drug therapies and co-morbidities such as diabetes or heart failure should be considered and accounted for when selecting one of the DOACs. These co-morbidities often introduce the potential for drug interactions depending on which drug therapy is used to manage them. Screening for potential drug interactions (e.g., strong Pg-P and CYP 3A4 inhibitors/inducers) and co-morbid conditions which can increase risk of bleeding (e.g., anemia, gastrointestinal bleeding, peptic ulcer disease). It is also important to consider patient preference for dosing frequency (see Table 22.3), diet restrictions, office visits for INR monitoring, and cost differences. In this patient, important considerations include his preference for a single-drug approach without the need for bridging with a parental agent for treatment of his acute VTE. If patient agrees to long-term oral anticoagulant therapy to reduce his risk of recurrent VTE, options without diet restrictions and with the least pill burden should be considered based on his history of non-adherence to multiple doses of warfarin and poor TTR. Fortunately, this patient does not have underlying co-morbidities and is not taking any concomitant drug therapy that would impact decision making when choosing a DOAC.

Key Points

- Long-term therapy is highly recommended to reduce the risk of recurrent VTE in patients presenting with an unprovoked VTE, especially in patients with a history of unprovoked VTE

- Underlying thromboembolic risk and bleeding risk is important to guide anticoagulant selection for treatment and prevention of recurrent VTE
- Consider specific patient characteristics such as renal function, risk factors for recurrent VTE, and bleeding risk (age, co-morbidities, history of non-adherence to follow-up or other medications), and patient preferences such as preferred dosing frequency, dietary needs, and bridging needs when selecting the most appropriate anticoagulant therapy

Self-Assessment Questions

1. A 75-year-old male presents to your anticoagulation clinic for a follow-up visit. PMH is significant for HTN (controlled), osteoarthritis, and recurrent VTE (recently diagnosed 3 months ago, previous 1st unprovoked event 2 years ago). His medications include warfarin and acetaminophen as needed for pain. His most recent vitals and labs are within normal limits and most recent CrCl is 50 mL/min. Patient is doing well on his current warfarin dose, however has been avoiding foods high in vitamin K content and he no longer wishes to avoid. He does not agree to have a consistent amount per week because this would be too difficult for him. Which of the following is the best management for this patient?

    (a) Discontinue warfarin and initiate apixaban which does not interact with foods high in vitamin K content
    (b) Discontinue warfarin because recommended duration of therapy is complete for this patient due to his high risk for major bleeding
    (c) Discontinue warfarin and initiate dabigatran because this therapeutic option is superior to warfarin
    (d) Continue warfarin therapy because this patient is not a candidate for direct oral anticoagulants

    The correct answer is A. The patient is a high risk for recurrent VTE given risk factors of age, sex, and history of VTE and bleeding risk is considered low given one risk factor of age, therefore long-term anticoagulation would be recommended. The direct oral anticoagulants are similar in efficacy to warfarin not superior. This patient is a candidate for direct oral anticoagulant.

2. Which of the following is the best management for an 80-year-old female diagnosed with an acute PE and a PMH significant for depression and previous unprovoked DVT (3 years ago). This patient presents with a calculated creatinine clearance of 58 mL/min and weight of 60 kg?

    (a) Initiate rivaroxaban 15 mg twice daily for 21 days then 20 mg daily
    (b) Initiate low molecular weight heparin + rivaroxaban 20 mg daily
    (c) Initiate apixaban 5 mg daily for 7 days then 2.5 mg daily
    (d) Initiate low molecular weight heparin + dabigatran 75 mg twice daily

The correct answer is A. This patient is presenting with an acute VTE which requires initial phase treatment with rapid-onset anticoagulant therapy. Initial parenteral anticoagulation is given before dabigatran and edoxaban. It is not given before rivaroxaban and apixaban. The recommended dose for dabigatran is 150 mg twice daily not 75 mg. The recommended dose for apixaban is 10 mg twice daily for 7 days then 5 mg twice daily for 6 months then patient can transition to 2.5 mg twice daily for long-term therapy to prevent recurrent VTE.

References

1. Galioto NJ, Danley DL, Van Maanen RJ. Recurrent venous thromboembolism. Am Fam Physician. 2011;83(3):293–300.
2. Kearon C. Long-term management of patients after venous thromboembolism. Circulation. 2004;110(9 Suppl 1):I10–8.
3. Nutescu EA, et al. Pharmacotherapy principles and practice. New York, NY: McGraw-Hill; 2013. p. 197–228.
4. Khan SR, Lim W, Dunn AS, et al. Antithrombotic therapy and prevention of thrombosis. In American College of Chest Physicians evidence-based clinical practice guidelines (9th ed). Chest. 2012;141(2):e195S–226S.
5. Prandoni P, Noventa T, Ghiraduzzi A, et al. The risk of recurrent venous thromboembolism after discontinuing anticoagulation in patients with acute proximal deep vein thrombosis or pulmonary embolism. A prospective cohort study in 1,626 patients. Haematologica. 2007;92:199–205.
6. Heit JA, Mohr DN, Silverstein MD, et al. Predictors of recurrence after deep vein thrombosis and pulmonary embolism: a population-based cohort study. Arch Intern Med. 2000;160:761–8.
7. Kearon C, Akl EA, Ornelas J, et al. Antithrombotic therapy for VTE disease: CHEST Guideline and Expert Panel Report. Chest. 2016;149(2):315–52.
8. Heidbuchel H, Verhamme P, Alings M, et al. European Heart Rhythm Association practical guide on the use of new oral anticoagulants in patients with non-valvular atrial fibrillation. Europace. 2013;15:625–51.
9. Kearon C, Ginsberg JS, Julian JA, et al. Comparison of fixed-dose weight-adjusted unfractionated heparin and low-molecular-weight heparin for acute treatment of venous thromboembolism. JAMA. 2006;296:935–42.
10. Burnett AE, Mahan CE, Vazquez SR, et al. Guidance for the practical management of the direct oral anticoagulants (DOACs) in VTE treatment. J Thromb Thrombolysis. 2016;41:206–32.

Chapter 23
Pulmonary Embolism (PE) with Thrombolytic Therapy

Justin M. Schmidt

Abstract Unfractionated heparin is the preferred anticoagulant while the effects of thrombolysis are evident. Oral anticoagulants are not recommended to be administered concurrently with thrombolytics and while direct oral anticoagulants have not been adequately studied after thrombolysis, use can be considered after the effects of thrombolysis are no longer present in select patients.

Keywords Pulmonary embolism • Thrombolytic • Fibrinolytic • Direct-acting oral anticoagulant

Case Introduction

A 65 y/o male was admitted and transferred to the medical intensive care unit 3 days ago after losing consciousness. He was hypotensive, tachycardic, tachypneic, and hypoxic on admission. Electrocardiogram revealed right bundle branch block (RBBB) and T-wave inversions. His initial NT-proBNP was 1524 pg/mL and his troponin I was 1.64 ng/mL. He was started on an unfractionated heparin (UFH) infusion protocol. A CT-angiogram revealed a saddle pulmonary embolus with extension into the main pulmonary arteries and right ventricular (RV) dilation (to view images of a CT of a saddle PE, follow this hyperlink). His BP was minimally responsive to fluids. It was decided to administer alteplase as an infusion (100 mg over 2 h) as a thrombolytic therapy. His UFH infusion was held prior to the infusion

---

J.M. Schmidt, PharmD, BCPS, BC-ADM
Midwestern University Chicago College of Pharmacy, 555 31st Street, Downers Grove, IL 60515, USA

Edward Hines Jr VA Hospital, 5000 S 5th Ave, Hines, IL 60141, USA
e-mail: jschmi@midwestern.edu

of alteplase and re-initiated 8 h after completion, once the aPTT decreased to 55 s (<2 × ULN). The heparin infusion has continued for an additional 3 days and his vitals have returned to normal. As the patient is nearing suitability for discharge, the issue of oral antithrombotic therapy arises. The patient has no kidney or liver disease, he is overweight (BMI 28), hypercoagulability workup is negative thus far and he has no known cancer.

Case Discussion

How Are Patients Who Receive Thrombolytics for VTE Different than Those Who Do Not?

Thromolytics are typically reserved for patients with massive or sub-massive pulmonary embolism (as opposed to those with low-risk PE). Massive PE is generally defined as a PE with sustained hypotension or bradycardia. Submassive PE refers to patients without hemodynamic instability, but with evidence of RV dysfunction or biomarkers suggesting myocardial tissue damage [1]. There is ongoing controversy regarding the use of thrombolytics in patients with submassive PE given more evenly matched risk and benefit, but the 2016 CHEST guidelines recommend against use of thrombolytics in patients without hypotension [2]. The case patient should be categorized as having a massive PE given his persistent hypotension. The patient also demonstrates RV dysfunction (RV dilation, elevated pro-BNP, new RBBB and T-wave inversions) and myocardial necrosis (elevated troponin I).

How Do Thrombolytics Affect Coagulation After Discontinuation?

Currently available thrombolytics are typically administered over 2 h or less for this indication. After discontinuation, the fibrinolytic and anticoagulant effects outlast the detectable serum concentration. aPTT levels less than twice the upper limit of normal (ULN) are commonly used to determine when it is safe to re-initiate anticoagulation (heparin is typically held during administration of thrombolytics in the United States, but commonly co-administered in Europe).

The 2016 CHEST guidelines recommend IV UFH for patients receiving thrombolytics [2]. This is likely due to the lack of data and experience with co-administration of other anticoagulants, the risk of hypotension compromising efficacy of subcutaneous and oral routes of administration and the availability of protamine to reverse the anticoagulant effects of UFH in the event of a bleed. The case patient's UFH infusion was discontinued during administration of the alteplase infusion and it was restarted 8 h later (the aPTT was <2 × ULN, indicating the therapeutic effects of alteplase were decreasing).

Is There Any Evidence Regarding the Use of Direct Oral Anticoagulants (DOACs) in Patients Receiving Thrombolysis?

Evidence regarding DOACs use after thrombolysis is limited. Phase III studies for DOACs excluded patients who recently received thrombolytics. An open-labelled retrospective cohort study evaluated apixaban and rivaroxaban after 50 mg alteplase over 2 h with IV UFH in 159 patients with predominantly submassive PE [3]. Approximately 24 h after the alteplase finished infusing, the UFH was discontinued and the oral anticoagulant was started. While the results of this study are promising, the design and size of the study will limit impact on guideline recommendations. This study would not apply to the case patient given that the case patient had a massive PE (under-represented in the study) and received 100 mg of alteplase while holding UFH.

Which Oral Anticoagulants Can Be Used After Thrombolysis?

Once a patient achieves hemodynamic stability and a reasonable amount of time has passed since thrombolysis (e.g., 24–48 h), oral anticoagulation initiation should be considered. Warfarin, dabigatran, rivaroxaban, apixaban, and edoxaban are all reasonable options. While there are limited data evaluating DOACs in patients experiencing massive PE and in those who receive thrombolysis, they have all proven effective in patients with less severe PE. The phase III study evaluating edoxaban evaluated a subgroup of patients with RV strain (evidenced by elevated NT-proBNP levels), and edoxaban was more effective than warfarin at preventing recurrent venous thromboembolism (3.3% vs. 6.2%, respectively, $p < 0.05$) [4]. The pulmonary embolism severity index (PESI) can help stratify short-term prognosis [5], and most patients receiving thrombolysis likely score in the intermediate to very high risk groups. Variables included in this tool include age, sex, comorbid disease states, measures of hemodynamic stability and mental status. This tool can help guide the timing of hospital discharge and follow-up. Traditionally, patients intermediate to very high risk PE have been hospitalized for at least 5 days during bridging with warfarin, whereas those with very low to low risk could be discharged with a low molecular weight heparin during this timeframe. Now that the case patient has achieved hemodynamic stability and is >24 h post-thrombolysis, Table 23.1 reviews the oral anticoagulant therapeutic options and the advantages and disadvantages of each.

Table 23.1 Advantages and disadvantages of oral anticoagulant therapy after PE and thrombolysis

Therapeutic option	Advantages	Disadvantages
Dabigatran	Limited monitoring	Would require two more days of LMWH, fondaparinux or UFH Lack of experience/data in this setting
Edoxaban	Limited monitoring	Would require two more days of LMWH, fondaparinux or UFH Lack of experience/data in this setting
Apixaban	Limited monitoring No additional/alternative anticoagulant required	Lack of experience/data in this setting
Rivaroxaban	Limited monitoring No additional/alternative anticoagulant required	Lack of experience/data in this setting
Warfarin	Greater experience/data in this setting	Would require bridging with LMWH, fondaparinux or UFH and additional monitoring/dietary requirements

Key Points

- Oral anticoagulants are not recommended to be administered concurrently with thrombolytics (unfractionated heparin is the preferred anticoagulant peri-thrombolysis).
- Oral anticoagulants can be used after the effects of thrombolysis are no longer present and sufficient time has passed to evaluate for bleeding (e.g., 24–48 h) as long as the patient is hemodynamically stable.
- While direct oral anticoagulants have not been adequately studied after thrombolysis, use in this setting is not contraindicated.

Self-Assessment Questions

1. A patient who experienced a massive pulmonary embolism is in the ICU having just received tenecteplase. Which of the following is true regarding the initiation of oral anticoagulation for this patient?

    (a) Oral anticoagulation can begin immediately given that the thrombolytic has already been administered
    (b) Oral anticoagulation can be started after the patient has achieved hemodynamic stability and is at least 24 h from administration of fibrinolysis
    (c) Oral anticoagulation should occur only upon discharge from this hospital
    (d) Oral anticoagulation is contraindicated in patients who have received thrombolytics

Correct Answer: B. Given concerns for bleeding with fibrinolysis after discontinuation and hemodynamic instability, it is reasonable to wait at least 24 h to start an oral anticoagulant. The 2016 CHEST guidelines recommend unfractionated heparin around the time of fibrinolysis given the above issues as well as the availability of a reversal agent. Administering an oral anticoagulant immediately is incorrect because it might be ineffective if absorption of the medication is compromised hypoperfusion. If, on the other hand, the perfusion is not compromised, there may be additive effects on the risk of bleed given persisting effects on aPTT and fibrinogen levels after thrombolytic discontinuation. Option C is incorrect because warfarin is commonly initiated in the hospital to hasten the ability to discontinue parenteral anticoagulation. There is no reason that DOACs would require outpatient initiation. Option D is not correct because, while these medications have not been evaluated in prospective RCTs in patients receiving thrombolysis for PE, their use is not specifically contraindicated.

2. Which of the following are true regarding the use of oral anticoagulants in patients receiving thrombolysis for massive PE? Choose all that apply.

    (a) Use of oral anticoagulants may be ineffective during periods of hemodynamic instability given compromise of intestinal blood flow
    (b) Oral anticoagulants without a reversal agent could pose additional bleeding risk if coadministered with a thrombolytic
    (c) Edoxaban has been studied in this setting and is safe and effective
    (d) Randomized controlled studies have established that unfractionated heparin is more safe and effective than oral anticoagulants during and shortly after thrombolysis
    (e) Given the short serum half-life of thrombolytics, oral anticoagulants should be started before thrombolytics to ensure that they are effective when serum concentrations are not detectable

Correct Answers: A and B. Theoretical concerns with administration of oral anticoagulants to patients with massive PE and thrombolysis include a lack of safety given added risk of bleed and lack of efficacy given lack of absorption. Option C and D are incorrect because there are no randomized controlled studies evaluating oral anticoagulants after thrombolysis for PE. Option E is incorrect because while the serum half-lives of thrombolytics are short, their effects are longer lasting.

References

1. Jaff MR, McMurtry MS, Archer SL, et al. Management of massive and submassive pulmonary embolism, iliofemoral deep vein thrombosis, and chronic thromboembolic pulmonary hypertension: a scientific statement from the American Heart Association. Circulation. 2011;123(16):1788–830. http://www.ncbi.nlm.nih.gov/pubmed/21422387
2. Kearon C, Akl EA, Ornelas J, et al. Antithrombotic therapy for VTE disease: CHEST Guideline And Expert Panel Report. Chest. 2016;149(2):315–52. http://journal.publications.chestnet.org/data/Journals/CHEST/934919/11026.pdf

3. Sharifi M, Vajo Z, Freeman W, et al. Transforming and simplifying the treatment of pulmonary embolism: "safe dose" thrombolysis plus new oral anticoagulants. Lung. 2015;193(3):369–74. http://www.ncbi.nlm.nih.gov/pubmed/25749665
4. Hokusai-VTE Investigators. Edoxaban versus warfarin for the treatment of symptomatic venous thromboembolism. N Engl J Med. 2013;369(15):1406–15. http://www.ncbi.nlm.nih.gov/pubmed/23991658
5. Aujesky D, Obrosky DS, Stone RA, et al. Derivation and validation of a prognostic model for pulmonary embolism. Am J Respir Crit Care Med. 2005;172(8):1041–6. http://www.ncbi.nlm.nih.gov/pubmed/16020800

Part V
Acute Coronary Syndrome (ACS)

Chapter 24
Patient on Oral Anticoagulant Presenting with ACS

Craig J. Beavers

Abstract Patients on oral anticoagulation potentially could present with acute coronary syndrome and providers needs to be aware of optimal management in this setting. Providers need to assess the type of anticoagulation the patient is on, assess the urgency of the procedure, and utilize bleeding avoidance strategies to mitigate risk.

Keywords PCI • Acute coronary syndrome • Bleeding avoidance • DOAC • Risk assessment • Bivalirudin

Case Introduction

A 60 year old male with a significant past medical history for hypertension, atrial fibrillation, and tobacco abuse presents to the emergency department at 3 PM with complaints of severe, substernal chest pain for the last 30 min. His ECG shows a 1 mm of ST-segment depression anteriorly. His troponins are elevated and he is given a diagnosis of a non-ST segment myocardial infarction (NSTEMI). His current vitals include a pulse of 70 beats per min, blood pressure is 114/71 mmHg, weight 76 kg, and height 180.3 cm. His serum creatinine is reported to be 1.03. He was given 324 mg of aspirin and nitroglycerin upon arrival. His home medications include apixaban 5 mg twice daily, last dose was at 8 AM, aspirin, and lisinopril.

C.J. Beavers, PharmD, BCPS-AQ Card, CACP
Cardiovascular Clinical Pharmacy Coordinator, University of Kentucky Healthcare,
Department of Pharmacy Practice and Science, College of Pharmacy, University of Kentucky, 800 Rose Street, Lexington, KY 40536, USA
e-mail: cjbeav2@uky.edu

Case Discussion

The use of a chronic oral anticoagulant (OAC) is common among patients who present with acute coronary syndrome (ACS). The exact frequency is unknown due to increasing rates of patients with venous thromboembolism (VTE) and atrial fibrillation (AF). Older estimates suggest anywhere from 5 to 7% of patients undergoing percutaneous coronary intervention (PCI) are receiving chronic OAC therapy [1]. However, data regarding the optimal management and outcomes for patients who present with ACS and who are on OAC are limited. Practitioners are faced with the tough position of limiting bleeding events without increasing thrombotic risks. The National Cardiovascular Disease Registry indicated that patients receiving warfarin at the time of PCI procedure had significantly increased in-hospital bleeding (elective PCI: adjusted odds ratio [OR] 1.26, urgent PCI: OR 1.42) and in-hospital mortality (elective PCI: 1.4% versus 0.6%, urgent PCI: 8.6% versus 4.5) compared to patients not receiving warfarin therapy [1]. Additional registry data has indicated that patients on warfarin with unstable angina (UA)/NSTEMI were less likely to undergo PCI (OR 0.80, 95% CI 0.75–0.86) or receive aspirin (OR 0.52, 95% CI 0.46–0.57) or clopidogrel (OR 0.53, 95% CI 0.50–0.56) [2]. Currently, there is no data on patients taking the direct oral anticoagulants (DOACs). Due to the data gaps and no clinical guidelines on the matter substantial variability exists on the management of these patients.

Considerations for the Management of a Patient Who Takes Chronic Warfarin Therapy Who Presents with ACS

For all patients presenting with ACS on warfarin, it is recommended to obtain an international normalized ratio (INR). If a patient presents needing an urgent PCI (ST-segment elevation myocardial infarction [STEMI] or high-risk NSTEMI), then it appears safe to do a PCI without additional anticoagulation when the INR is 2–3 [3]. There is no data for a patient who presents with an INR >3 thus an individualized strategy should be devised. It may be impractical in STEMI patients to attempt vitamin K antagonist reversal due to the need to avoid delays in door-to-balloon time [4]. If a patient has UA/NSTEMI and PCI can be delayed, then expert consensus advises the INR be ≤1.8 when femoral access is to be used [5]. Alternatively, if radial access is to be used then the INR should not exceed greater than 2.2 [4]. If a patient has an INR <2, it would be appropriate to consider use of recommended ACS intravenous anticoagulation (e.g., heparin, bivalirudin) in the lab. If a patient with UA/NSTEMI has an elevated INR and needs to go to procedure earlier (within 24–48 h), then administration of vitamin K, fresh frozen plasma, or factor products can be considered if the benefits outweigh the risk [5]. Should an UA/NSTEMI patient not require

Table 24.1 Management of VKA during percutaneous coronary intervention (PCI)

Obtain an international normalized ratio (INR)
It appears safe to perform PCI without additional anticoagulation when the INR is 2–3 in patients presenting for urgent PCI (STEMI and high-risk NSTEMI)
An individualized strategy should be devised for people with an INR >3
It may be impractical to reverse VKA due to urgency of STEMI or high-risk NSTEMI
Preference should be given to using radial access
Expert consensus advises the INR be ≤1.8 when femoral access is to be used for UA/NSTEMI PCI
If a patient has an INR <2, it would be appropriate to consider use of recommended ACS intravenous anticoagulation (e.g., heparin, bivalirudin) in the lab

PCI it is prudent to perform a risk/benefit analysis based on anticoagulation indication to determine if warfarin should be continued in addition to dual antiplatelet therapy (DAPT), if it can be stopped in favor of DAPT, or if the OAC can be continued without DAPT. See Table 24.1 for a review of consideration for the management of VKA during PCI.

Considerations for the Management of a Patient Who Takes Chronic DOACs (Apixaban, Dabigatran, Edoxaban, and Rivaroxaban)

Currently, there is no data on the management of patients on DOACs around the time of PCI. There is no laboratory measure to monitor the degree of anticoagulation with these agents at presently. It is critical for providers to determine the timing of the last dose of these agents in conjunction with renal function assessed through creatinine clearance. If a DOAC was administered in the last 4–6 h it would be at peak concentrations and potentially place the patient at increased risk of bleeding. Limited, mixed data does not provide clear indication if PCI can be performed while on a DOAC alone [6]. Thus, in emergent situations, it is recommended by expert consensus to give additional heparin or bivalirudin as bailout when needed if thrombosis develops during PCI in these scenarios [7]. Furthermore, the decision to continue or stop the DOAC should be individualized [5]. Like warfarin, if a UA/NSTEMI patient does not require PCI it is prudent to perform a risk/benefit analysis (history of recent venous thromboembolism, high CHA_2DS_2-VASc, hypercoagulable disorder, history of recent bleeding, poor renal function, etc.) based on anticoagulation indication to determine if the DOAC should be continued in addition to dual antiplatelet therapy (DAPT), if it can be stopped in favor of DAPT, or if the OAC can be continued without DAPT.

Table 24.2 Bleeding avoidance strategies

Pharmacology	Bivalirudin, Lower dose heparin, Judicious use of glycoprotein IIb/IIIa
Procedure	Radial access, Smaller sheath size, Flouro guided access, Ultrasound guide access, Bleeding risk stratification
Technology	Vascular closure device

Global Considerations in this Population

Expert consensus recommends that patients on oral anticoagulation around PCI be managed with implementation of various bleeding avoiding strategies (Table 24.2) [8]. In patients on an OAC it is preferred that radial access be used. Due to the lower risk of bleeding, preference is given toward using bivalirudin as the agents of choice for intravenous anticoagulation [7]. It is also recommend that clopidogrel be the preferred antiplatelet for use in ACS for patients on an OAC, especially if the patient is going to require DAPT plus the OAC. The use of glycoprotein IIb/IIIa inhibitors should be avoided if possible [7]. In addition, the patient should be loaded with the P2Y12 inhibitor during or after angiography [7]. Data surrounding the role of intravenous P2Y12 cangrelor in this population is lacking but could be appealing given its rapid onset and offset. Finally, standard reversal practices should be followed for patient on an OAC who develops bleeding during or after PCI including un-activated 4-factor prothrombin complex concentrate products for warfarin, idarucizumab for dabigatran, and un-activated 4-factor prothrombin complex concentrate for the factor Xa inhibitors (See Table 42.2 for review of reversal agents) [5, 7].

Key Points

- It is increasingly common that patients on an OAC present with ACS events and potentially require PCI
- This patients are at an increased risk of bleeding events and mortality
- Limited data and expert consensus guide decision making for these situations
- Providers need to evaluate the urgency of the procedure, the risk/benefit of continuing OAC therapy, and the risk/benefit of performing PCI while on the OAC.
- For patients receiving warfarin the INR should be measured
- Procedures should be performed via radial access, if able, bleeding avoidance strategies should be used, and clopidogrel should be the antiplatelet of choice until more data is available
- Standard reversal procedures should be followed if a patient on an OAC develop bleeding during or after PCI

Self-Assessment Questions

1. A 65 yo female with history of recurrent DVT on warfarin 5 mg daily presents to your emergency department for an ST-segment Elevation Myocardial Infraction (STEMI). Her INR was collected by point of care in the emergency department and was reported to 2.4 and all other labs are within normal limits. She is taken emergently to the catheterization laboratory. As a provider on the STEMI response team, you are asked your opinion on how to manage this patient.

    (a) Perform catheterization with radial access, reverse the warfarin using 4-factor prothrombin complex concentrate, utilize bivalirudin, and assure patient is loaded on clopidogrel 600 mg followed by 75 mg daily
    (b) Perform the catheterization with femoral access, perform the cath on warfarin with bailout heparin, administer glycoprotein II/IIIa inhibitor, and assure patient is loaded on clopidogrel 600 mg followed by 75 mg daily
    (c) Perform the catheterization with radial access, perform the cath on warfarin with bailout bivalirudin, and assure patient is loaded after catheterization on clopidgorel 600 mg followed by 75 mg daily
    (d) Perform the catheterization with femoral access, perform the cath on warfarin with bailout bivalirudin, and assure patient is loaded during the procedure with prasugrel 60 mg followed by 10 mg daily

    Answer: The correct answer would be C. Given the limited data, it appears safe in urgent situations to perform the catheterization on warfarin since the patient's INR is 2–3. This would make answer A incorrect. Based on expert consensus, it is preferred that the patient use bivalirudin and radial access, which are a bleeding avoidance strategies, and clopidogrel in these situations. This would make answers B and D incorrect. Finally, experts recommend avoiding glycoprotein IIb/IIIa inhibitors which would also make B incorrect.

2. Which of the following statements would be true regarding managing a patient on apixaban who presents with an ACS event?

    (a) It is best to collect an INR and aPTT level in order to assess the degree of anticoagulation
    (b) The majority of data with DOAC suggest using bivaliurdin infusion upon presentation and during percutaneous coronary intervention
    (c) The patient should have an INR <1.8 in order to perform the procedure via femoral access
    (d) The decision to continue or stop apixaban should be individualized based on risk/benefit

    Answer: The correct answer is D. Apixaban cannot be monitored via INR or aPTT values and provide no use when making decisions regarding the PCI procedure and thus makes answer A incorrect. There currently is limited data to guide providers regarding the best means of management; however, expert consensus states additional anticoagulation should be considered bailout if the OAC has been recently administered. This makes B is incorrect as this would not be bailout use. Expert consensus also indicates that radial artery access in preferred. Since you cannot monitor the factor Xa inhibitors by INR, the only time it would be ideal to consider femoral access is if the apixaban has been withheld for 24–48 h. Thus, answer C is not correct.

References

1. Faxon DP, Eikelboom JW, Berger PB, et al. Antithrombotic therapy in patients with atrial fibrillation undergoing coronary stenting: a North American perspective-executive summary. Circ Cardiovasc Intcrv. 2011;4:522–34.
2. Aggarwal A, Dai D, Rumsfeld JS, et al. Impact of home warfarin use on the treatment and outcomes of patients undergoing percutaneous coronary intervention. Am J Cardiol. 2008;101:1413–7.
3. Karjalainen PP, Vikman S, Niemela M, et al. Safety of percutaneous coronary intervention in stable coronary artery disease patients. EuroIntervention. 2013;8:1052–60.
4. Dunn SP, Holmes DR, Moliterno DJ. Drug-drug interactions in the cardiovascular catheterizations and interventions. J Am Coll Cardiol Intv. 2012;5:1195–208.
5. Naidu SS, Aronow HD, Box LC, et al. SCAI expert consensus statement: 2016 best practices in the cardiac catheterization laboratory: (endorsed by the Cardiological Society of India, and Sociedad Latino Americana de Cardiologica Intervencionista; affirmation of value by the Canadian Association of Interventional Cardiology-Association Canadienne de Cardiologie d'intervention). Catheterization and Cardiovascular Int erventions 2016: online before print. http://www.scai.org/Guidelines/default.aspx
6. Mallidi JR, Lotfi AS. Management of STEMI in patients on NOACs and undergoing primary PCI. 2015. http://www.acc.org/latest-in-cardiology/articles/2015/10/22/10/43/management-of-stemi-in-patients-on-noacs-and-undergoing-primary-pci. Accessed 1 May 2015.
7. Lip GYH, Windecker S, Huber K, et al. Management of antithrombotic therapy in atrial fibrillation patients presenting with acute coronary syndrome and/or undergoing percutaneous coronary or valve interventions: a joint consensus document of the European Society of Cardiology Working Group on Thrombosis, European Heart Rhythm Association (EHRA), European Association of Percutaneous Cardiovascular Intervention (EAPCI), and the European Association of Acute Cardiac Care (ACCA) endorsed by the Heart Rhythm Society (HRS) and Asia-Pacific Heart Rhythm Society (APHRS). Eur Heart J. 2014;35(45):3155–79.
8. Daureman HL, Rao SV, Resnic FS, Applegate RJ. Bleeding avoidance strategies: consensus and controversy. J Am Coll Cardiol. 2011;58:1–10.

Chapter 25
Oral Anticoagulant Therapy Post-Percutaneous Coronary Intervention

Craig J. Beavers

Abstract Patients who are on oral anticoagulation who receive a stent via PCI represent a challenging patient population. A multitude of pharmacotherapy considerations must be evaluated to design a regimen that reduces bleeding and prevents thrombosis.

Keywords Percutaneous coronary intervention • PCI • Bleeding • Stent • Triple therapy • DOAC • Dual antiplatelet therapy • DAPT

Case Introduction

The same patient from case 24 has moved from the catheterization laboratory to the floor. He was administered cangrelor as the P2Y12 agent in the lab and received a drug-eluting stent to his proximal LAD. They left him on his apixaban and didn't use any bailout bivalirudin or heparin. The team is now debating long-term management of his oral anticoagulant (OAC) and dual antiplatelet therapy (DAPT).

Case Discussion

What factors need to be considered when developing a plan regarding this patient post-PCI regimen?

C.J. Beavers, PharmD, BCPS-AQ Card, CACP
Cardiovascular Clinical Pharmacy Coordinator,
University of Kentucky Healthcare, Department of Pharmacy Practice and Science,
College of Pharmacy, University of Kentucky, 800 Rose Street,
Lexington, KY 40536, USA
e-mail: cjbeav2@uky.edu

© Springer International Publishing AG 2017
K. Kiser (ed.), *Oral Anticoagulation Therapy*,
DOI 10.1007/978-3-319-54643-8_25

Estimate Bleeding Risk Versus Risk of Ischemia

Careful decision making must occur in the management of patients who require DAPT in addition to an OAC, also known as triple therapy (TT). Evidence suggests the bleeding risk in these patients is increased two to threefold [1]. One of the first considerations should be does the patient still have an indication for the OAC [2]. If it is safe to stop the OAC, then it should be contemplated. It is clear from historical data that DAPT is superior over warfarin for prevention of ischemic events associated with stent placement [3]. When applicable, it may be prudent to utilize risk scores to characterize the risk of ischemic (stroke, myocardial infarction, stent thrombosis) events versus bleeding to aid in decision making. In atrial fibrillation (AF) patients, the utilization of the CHA_2DS_2-VASc and HASBLED for risk assessment, as outlined in Chap. 2, can be used for assessment. For patients with venous thromboembolism (VTE), the DASH score (D-dimer abnormal, age ≤50 years, male patient, and hormone use at VTE onset) and the American College of Chest Physicians bleeding score can be used [4, 5]. However, there are some limitations with these scorings systems as some of the same hazards exist in the thrombosis and bleeding models [2]. Furthermore, the scoring systems were not devised for patients on an OAC plus DAPT or they estimate an annualized versus a short-term risk. The patient in the case has a CHA_2DS_2-VASc score of 4 (4.0% annualized risk) and a HASBLED score of 2 (1.88% annualized risk) indicting a higher risk of thrombosis versus bleeding. It would be prudent to consider the use of OAC in addition to the DAPT.

Selection of Regimen

If it is decided the patient needs to remain on an OAC in addition to DAPT, then consideration of the pharmacotherapy regimen needs to occur to minimize both ischemic events and bleeding. The current available evidence is limited in terms of large, prospective, adequately powered randomized trials and is mostly derived from observational studies, smaller trials, and expert consensus. When considering an OAC a provider must contemplate utilization of warfarin versus the direct oral anticoagulants (DOACs), such as apixaban, dabigatran, edoxaban, rivaroxaban, in conjunction with DAPT [2, 6, 7]. The efficacy and safety of DOACs in patients with histories of AF or VTE who have had PCI are lacking. However, data of these agents in patients who lack AF or VTE but had a recent ACS demonstrated increased risk of bleeding when added to DAPT [8–10]. Given this reason, most experts currently recommend to avoid the use of DOACs in this setting until there is more data in AF and VTE patients. Preferential consideration should be given to warfarin with a lower intensity INR. Ideally the INR range should be 2–2.5 [1]. Similarly to the DOACs, it is preferred to avoid the newer P2Y12 inhibitors, such as prasugrel and ticagrelor, due to limited evaluation in this population and increased bleeding risk.

Finally, it is preferred that aspirin be used at the 81 mg dose also to reduce bleeding risk while providing optimal ischemic protection. The patient in the case is currently on warfarin so it would be ideal to leave him on warfarin but change his goal INR range to be 2–2.5. There are trials underway looking at using the DOACs in this population.

Double Versus Triple Therapy

Due to the substantial increase risk of bleeding, it has been theorized removing a component of the TT might reduce the bleeding. Removing aspirin has been investigated in the prospective, open-label, multi-center. What is the Optimal Antiplatelet and Anticoagulant Therapy in Patients with Oral Anticoagulation and Coronary Stenting (WOEST) trial. In this trial a total of 573 patients on warfarin were randomized to aspirin plus clopidogrel or clopidogrel alone. The trial demonstrated lower overall bleeding at 12 months, which was the primary endpoint, in the patients on clopidogrel alone versus DAPT (hazard ratio, 0.36; 95% confidence interval, 0.26–0.50, $p < 0.01$) [11]. There was no increased rate of thrombotic events; however, this was a secondary endpoint and trial was not powered to look at these events. This trial provides promise regarding this strategy. The one potential concern related to dropping aspirin would be the chance of no antiplatelet protection if the patient was a clopidogrel non-responder and it would be prudent to assess this should the aspirin be removed. Several trials are underway looking at the use of DOACs with some of the novel antiplatelets alone. For the patient in the case, it could be considered to drop the aspirin therapy but it might be wise to assure the patient is a clopidogrel responder via P2Y12 assay. If the patient were a clopidogrel non-responder it would be reasonable to one of the new anti-platelets in this instance.

Duration of Therapy of DAPT

In patients who may need TT the duration of therapy needs to be addressed. If patients received a second generation drug-eluting stent (DES), which is the most common type of stents utilized currently, the 2016 American College of Cardiology/American Heart Association Dual Antiplatelet Therapy Guidelines recommend 12 months of DAPT therapy in patients with an ACS event and 6 months of DAPT in patients with stable, elective PCI, generally [1]. If a patient were to get a bare-metal stent (BMS), DAPT can be continued for a minimum of 1 month in the elective setting or up to 12 months post-ACS [1]. Experts recommend shortening the duration to 6 months in the post-ACS population when the patient is on TT irrespective of stent type [7]. It is unclear the optimal management of these patients with the use of the novel biodegradable stents. It would be reasonable to continue DAPT for a minimum of 6 months in the patient from the case if they were to remain on TT.

Other Considerations

If TT is utilized, experts recommend for more frequent INR monitoring and methods to assure there is a time in therapeutic range is ≥80%. Finally, given the use of TT it is prudent to assure the patient is on some form of gastrointestinal prophylaxis (GI). If GI prophylaxis is used it would be prudent to use a proton pump inhibitor and to avoid omeprazole and esomeprazole due to drug-drug interaction.

Key Points

- The use of TT increases the risk of bleeding two to threefold
- It is critical for providers to consider the need for an OAC, the selection of the type of anticoagulation, degree of anticoagulation, antiplatelet selection, and duration of antiplatelet therapy (See Table 25.1 for review)
- At the current time, experts recommend utilization of warfarin therapy when an OAC is needed with a goal INR 2–2.5
- It is prudent to avoid the use of the more potent antiplatelet agents, such as ticagrelor or prasugrel
- Efforts should be made to assure the patient has close follow-up and is considered for gastrointestinal prophylaxis

Self-Assessment Questions

1. A 70-year-old female patient who is on warfarin for a DVT, which occurred 12 months ago after a knee surgery, presents to the emergency department for an NSTEMI. She is taken to the cath lab and has a drug-eluting stent placed into the right coronary artery. Which of the following is true regarding the best management of this patient?

    (a) Switch the patient to apixaban 10 mg twice daily for 7 days followed by 5 mg twice daily plus clopidogrel 75 mg daily and aspirin 81 mg daily
    (b) Keep the patient on warfarin with a goal INR 2–2.5 as well as starting clopidogrel 75 mg daily, aspirin 81 mg daily, and omeprazole 20 mg daily
    (c) Keep the patient on warfarin with a goal INR 2–2.5 as well as starting ticagrelor 90 mg twice daily and aspirin 81 mg daily, and pantoprazole 40 mg daily
    (d) Stop warfarin and start patient on ticagrelor 90 mg twice daily and aspirin 81 mg daily

    ANSWER: Answer D is the best choice. Based on lack of data and expert opinion, it preferred to avoid apixaban due to the potential for increased risk of bleeding

Table 25.1 Key clinical considerations in triple therapy post PCI [6]

Issue	Vitamin K antagonist (VKA)	Direct oral anticoagulant (DOAC)
Initial antithrombotic treatment	TT (low-dose aspirin (ASA)[a,b], clopidogrel, VKA)	TT (low-dose ASA, clopidogrel, DOAC)
Duration of TT	Elective setting + BMS: 1 month Elective setting + new-generation DES: 6 months[c] ACS setting + BMS/new generation DES: 6 months[d]	Elective setting + BMS: 1 month Elective setting + new-generation DES: 6 months[c] ACS setting + BMS/new generation DES: 6 months[d]
Intensity of OAC during TT	Reduced[e]	Reduced[f]
Special care during TT	Frequent INR monitoring[g] Attention to high quality OA[i] Routine gastric protection[j]	Frequent laboratory monitoring[h] Routine gastric protection
Subsequent antithrombotic treatment[m]	VKA[k,l]+ single antiplatelet agent[m]	DOAC[l,n]+ single antiplatelet agent[m]

TT triple therapy, *ACS* acute coronary syndrome, *DES* drug-eluting stent, *EES* everolimus-eluting stent, *ZES* zotarolimus-eluting stent, *BMS* bare-metal stent, *INR* International Normalized Ratio, *CBC* complete blood count, *Hgb* hemoglobin, *PPI* proton pump inhibitor, *TTR* time in therapeutic range

[a]75–100 mg/day
[b]May be omitted in selected patients at high risk of bleeding, and low risk of stent thrombosis
[c]One month only maybe considered when the risk of bleeding is highly increased, and a new-generation EES or ZES has been implanted
[d]One month only may be considered when the risk of bleeding is highly increased, and either BMS or a new-generation EES or ZES has been implanted
[e]INR range 2.0–2.5
[f]Lower dose of DOAC: dabigatran 110 mg BID, rivaroxaban 15 mg daily, apixaban 2.5 mg twice daily, edoxaban 30 mg daily
[g]Every 2 weeks
[h]Creatinine clearance, CBC, and HgB every 4 weeks
[i]Average TTR >70%
[j]Preferably with PPI not interfering with clopidogrel metabolism (e.g., pantoprazole, dexlansoprazole)
[k]After the initial course of 1–6 months of TT has been completed standard INR range may be resumed (unless other indications for reduced are present)
[l]VKA/DOAC monotherapy may be considered after BMS implantation in elective setting, especially when bleeding risk is highly increased
[m]Either low-dose aspirin (75–100 mg/day) or clopidogrel, depending on the individual risk of bleeding, especially gastrointestinal, and stent thrombosis
[n]Standard DOAC dose may be resumed (unless other indications for reduced dose are present)

which makes answer A incorrect. Answer B is incorrect due to the fact there is drug-drug interaction with clopidogrel and omeprazole. If a PPI is use then it is preferred to use an agent that does not inhibit CYP2C19. Answer C is incorrect due to lack of data and potential for increased bleeding with the more potent antiplatelet agents. Answer D is correct because the patient had a provoked reason for a DVT which typically only requires 3–6 months of treatment. It would be ideal to stop the OAC and put on DAPT alone. Furthermore, there is data with aspirin alone to prevent recurrent VTE.

2. Please select the following response(s) regarding triple therapy that is/are true:

   (a) It is important to utilize aspirin doses of <100 mg
   (b) It is critical for the patient to keep on triple therapy for at least 12 months after any stent placement for elective and urgent procedures
   (c) The risk of bleeding is lower and ischemic events are higher when aspirin is dropped from triple therapy
   (d) It critical to genetically test patients to determine if there would be any issues with warfarin metabolism

ANSWER: The only answer which is correct would be A. It is important to assure the lowest dose of aspirin is used to limit bleeding, specifically gastrointestinal bleeding. Answer B is wrong since patients with elective PCI, patients on TT, or bare-metal stent placement could allow for shorter duration of therapy. Answer C is incorrect since the WOEST trial demonstrated lower bleeding with no increase in ischemic events. However, it must be noted that the trial was not powered to look at ischemic events. Finally, answer D is incorrect as there is currently no recommendation per any guidelines to genetically test patients for warfarin metabolism.

References

1. Levine GN, Bates ER, Bittl JA, et al. 2016 ACC/AHA guideline focused update on duration of dual antiplatelet therapy in patients with coronary artery disease: a report of the American College of Cardiology/American Heart Association task force on clinical practice guidelines. J Am Coll Cardiol. 2016. pii: S0735-1097(16)01699-5.
2. Capodanno D, Angiolillo DJ. Management of antiplatelet and anticoagulant therapy in patients with atrial fibrillation in the setting of acute coronary syndromes or percutaneous coronary interventions. Circ Cardiovasc Interv. 2014;7:113–24.
3. Lean MB, Baim DS, Popma JJ, et al. A clinical trial comparing three antithrombotic-drug regimens after coronary artery stenting. N Engl J Med. 1998;339(23):1665–71.
4. Tosetto A, Iorio A, Marcucci M, et al. Predicting disease recurrence in patients with previous unprovoked venous thromboembolism: a proposed prediction score (DASH). J Thromb Haemost. 2012;10(6):1019–25.
5. Kearon C, Akl EA, Comerota AJ, et al. Antithrombotic therapy for VTE disease: antithrombotic therapy and prevention of thrombosis, 9th ed: American College of Chest Physicians evidence-based clinical practice guidelines. Chest. 2012;141(2 Suppl):e419S–94S.
6. Rubboli A, Faxon DP, Airaksinen KEJ, et al. The optimal management of patients on oral anticoagulation undergoing coronary artery stenting. Thromb Haemost. 2014;113:1080–7.
7. Lip GYH, Windecker S, Huber K, et al. Management of antithrombotic therapy in atrial fibrillation patients presenting with acute coronary syndrome and/or undergoing percutaneous coronary or valve interventions: a joint consensus document of the European Society of Cardiology Working Group on Thrombosis, European Heart Rhythm Association (EHRA), European Association of Percutaneous Cardiovascular Interventions (EAPCI) and European Association of Acute Cardiac Care (ACCA) endorsed by Heart Rhythm Society (HRS) and Asia-Pacific Heart Rhythm Society (APHRS). Eur Heart J. 2014;35(45):3155–79.

8. Oldgren J, Budaj A, Granger CB, et al. Dabigatran vs. placebo in patients with acute coronary syndromes on dual antiplatet therapy: a randomized, double-blind, phase II trial. Eur Heart J. 2011;32(22):2781–9.
9. Alexander JH, Lopes RD, James S, et al. Apixaban with antiplatelet therapy after acute coronary syndrome. N Engl J Med. 2011;365:699–708.
10. Mega JL, Braunwald E, Wiviott SD, et al. Rivaroxaban in patients with recent acute coronary syndrome. N Engl J Med. 2012;366:9–19.
11. Dewilde WJ, Oirbans T, Verheugt FW, et al. Use of clopidogrel with or without aspirin in patients taking oral anticoagulants therapy and undergoing percutaneous coronary intervention: an open-label, randomized, controlled trial. Lancet. 2013;381:1107–15.

Chapter 26
ST-Segment Elevation Myocardial Infarction (Lytic Candidate) on Oral Anticoagulant

Craig J. Beavers

Abstract Patients on oral anticoagulation who present with a ST-segment myocardial infarction and require fibrinolytics therapy represent a high patient population. With limited evidence to guide management, providers must assess risk versus benefit and attempt to mitigate bleeding events.

Keywords Fibrinolytics • STEMI • Bleeding • Door-to-needle • Risk assessment Hemorrhage

Case Introduction

A 55-year-old man with history of Factor V Leiden on warfarin presents to a rural emergency department with a ST-segment elevation myocardial infarction (STEMI). Due to severe weather, the hospital is not going to be able airlift him to a hospital with percutaneous coronary intervention (PCI) capability and it would take 2 h via ambulance. The team is considering fibrinolytic therapy. His INR was determined to be 2.3 via point of care testing in the emergency department. He has normal renal function, is 77 kg, and has an additional past medical history of dyslipidemia. His current blood pressure is 110/78 mmHg.

Case Discussion

Based on the 2013 American College of Cardiology Foundation/American Heart Association Guideline for the Management of STEMI, the preferred means of reperfusion is by PCI within a timely manner [1]. If a STEMI patient arrives to a

---

C.J. Beavers, PharmD, BCPS-AQ Card, CACP
Cardiovascular Clinical Pharmacy Cooridnator, University of Kentucky Healthcare,
Department of Pharmacy Practice and Science, University of Kentucky, College of Pharmacy,
800 Rose Street, Lexington, KY 40536, USA
e-mail: cjbeav2@uky.edu

Table 26.1 Recommended dosing for fibrinolytic agents in myocardial infarction

Medication	Full dose
Alteplase (tPA)	15 mg intravenous (IV) bolus, followed by 0.75 mg/kg IV infusion over 30 min (up to 50 mg), followed by 0.5 mg/kg IV infusion over 60 min (up to 35 mg)
Reteplase (r-PA)	10 units + 10 units IV bolus given 30 min apart
Tenecteplase (TNK-tPA)	Give the following as a single IV bolus: 30 mg if <60 kg 35 mg if 60 to <70 kg 40 mg if 70 to <80 kg 45 mg if 80 to <90 kg 50 mg if ≥90 kg

non-PCI capable hospital and is not able to be transferred to a PCI capable hospital, then the guidelines recommend the patient be given fibrinolytic therapy [1] (Table 26.1). Due to the increased risk of hemorrhagic events, there are several absolute and relative contraindications to fibrinolytic therapy in STEMI. Among the relative contraindications is the use of oral anticoagulant (OAC) therapy. Due to growing use of OAC in patients with high cardiovascular risk there is an escalating potential they may need fibrinolytic therapy [2]. There is limited guidance on how to best manage these patients. Data from patients on warfarin who received fibrinolytic therapy frequently have major bleeding events. One study demonstrated 7/36 (19%) of these patients developed major bleeding or intracranial haemorrhage (ICH) with only one of the ICH being fatal [3]. This is a marked increase in bleeding compared to Thrombolysis in Myocardial Infarction (TIMI) major bleeding noted in the alteplase in myocardial infarction clinical trial which was reported to be 2.3% [4]. Another study found patients on OAC, specifically warfarin, who received fibrinolytics for STEMI trended toward having more serious bleeding [5]. Risk factors associated with bleeding included age, aspirin use, and previous fibrinolytic use [5]. Two additional analyses found patients on warfarin who were age 65 or older and received fibrinolytics therapy appeared to be at an increased risk of bleeding when INR values were over 3 [3, 6].

As alluded, there is limited data to guide providers in the management of these patients (Table 26.2). Anytime fibrinolytics are considered it is critical that a risk/benefit analysis be performed. For patients on warfarin, providers can extrapolate from the stroke literature and use the barometer of an INR >1.7 as a cut point as a contraindication for lytic therapy [7]. For patients on the direct oral anticoagulants (DOACs), such as apixaban, dabigatran, edoxaban, or rivaroxaban, it would be prudent to determine the time of the last dose and assure the patient does not have any reason for impaired clearance [7]. The patient could be considered contraindicated to fibrinolytic therapy should they have had recent exposure (within 6–12 h) to their DOAC. However, despite these recommendations, some experts recommend not withholding fibrinoyltic therapy to patients on an OAC [6]. If the use fibrinolytic is decided, there should be an effort to assure blood pressure is

Table 26.2 Considerations before using fibrinolytic therapy in myocardial infarction

Perform a thorough risk/benefit analysis
If patient is on warfarin, an INR >1.7 can be used as cut point for relative contraindication
Determine time of last dose of anticoagulation, especially for patients on DOACs
Assess patients renal function to assure appropriate clearance
If fibrinolytics are given, assure blood pressure is adequately controlled and patient is closely monitored
It is not recommend to provide reversal of the anticoagulation since the door to need time is short

Table 26.3 Monitoring parameters for fibrinolytic therapy

• Blood pressure
• Serum cardiac biomarkers
• Complete blood count
• Prothrombin time/INR
• aPTT
• ECG
• Evidence of gastrointestinal bleeding
• Signs of hematuria or gingival bleeding
• Acute changes in mental status

controlled to prevent risk of ICH [1]. In the United States, the only fibrinolytics in use are the fibrin specific agents, which include alteplase, tenecteplase, and reteplase. Typically with these agents it recommended to give anticoagulation therapy [1]. However, if a patient was on OAC it would be prudent to withhold this therapy. Given the unknown risk/benefit as well as the short door to needle time of 30 min for fibrinolytic therapy; there is no recommendation for reversal of OAC therapy prior to administration of the fibrinolytic. However, if patient receives fibrinolytic therapy while on OAC and bleedings occurs then standard reversal practices should be implemented. Finally, it is unknown in terms of benefit/risk in this population if half-dose fibrinolytic therapy could be administered to bridge the patient to PCI [8]. However, this strategy could be considered to reduce risk of bleeding while treating myocardial ischemia. Any patient on OAC who receives fibrinolytics should receive close monitoring during and after administration of therapy for up to 48 h (Table 26.3).

The patient in the case has an INR of 2.3 which could potentially put him at risk of bleeding. His blood pressure is under control and he is relatively young with limited co-morbidities. If a conservative strategy is selected, then the patient would be contraindicated to therapy. However, the team decided to administer half-dose fibrinolytics in preparation to send him to the nearest PCI capable hospital. The patient was closely monitored during and after the administration of fibrinolytic therapy.

Key Points

- Ideally transfer the patient to the closest PCI capable facility
- Administration of fibrinolytics to patients on OAC increases the risk of major bleeding including ICH
- There is limited data on the optimal management of patient on OAC who need fibrinolytics for a STEMI
- A risk/benefit analysis should occur before the administration of fibrinolytic therapy
- In a conservative management approach, all patients on OAC would be contraindicated to fibrinolytics
- If it is decided to administer fibrinolytics, the patients' blood pressure should be controlled and the patient should be monitored during and after administration

Self-Assessment Questions

1. A 70-year-old patient on dabigatran for atrial fibrillation, history of stroke with previous fibrinolytic therapy as treatment, and diabetes is admitted for the management of a STEMI at his local hospital. His hospital is PCI capable but only has one cath lab which currently has another patient who had STEMI occupying it. It is likely the case will not be finished in order to reach the door-to-balloon time within 90 min requirement. The patient has normal renal function, blood pressure of 190/85 mmHg, weight is 70 kg, and the patient took dabigatran 12 h ago. How should the emergency department proceed with this patient if they were to consider fibrinolytic therapy?

    (a) Start the patient on nicardipine in order to control blood pressure and administer 50 mg alteplase while waiting for the cath lab to open
    (b) Start the patient on nicardipine in order to control blood pressure and administer 15 mg intravenous bolus of alteplase over 1–2 min, followed by 50 mg over 30 min, then 35 mg over 1 h
    (c) Start the patient on nicardipine in order to control blood pressure, administer idarucizumab to reverse the dabigatran, and administer 15 mg intravenous bolus of alteplase over 1–2 min, followed by 50 mg over 30 min, then 35 mg over 1 h
    (d) Given the patients age, co-morbidities, use of anticoagulation therapy, and history of previous administration of fibrinoyltics, the patient would be an increased risk of bleeding and should be contraindicated to therapy

    ANSWER: The correct answer is D. The patient has a variety of risk factors which would put them at increased risk of bleeding including ICH. It would be more prudent to withhold fibrinolytic therapy. Answer A or B would be an appropriate consideration in a patient who was healthy and had not had fibrinolytic therapy previously. Answer C is would be incorrect at this time as there is no data on the risk/benefit of administration of fibrinolytic therapy with concurrent reversal of anticoagulation.

2. Which of the following is NOT considered a parameter to monitor after administration of fibrinolytic therapy in a patient on OAC?

   (a) Complete blood count
   (b) Blood pressure
   (c) D-dimer
   (d) ECG

ANSWER: The correct answer is C. All of the other answers, as indicated in the Table 26.3 in the text, are critical to be monitored for at least 48 h after administration of fibrinolytics to patients on OAC. Answer A is critical to assess to assure the patient his not developing a new bleeding event post-infusion of fibrinolytics. Answer B is critical to assure the patient has adequate control to prevent conversion to an ICH. Answer D is critical to assure the patient is not developing a new or recurrent MI.

References

1. O'Gara PT, Kushner FG, Ascheim DD, et al. 2013 ACCF/AHA guideline for the management of ST-elevation myocardial infarction. J Am Coll Cardiol. 2013;61(4):e78–e140.
2. Lip GYH, Windecker S, Huber K, et al. Management of antithrombotic therapy in atrial fibrillation patients presenting with acute coronary syndrome and/or undergoing percutaneous coronary or valve interventions: a joint consensus document of the European Society of Cardiology Working Group on Thrombosis, European Heart Rhythm Association (EHRA), European Association of Percutaneous Cardiovascular Intervention (EAPCI), and the European Association of Acute Cardiac Care (ACCA) endorsed by the Heart Rhythm Society (HRS) and Asia-Pacific Heart Rhythm Society (APHRS). Eur Heart J. 2014;35(45):3155–79.
3. Sarrinen S, Puolakka J, Boyd J, et al. Warfarin and fibrinolysis-a challenging combination: an observational cohort study. Scand J Trauma Resusc Emerg Med. 2011;19:21.
4. Bovill E, Terrin M, Stump D, et al. Hemorrhagic events during therapy with recombinant tissue-type plasminogen activator, heparin, and aspirin for acute myocardial infarction: results of the thrombolysis in myocardial infarction (TIMI) phase II trial. Ann Intern Med. 1991;115(4):256–65.
5. Stanley AG, Fletcher S, Tan A, Barnett DB. Is warfarin a contraindication to thrombolysis in acute ST elevation myocardial infarction? Heart. 2006;92(8):1145–6.
6. Brass L, Lichtman J, Wang Y, et al. Intracranial haemorrhage associated with thrombolytic therapy for elderly patients with acute myocardial infarction: results from the cooperative cardiovascular project. Stroke. 2000;31:1802–11.
7. Demaerschalk BM, Kleindorfer DO, Adeoye OM, et al. Scientific rationale for the inclusion and exclusion criteria for intravenous alteplase in acute ischemic stroke: a statement for healthcare professionals from the American Heart Association/American Stroke Association. Stroke. 2016;47:581–641.
8. Larson DM, Duval S, Sharkey SW, et al. Safety and efficacy of a pharmaco-invasive reperfusion strategy in rural ST-elevation myocardial infarction patients with expected delays due to long-distance transfers. Eur Heart J. 2012;33(10):1232–40.

Chapter 27
ACS with Bypass Surgery

Craig J. Beavers

Abstract Patient who require coronary artery bypass grafting while on oral anticoagulation need advanced care management. Considerations must occur regarding proper timing of session for surgery, need to bridge, and appropriate time to resume therapy safely.

Keywords Coronoary artery bypass graft • CABG • DOAC • Bridging • Reversal • Valves • Heparin

Case Introduction

A 49-year-old female presents to the hospital with an NSTEMI. Her coronary angiography has indicated that she has three vessel diseases and will need to undergo coronary artery bypass surgery (CABG) within the next 24–48 h. Her past medical history includes atrial fibrillation (AF) for which she takes rivaroxaban 20 mg daily. Other past medical history includes type 2 diabetes, hypertension, hyperlipidemia, obesity, and gastroesophageal reflux disease. She has a creatinine clearance of 85 mL/min, no drug allergies, and weighs 100 kg. Her ejection fraction is estimated to be 55%. She has a hemoglobin of 10 mg/dL.

Case Discussion

In the continuum of bleeding risk for invasive procedures, CABGs are deemed to be high risk [1]. Thus for patients on oral anticoagulation (OAC) it is paramount to develop strategies to mitigate the additional bleeding risk conferred by these agents

---

C.J. Beavers, PharmD, BCPS-AQ Card, CACP
Cardivascular Clinical Pharmacy Coorindator, University of Kentucky Healthcare,
Department of Pharmacy Practice and Science, University of Kentucky, College of Pharmacy,
800 Rose Street, Lexington, KY 40536, USA
e-mail: cjbeav2@uky.edu

but limit thrombotic risk. Generally, CABGs occur electively or in an urgent/emergent manner and the strategies differ in each setting.

Elective CABG Considerations

An elective CABG provides opportunity to plan for anticoagulation interruption and bridging if required. Any time anticoagulation is interrupted there is the potential for an increased risk in thrombotic events to occur and this must be considered in the decision. The major thrombotic risk factors to consider in this situation include history of AF, prosthetic heart valves, and recent venous thromboembolism (VTE). In patients with AF, the CHA_2DS_2-VASc can be used to estimate thrombotic risk, as described in Case 1 [2]. There is no specific risk score for valve patients or patients with VTE; however, these patients are deemed to be at the highest risk for thrombotic events within in the first 3 months of valve placement or VTE event [2]. One could consider using the CHEST scoring system to determine degree of periprocedural thrombotic risk to deem if patient needs bridging [3]. If it is decided that anticoagulation is to be held for surgery then the period with no anticoagulation should be as short as possible [4]. For patients on warfarin who are having a high risk elective procedure, it is recommended to stop therapy 5 days before procedure based on the pharmacokinetics/pharmacodynamics of the medication [4]. It is prudent to obtain prothrombin time (PT)/international normalized ratio (INR) level on the day before surgery to assure return of normal coagulation. If INR is above 1.5, it is recommended to administer 1–2 mg of vitamin K by mouth and re-check the INR the day of surgery [4, 5]. If a patient is on warfarin and is at high risk of thrombosis necessitating bridging (patients with mechanical heart valves or recent VTE), then use of low molecular weight heparin (LMWH) or unfractionated heparin (UFH) at therapeutic doses can be utilized [6]. If a patient is at low/moderate risk of thrombosis and a higher risk of bleeding, then degree of bridge anticoagulation can be reduced [6]. Bridging therapy is generally started when INR has dropped below two which on average would occur on about 3 days before procedure [6]. If LMWH is used, it is ideally stopped 24 h before the procedure to allow adequate elimination whereas intravenous UFH is stopped about 5 h before procedure [6] given a CABG is considered a high-bleeding risk procedure. Post-procedure, both LMWH and UFH are re-started when it is felt adequate hemostasis is reached at the dose prior to the procedure and continued until INR is at goal [6]. Often in CABG this is approximately 48–72 h after surgery [7]. Generally, the direct oral anticoagulants (DOACs) can be stopped about 2–3 days prior to procedure with normal renal function [2, 4, 5] and do not require bridging if the patient goes to procedure close to near the washout time (Table 27.1). If the patient has an extended period of time after the DOAC therapy has had clearance, then IV UFH or LWMH can be considered. Unlike warfarin, there is no means to monitor these agents to assure restoration of hemostasis [5]. Post- surgery, given the quick onset of action of the DOACs, there is rarely a need for bridging therapy when re-starting these agents [4, 5].

Table 27.1 Direct oral anticoagulant interruptions suggestions [7]

Drug and renal function	Low bleeding risk surgery (2 or 3 drug ½ lives between last dose and surgery	Resumption of therapy after lower bleeding risk surgery	High bleeding risk surgery (4 or 5 drug ½ lives between last dose or surgery)	Resumption of therapy after higher bleeding risk surgery
Dabigatran CrCl > 50 mL/min	Last dose 2 days before procedure	Resume on day after procedure (24 h post-operative)	Last dose 3 days before procedure	Resume 2–3 days after procedure (48–72 h post-operative)
Dabigatran CrCl 30–50 mL/min	Last dose 3 days before procedure	Resume on day after procedure (24 h post-operative)	Last dose 2 days before procedure	Resume 2–3 days after procedure (48–72 h post-operative)
Rivaroxaban CrCl > 50 mL/min	Last dose 2 days before procedure	Resume on day after procedure (24 h post-operative)	Last dose 3 days before procedure	Resume 2–3 days after procedure (48–72 h post-operative)
Rivaroxaban CrCl 30–50 mL/min	Last dose 2 days before procedure	Resume on day after procedure (24 h post-operative)	Last dose 3 days before procedure	Resume 2–3 days after procedure (48–72 h post-operative)
Rivaroxaban CrCl 15–29.9 mL/min	Last dose 3 days before procedure	Resume on day after procedure (24 h post-operative)	Last dose 4 days before procedure	Resume 2–3 days after procedure (48–72 h post-operative)
Apixaban CrCl >50 mL/min	Last dose 2 days before procedure	Resume on day after procedure (24 h post-operative)	Last dose 3 days before procedure	Resume 2–3 days after procedure (48–72 h post-operative)
Apixaban CrCl 30–50 mL/min	Last dose 3 days before procedure	Resume on day after procedure (24 h post-operative)	Last dose 4 days before procedure	Resume 2–3 days after procedure (48–72 h post-operative)
Edoxaban CrCl > 50 mL/min	Last dose 2 days before procedure	Resume on day after procedure (24 h post-operative	Last dose 3 days before procedure	Resume 2–3 days after procedure (48–72 h post-operative)

Urgent/Emergent CABG Considerations

In urgent/emergent situations there is more of a need to reverse the anticoagulation therapy in order to prevent or treat perioperative bleeding. For patients on warfarin who require immediate reversal of therapy it is recommend that the patient receive un-activated four factor prothrombin complex concentrate (PCC) or plasma products in conjunction with vitamin K. It should be noted the use of these products can increase the risk of thrombosis. Vitamin K alone can be used if the patient has urgent, versus emergent, need for surgery that will occur within 1–2 days [4]. For patients who are on dabigatran the use of idarucizumab can be considered for emergent situations. Idarucizumab is a humanized monoclonal antibody that neutralizes dabigatran in a dose-dependent manner [8]. It was approved by the Food and Drug Administration based on the Reversal Effects of Idarucizumab on Active Dabigatran (REVERSE-AD) trial which demonstrated that administration of two doses of 2.5 g of idarucizumab provided normalization of hemostasis with limited risk of thrombosis [8]. If idarucizumab is used, providers should assess signs of bleeding and monitor routine hemostatic laboratory parameters to assure bleeding has decreased or ceased. At the moment it is not clear if additional doses provide benefit and consideration can be given to using other means to reverse coagulation at this point. At the time of this writing, there is no specific antidote for the factor Xa inhibitors (apixaban, edoxaban, or rivaroxaban) but there are promising options in the pipeline [9]. For these agents, expert consensus suggests administration of un-activated four factor PCC based on experimental models [5]. If any patient on OAC develops a bleed peri-operatively, it is critical to provide additional support as needed with packed red blood cells, platelets, and fresh frozen plasma.

In this patient case, she has a CHA_2DS_2-VASc score of 4 which would be considered moderate to high risk of thrombosis; however, this risk is an annualized risk versus an acute risk. Given the fact the patient is on rivaroxaban with good renal function, it would be preferred to stop rivaroxaban at least 48 h before the surgery. Since this is an NSTEMI it would be preferred to delay the procedure for 48 h to allow the rivaroxaban to clear. Since rivaroxaban has a quick onset of action it can be resumed as soon as adequate hemostasis has been achieved. There would be no need for bridging therapy.

Key Points

- For patients needing an elective CABG, providers should evaluate the risk of thrombosis and devise a plan for cessation and resumption of anticoagulation therapy as well as need for bridging therapy
- Warfarin therapy is generally stopped 5 days prior to elective surgery and an INR is checked the day before. If INR >1.5 then vitamin K 1–2 mg is administered with a repeat INR on the day of surgery
- Patients who have mechanical heart valves or recent VTE pose the highest risk and should be bridged 48–72 h pre-procedure with LMWH or UFH and can be resumed post-procedure when hemostasis is achieved
- Patient on DOAC should have therapy stopped about 48 h prior to procedure and they can be resumed post-procedure without bridging when hemostasis is achieved
- Patients presenting for an emergent CABG on warfarin or a factor Xa inhibitor can be administered un-activated four factor PCC to reversal anticoagulation.
- If CABG is more urgent (occurring in 1–2 days) then vitamin K can be given for reversal of warfarin

27 Acute Coronary Syndrome (ACS) with Bypass Surgery

- Patient on dabigatran needing emergent CABG can be administered idarucizumab 2.5 mg every 15 min for two doses
- If bleeding occurs, support measures with blood products should be provided

Self-Assessment Questions

1. Which of the following would be true regarding the emergent management of a patient going to a CABG on dabigatran?
   (a) The patient should be administered vitamin K
   (b) The patient should be administered un-activated four-factor prothrombin complex concentrate
   (c) The patient should be administered idarucizumab 2.5 mg once
   (d) The patient should be administered idarucizumab 2.5 mg twice 15 min apart

   ANSWER: The correct answer is D. Based on the REVERSE-AD trial, administration of idarucizumab 2.5 mg 15 min apart normalized hemostasis in patient on dabigatran and provided reversal for emergent surgery. Answer A is incorrect as vitamin K has no impact on dabigatran. Answer B is in correct since animal models have demonstrated minimal effects of four factor PCC on dabigatran. Answer C is incorrect since there is no evidence regarding the impact of administration of 2.5 mg idarucizumab on hemostatic parameters.

2. A 68-year-old male patient with a mechanical mitral valve on warfarin and history of atrial fibrillation is going to have an elective CABG and aortic valve replacement in 1–2 weeks. The patient is currently on warfarin with an INR of three. His SCr is 1.05 and his weight is 80 kg. Which of the following would be the most ideal plan regarding his anticoagulation management?
   (a) Stop warfarin 24–48 h prior to the CABG and restart 12 h after surgery
   (b) Stop warfarin 5 days before CABG and restart 48 h after surgery
   (c) Stop warfarin 5 days before CABG, check an INR daily, start UFH when INR <2.5 stop heparin 5–6 h before surgery, and then restart UFH as a bridge to warfarin 48–72 h after surgery until INR at goal
   (d) Give vitamin K 24–48 h before surgery, check an INR before procedure and give un-activated 4-factor PCC prior if INR >2, restart warfarin 12 h after surgery

   ANSWER: The correct answer would be C. A patient with a mechanical valve and atrial fibrillation is at a high risk of thrombosis and it is recommended the patient be bridged in the peri-procedural period. Thus it is recommended that therapy be stopped 5 days before surgery and INRs check daily. The patient can be bridged with LMWH or UFH once the INR is <2. Unfractionated heparin and warfarin can be restarted once haemostasis is achieved post-procedure. The UFH bridge should remain until the INR is at goal. Answer A is not correct since the response more describes the pharmacokinetic and pharmacodynamics principles of a DOAC. Warfarin generally requires 4–5 days of washout for normalization of hemostasis. Answer B is not correct since there is no mentioning of bridging. Answer D is incorrect due to the fact the patient is going to have an elective procedure. It would be ideal to let the INR drift down versus using a reversal agent due to the risk of thrombosis. In addition, there is no bridging mentioned in this option.

References

1. Spyropoulos AC, Douketis JD. How I treat anticoagulated patients undergoing an elective procedure or surgery. Blood. 2012;120:2954–62.
2. Baron TH, Kamath PS, McBane RD. Management of antithrombotic therapy in patients undergoing invasive procedures. N Engl J Med. 2013;368:3113–24.
3. Douketis JD, Spyropoulos AC, Spencer FA, et al. Perioperative management of antithrombotic therapy. Chest. 2012;141(2 Suppl):e326S–50s.
4. Ortel TL. Perioperative management of patients on chronic antithrombotic therapy. Blood. 2012;120:4699–705.
5. Faraoni D, Levy JH, Albaladejo P, et al. Updates in the perioperative and emergency management of non-vitamin K antagonist oral anticoagulants. Crit Care. 2015;19(1):203.
6. Rechenmacher SJ, Fang JC. Bridging anticoagulation: primum non nocere. J Am Coll Cardiol. 2015;66(12):1392–403.
7. Quality Improvement Organization. Management of anticoagulation in the peri-procedural period. 2014. http://qio.ipro.org/wp-ontent/uploads/2012/12/MAP2014_5_01.pdf. Access 8 May 2016.
8. Pollack CV, Reilly PA, Eikelboom J, et al. Idarucizumab for dabigatran reversal. N Engl J Med. 2015;375:511–20.
9. Smythe MA, Trujillo T, Fanikos J. Reversal agents for use with direct and indirect anticoagulants. Am J Health Syst Pharm. 2016;73(10 Suppl 2):S27–48.

Part VI
Drug Interactions

Chapter 28
Anticoagulant Drug-Drug Interactions with CYP 3A4 Inhibitors

Lea E. dela Pena

Abstract Cytochrome P450 is a group of enzymes that metabolize many medications; understanding which CYP P450 isoenzyme(s) a particular medication may inhibit will help the clinician recognize the potential implications the drug interaction may have with anticoagulants. Warfarin is particularly affected by the CYP2C9, 3A4, and 1A2 isoenzymes; however, DOACs are relatively new to market so all possible drug interactions have not been identified. Using appropriate drug information resources is a valuable tool for the clinician to look up possible interactions.

Keywords Cytochrome P450 • CYP2C9 • CYP3A4 • CYP1A2 • CYP 3A4 inhibitors • Azole antifungals • Clarithromycin • Gemfibrozil • Cimetadine • Ritonavir • Warfarin R- and S-enantiomers • P-glycoprotein (P-gp)

Case Introduction

A 55 year old female patient with past medical history significant for recurrent DVT, type 2 diabetes, dyslipidemia, obesity, and recurrent yeast infections presents to her gynecologist's office with complaints of vaginal itching and white vaginal discharge × 3 days. She requests a prescription for oral fluconazole 150 mg for presumed vulvocandidiasis. She has had several episodes of vulvovaginal candidiasis over the last few years so her physician is considering putting her on a weekly regimen to prevent future occurrences. Her current medications include metformin, insulin glargine, pravastatin, and warfarin.

L.E. dela Pena, PharmD, BCPS
Midwestern University Chicago College of Pharmacy,
555 W 31st St, Downers Grove, IL 60515, USA
e-mail: ldelap@midwestern.edu

Case Discussion

Drug interactions play an important role when using anticoagulant medications. Certain interactions may put a patient at risk for thrombosis or at risk for bleeding, neither of which is a desirable outcome. Clinicians should be aware of the major types of interactions that may come into play with the anticoagulant medication a particular patient is using.

Cytochrome P450 is a group of enzymes that metabolize many medications. These enzymes are primarily located in the liver. While there are several different enzymes within the CYP450 group, only a handful have been identified as having a major effect on the metabolism of medications; these are CYP1A2, CYP2C9, CYP2C19, CYP2D6, and CYP3A4. Drugs can be metabolized by one or more P450 enzyme. Drugs that inhibit this pathway reduce P450 activity, which results in slower substrate metabolism and increased effect of the substrate; drugs that induce this pathway will increase P450 activity, which results in faster substrate metabolism and decreased effect of the substrate [1]. The effects of inhibitors are usually seen quickly whereas the effects of inducers may be delayed. The following drugs are inhibitors of CYP3A4 [1]:

- Clarithromycin
- Azole antifungals (e.g., ketoconazole, itraconazole, fluconazole)
- Gemfibrozil
- Cimetadine
- Ritonavir

Treatment of recurrent vulvovaginal candidiasis can be accomplished with either oral or topical regimens. For oral fluconazole, the dosing regimen would be 150 mg po daily × 3 days, then 150 mg po weekly × 6 months [2]. Fluconazole is considered a moderate CYP3A4 inhibitor, unlike ketoconazole or itraconazole which are considered strong CYP3A4 inhibitors. Topical regimens with other azole antifungals are given daily for one to seven nights, then weekly for 6 months [2]. If another non-interacting medication is appropriate to use, that would be ideal. Topical administration would be less likely to cause an interaction since the medication is not systemically absorbed. However, the patient may have a preference for oral vs. topical administration so it would be prudent to ask her which she would like.

What is the concern of using fluconazole with anticoagulant medications?

Warfarin

Warfarin is manufactured as a racemic mixture of R- and S-enantiomers. The S-enantiomer of warfarin is the more potent isomer and is primary metabolized through CYP2C9. The R-enantiomer of warfarin is the less potent isomer and is primarily metabolized through CYP1A2 and CYP3A4 [3]. Fluconzaole is an inhibitor of the CYP3A4 enzyme. Inhibition of this CYP P450 enzyme decreases their ability to inactivate warfarin which can lead to a prolonged clinical effect, increased INR levels for patient, and put that patient at risk for bleeding. For patients taking concomitant warfarin, even a single dose of oral fluconazole can cause clinically meaningful elevations in the INR and/or cause bleeding which necessitates the holding of warfarin for at least one dose [4]. Clinicians will need to closely monitor INR levels in patients on both fluconazole and warfarin together and adjust the dose of warfarin if needed [5]. Patients will respond differently to these types of drug interactions so it is important for the clinician to take an individualized approach to adjusting the warfarin dose, if needed, instead of a one size fits all approach.

Direct Oral Anticoagulants (DOACs)

The effect of the P450 enzyme system on the metabolism of the DOACs is highly variable. Dabigatran and edoxaban are not metabolized via the P450 system so inhibitors or inducers of P450 enzymes should not have an interaction with either dabigatran or edoxaban. In contrast, rivaroxaban and apixaban are both metabolized by CYP3A4, and are thus potentially subject to interacting with inhibitors and/or inducers of 3A4; however, over half of the metabolism of these drugs is through other pathways that do no not involve 3A4, which would control the impact of any interaction [6]. The DOACs are substrates for the P-glycoprotein (P-gp) system which pumps drugs out of cells; P-gp is found in the gastrointestinal tract, liver, pancreas, kidney, and brain. Similar to CYP3A4, drugs that inhibit the P-gp system increase the absorption of P-gp substrates, whereas drugs that induce the P-gp system decrease the absorption of P-gp substrates [6]. Some drugs can be both inhibitors/inducers of P-gp as well as CYP3A4 (discussed in Chap. 30). In combination with a DOAC, unless a strong 3A4 inhibitor is prescribed or a strong 3A4 inhibitor in combination with a P-gp inhibitor, most clinicians would just closely monitor the patient; the exception would be in the setting of reduced renal function, dose adjustments may be warranted.

Since these medications are relatively new to the market, there aren't as many reports of drug interactions as there are with warfarin. As more patients are exposed to DOACs, more interactions can be expected to be reported through post-marketing surveillance. It is important for the clinician to check numerous drug information resources, such as Micromedex, Facts and Comparisons, or LexiComp, as well as the package insert, when confronted with a potential drug interaction. It would also be prudent to conduct a literature search to determine if any recent case reports have been published in regards to specific drug interactions. One study suggests that although there is a potential interaction between fluconazole and rivaroxaban, these two medications may be administered together with caution [7]. Patients should be instructed to monitor for any unusual bleeding or bruising while on concomitant therapy and to report any findings to their health care provider. No published studies are available regarding an interaction between fluconazole and either dabigatran, apixaban, or edoxaban.

Key Points

- Understanding which CYP P450 isoenzyme(s) a particular medication may inhibit will help the clinician recognize the potential implications the drug interaction may have with anticoagulants.
- Warfarin is particularly affected by the CYP2C9 (which will be discussed in Chap. 30), 3A4, and 1A2 isoenzymes.
- The DOACs are relatively new to market so not all potential drug interactions have been identified. Clinicians should consult different drug information resources if a drug interaction is suspected.

Self-Assessment Questions

1. A 66 year old female patient presents to the emergency department with an acute DVT. Her past medical history is significant for osteopenia and GERD. She is currently on calcium citrate, vitamin D, and cimetidine. Which of the following anticoagulants would have a clinically significant interaction with any of her current medications?

   (a) Warfarin
   (b) Apixaban
   (c) Edoxaban
   (d) Dabigatran

   The correct answer is A. Although cimetidine is a CYP3A4 inhibitor, it is only moderate, not strong, so there is no clinically significant interaction with the listed DOACs at this time, which makes answers B, C, and D incorrect. Caution should still be used if a DOAC is used with cimetidine; patients should be told to report any unusual bleeding or bruising to their health care provider. Cimetidine can increase the INR if taken concomitantly with warfarin. An alternative H2 receptor antagonist that does not go through CYP3A4 should be used if possible, such as famotidine, ranitidine, or nizatidine. If a patient insists on using cimetidine with warfarin, the INR should be monitored closely and warfarin doses adjusted as necessary.

2. A 68 year old male patient with history of atrial fibrillation and hypertension presents to his primary care physician's office due to worsening productive cough, fever, and nasal congestion × 6 days. He is currently taking metoprolol as well as dabiagran for stroke prevention. He is diagnosed with community acquired pneumonia and his physician prescribes a 7 day course of clarithromycin. Which of the following anticoagulant medications is expected to have a clinically significant interaction with clarithromycin?

   (a) Warfarin
   (b) Dabigatran

(c) Rivaroxaban
(d) Apixaban
(e) Edoxaban

The correct answer is A. The administration of warfarin and clarithromycin can result in an increased INR level so close monitoring and dosage adjustments of warfarin will be needed. Clarithromycin is not considered a strong inhibitor of CYP 3A4 so the listed DOACs are fine to use. Clinical monitoring for any unusual bleeding or bruising would be prudent for any of the anticoagulant medications.

References

1. Lynch T, Price A. The effect of cytochrome P450 metabolism on drug response, interactions, and adverse effects. Am Fam Physician. 2007;76:391–6.
2. Sobel JD. Recurrent vulvovaginal candidiasis. Am J Obstet Gynecol. 2016;214:15–21.
3. Coumadin [package insert]. Princeton, NJ: Bristol-Myers Squibb Company; 2015.
4. Turrentine MA. Single-dose fluconazole for vulvovaginal candidiasis: impact on prothrombin time in women taking warfarin. Obstet Gynecol. 2006;107:310–3.
5. Ageno W, Gallus AS, Wittkowsky A, et al. Oral anticoagulant therapy: antithrombotic therapy and prevention of thrombosis, 9th ed: American College of Chest Physicians evidence-based clinical practice guidelines. Chest. 2012;141(2 Suppl):e44S–88S.
6. Fitzgerald JL, Howed LG. Drug interactions of direct-acting oral anticoagulants. Drug Saf. 2016;39(9):841–5.
7. Mueck W, Kubitza D, Becka M. Co-administration of rivaroxaban with drugs that share its elimination pathways: pharmacokinetic effects in healthy subjects. Br J Clin Pharmacol. 2013;76:455–66.

Chapter 29
Significance of P-glycoprotein (P-gp) Drug-Drug Interactions

Dave L. Dixon

Abstract This case describes the P-glycoprotein (P-gp) transport system and the significance of potential drug-drug interactions with P-gp inhibitors and inducers.

Keywords P-glycoprotein • Drug-drug interactions • Anticoagulants • Apixaban • Dabigatran • Edoxaban • Rivaroxaban

Case Introduction

A 57-year-old African-American male presents for follow-up visit to check his INR. He has no new complaints. He was started on warfarin 3 months ago for stroke prophylaxis (non-valvular atrial fibrillation) and has had erratic INRs despite adequate adherence, a consistent diet, and frequent clinic follow-up. Other past medical history includes HIV, hypertension, stage 3 CKD (SCr 1.9 mg/dL; CrCl 35 mL/min; Weight 58 kg), hyperlipidemia, and NSTEMI (3 years ago). His current medications include metoprolol succinate, lisinopril, chlorthalidone, ritonavir, atazanavir, tenofovir/emtricitabine, aspirin, warfarin and rosuvastatin. He reports no recent diet changes or signs/symptoms of any bleeding. His INR today is 1.7. The physician decides to switch him to a target-specific oral anticoagulant (DOAC) and asks for your assistance in selecting an agent that will not interact with his current medications.

Case Discussion

What is the P-gp transport system and what is the clinical significance of P-gp-mediated drug interactions?

D.L. Dixon, PharmD, BCACP, FNLA, FCCP, FACC
Department of Pharmacotherapy and Outcomes Science, VCU School of Pharmacy,
410 N. 12th St., PO Box 980533, Richmond, VA 23298-0533, USA
e-mail: dldixon@vcu.edu

Table 29.1 P-gp inhibitors and inducers

Characteristic	Medications			
P-gp inhibitors	Amiodarone[b]	Azithromycin[b]	Carvedilol	Clarithromycin[a]
	Conivaptan[a]	Cyclosporine	Diltiazem[b]	Dronedarone[b]
	Erythromycin[b]	Itraconazole[a]	Ketoconazole[a]	Ritonavir[a]
	Quinidine[b]	Ranolazine[b]	Verapamil[b]	
P-gp inducers	Carbamazepine[c]	Phenytoin[c]	Rifampin[c]	St. John's wort[a]

Ref: http://www.fda.gov/Drugs/DevelopmentApprovalProcess/DevelopmentResources/DrugInteractionsLabeling/
[a]Strong CYP3A4 inhibitor
[b]Weak-moderate CYP3A4 inhibitor
[c]CYP3A4 inducer

P-gp Transport System

Two types of transporters, adenosine triphosphate (ATP)-binding cassette and solute carrier, manage the transport of medications in and out of cells [1]. The most relevant transporter system to anticoagulants is p-glycoprotein (P-gp), which is located in the small intestine, blood-brain barrier, liver, and kidneys [1]. As such, drugs that interact with P-gp can affect the absorption, metabolism, and elimination of other agents. Interestingly, many drugs that impact P-gp also interact with CYP3A4, which can increase the potential for a more clinically significant drug-drug interaction (see Table 29.1).

P-gp-Mediated Drug Interactions

It is well established that many commonly used drug classes are P-gp substrates, while others inhibit or induce P-gp [1]. These include many different drug classes, such as antiarrhythmics, antibiotics, antifungals, antihypertensives, antiplatelets, and statins. Furthermore, each of the DOACs are substrates for P-gp, which has brought more attention to P-gp-mediated drug interactions [1]. P-gp inhibition can increase the concentration of DOACs and the risk of bleeding, while P-gp induction can decrease the effectiveness of these agents. It is difficult, however, to accurately predict the potential significance of a P-gp-mediated drug interaction because of individual variations in expression of the gene that codes for P-gp [1]. Further research is warranted to better understand patient-specific differences in the expression and functionality of P-gp. With that said, there is a greater likelihood for significant drug-drug interactions with those drugs that are substrates for P-gp and metabolized by CYP3A4 (see Table 29.2 for summary of P-gp mediated drug-drug interactions with DOACs).

Table 29.2 Anticoagulants and P-gp-mediated drug-drug interactions

Anticoagulant	Interaction characteristics	US package insert recommendations
Apixaban [3]	Strong CYP3A4 and P-gp inducers	Avoid combination and consider alternative agents
	Strong CYP3A4 and P-gp inhibitors	If currently taking 5 mg twice daily, reduce dose to 2.5 mg twice daily If currently taking 2.5 mg twice daily, avoid combination and consider alternative agents
	Weak-moderate CYP3A4 and P-gp inhibitors	No dose adjustment recommended
Dabigatran [4]	P-gp inducers	Avoid combination and consider alternative agents
	P-gp inhibitors	Atrial fibrillation: Consider reducing dose to 75 mg twice daily if used with dronedarone or ketoconazole in patients with CrCl 30–50 mL/min. Avoid in patients with CrCl <30 mL/min VTE: Avoid in any patient with CrCl <50 mL/min
Edoxaban [5]	P-gp inhibitors	Atrial fibrillation: Do not reduce dose VTE treatment: Reduce dose to 30 mg daily
	P-gp inducer (specific only to rifampin)	Avoid use with rifampin and consider alternative agents
Rivaroxaban [2]	Strong CYP3A4 and P-gp inducers	Avoid combination and consider alternative agents
	Strong CYP3A4 and P-gp inhibitors	Avoid combination and consider alternative agents
	Moderate CYP3A4 and P-gp inhibitors	Consider alternative agent with CrCl 15–80 mL/min Use only if benefit outweighs potential risk

Warfarin and P-gp

Warfarin has many drug-drug interactions that add to the difficulty of maintaining a therapeutic INR. However, it is important to note that while the DOACs are substrates for P-gp, warfarin is not. While there is evidence that warfarin may inhibit P-gp in the liver, there is no evidence that P-gp affects the absorption of warfarin. Additionally, warfarin is well absorbed in the gut, which prevents any likely interaction with P-gp [1].

Which DOAC Would Be Preferred in this Patient?

- Ritonavir is both an inhibitor of P-gp and a strong inhibitor of CYP3A4.
  - Rivaroxaban is not recommended and an alternative agent should be considered [2].

- The apixaban dose in this patient would be 2.5 mg twice daily given his weight is ≤60 kg and SCr is ≥1.5, however, a 50% dose reduction is warranted when used in a P-gp and strong CYP3A4 inhibitor. As such, apixaban is not recommended and an alternative agent should be considered [3].
- Dabigatran is an option given the patient's CrCl is >30 mL/min, however, there is no clear guidance regarding dosing [4]. A conservative approach would include using the lower dose, 75 mg twice daily, given the patient's renal function.
- Edoxaban is also an option since it is minimally metabolized by CYP3A4. The appropriate dose based on this patient's renal function would be 30 mg once daily [5].

Key Points

- Many drugs are substrates, inhibitors, or inducers of P-gp, including the DOACs.
- Drugs that are substrates for P-gp and are significantly metabolized by CYP3A4 are of greatest concern.
- The clinician should carefully review patient profiles for potential drugs that may enhance or reduce the effectiveness of DOACs.

Self-Assessment Questions

1. A 68-year-old female has been taking apixaban 5 mg twice daily since her pulmonary embolism 1 month ago. She has no other significant past medical history and takes no other medications. Her renal and hepatic function is stable. Today, she is diagnosed with community-acquired pneumonia. Which of the following macrolide antibiotics would be LEAST preferred in this patient?

    (a) Azithromycin
    (b) Clarithromycin
    (c) Erythromycin
    (d) All of the above

    The correct answer is B. While each of these macrolides are P-gp inhibitors, only clarithromycin is also a potent CYP3A4 inhibitor. This is problematic since apixaban relies heavily (75%) on CYP3A4 metabolism. A dose reduction would be necessary while the patient was on clarithromycin and could confuse the patient about their dosing. Answers A and C would be more reasonable choices considering that azithromycin and erythromycin are only weak-moderate CYP3A4 inhibitors and would not require any changes in the patient's apixaban dose.

2. A 73-year-old male is admitted from a skilled nursing facility and diagnosed with a major bleed. He has had paroxysmal atrial fibrillation for the past 3 years

and was being anticoagulated with rivaroxaban. Records from the skilled nursing facility show a new medication was started 10 days ago. Other past medical history includes diabetes, peripheral neuropathy, prostate cancer, GERD, and urinary incontinence. His renal and hepatic function is normal. Which of the following medications was MOST likely added to his drug regimen and may have increased the effectiveness of the rivaroxaban?

(a) Carbamazepine
(b) Carvedilol
(c) Amiodarone
(d) Ketoconazole

The correct answer is D. Rivaroxaban is heavily metabolized by CYP3A4 and is a substrate for P-gp. Strong CYP3A4 and P-gp inhibitors, such as ketoconazole, can increase the effectiveness of rivaroxaban and increase the risk of adverse bleeding events. Answer A is a P-gp and CYP3A4 inducer and would decrease the effectiveness of rivaroxaban and increase the risk of stroke, but not bleeding. Answers B and C also inhibit P-gp but are weak-moderate CYP3A4 inhibitors and may be used safety in most patients where the benefit outweighs the risk.

References

1. Wessler JD, Grip LT, Mendell J, Giugliano RP. The P-glycoprotein transport system and cardiovascular drugs. J Am Coll Cardiol. 2013;61(25):2195–502.
2. Xarelto® [package insert]. Titusville, NJ: Janssen Pharmaceuticals, Inc.; 2011.
3. Eliquis® [package insert]. New York, NY: Bristol-Myers Squibb Company and Pfizer Inc.; 2012.
4. Pradaxa® [package insert]. Ridgefield, CT: Boehringer Ingelheim Pharamcueticals, Inc.; 2010.
5. Savaysa® [package insert]. Tokyo, Japan: Daiichi Sankyo Co., Ltd.; 2015.

Chapter 30
Considerations with Pharmacodynamic Drug-Drug Interactions

Jill S. Borchert

Abstract A case in which new medications pose a risk of a pharmacodynamic drug-drug interaction with anticoagulants is discussed. The case reviews possible mechanisms of pharmacodynamic interactions, provides examples of the interactions and discusses clinical aspects to consider when evaluating pharmacodynamic interactions.

Keywords Pharmacodynamic • Drug interaction • Pharmacodynamic drug-drug interaction • Anticoagulant • Warfarin • Direct oral anticoagulant

Case Introduction

A 48 year-old woman presents to the clinic for anticoagulation follow-up and INR monitoring and mentions she is taking several new medications. Her INR has been within therapeutic range for the last few visits. She mentions that she was diagnosed with diabetes by her primary care physician (PCP). She did not start taking the diabetes medication prescribed by her physician and instead started an exercise program. However, this has been making her lower back hurt so she occasionally takes ibuprofen 200 mg 1–2 tablets as needed for pain. Her mood has been "down" ever since her DVT and the diagnosis of diabetes has made her more depressed; therefore, her PCP started escitalopram 10 mg PO daily. Lastly, she read online that diabetes can increase her risk of a heart attack so she started taking aspirin 325 mg PO daily. Her past medical history is significant for deep vein thrombosis (first-event, 3 months ago) and new diagnoses of type 2 diabetes and depression. Her last labs indicated an elevated fasting glucose and A1C, but all other labs were within normal limits. She is a non-smoker. Medications at her last anticoagulation clinic visit: warfarin 4 mg PO daily, calcium 600 mg PO daily.

J.S. Borchert, PharmD, BCACP, BCPS, FCCP
Midwestern University Chicago College of Pharmacy,
555 31st Street, Downers Grove, IL 60515, USA
e-mail: jborchert@midwestern.edu

© Springer International Publishing AG 2017
K. Kiser (ed.), *Oral Anticoagulation Therapy*,
DOI 10.1007/978-3-319-54643-8_30

Case Discussion

Do Any of this Patient's New Medications Pose a Risk of a Pharmacodynamic Drug-Drug Interaction?

A pharmacodynamic interaction is one in which there is an additive or antagonistic effect of one drug on another drug's pharmacologic effects. All three of this patient's new medications (ibuprofen, escitalopram, and aspirin) pose a potential for a pharmacodynamic interaction [1, 2]. These medications have potential antiplatelet effects. While warfarin is an anticoagulant and not an antiplatelet medication, this pharmacodynamic interaction may increase the risk of bleeding. Further, both non-steroidal anti-inflammatory agents (NSAIDs) and aspirin independently may injury the gastrointestinal (GI) mucosa providing another pharmacodynamic mechanism for the potential increased risk of bleeding. NSAIDs, aspirin and escitalopram generally do not cause clinically significant alterations in the INR. Table 30.1 outlines examples of pharmacodynamic interactions with warfarin [2, 3].

What Is the Mechanism of These Pharmacodynamic Drug-Drug Interactions and What Is the Impact on Bleeding Risk?

Low doses of aspirin selectively inhibit cyclooxygenase (COX)-1 and inhibit thromboxane A2 production [4]. Inhibition of COX-1 on the platelet causes an antiplatelet effect; however, the COX-1 enzyme also is present in the GI mucosa and the integrity of the GI mucosa can be diminished with aspirin [5]. In a population-based, retrospective case-control study, combination of aspirin with warfarin increased the risk of GI bleeding by approximately 6.5-fold compared to matched controls [6]. In general, lower doses of aspirin are as effective and pose a lower bleeding risk than higher doses [7]. Nonetheless, low-dose aspirin remains associated with an increased risk for GI complications [5].

Table 30.1 Examples of pharmacodynamic interactions with warfarin [2, 3]

Food, drug or class	Mechanism
Aspirin and NSAIDS	Antiplatelet, direct gastrointestinal injury
P2Y12 inhibitors (e.g. clopidogrel)	Antiplatelet
SSRIs	Altered platelet function
Thyroid replacement (e.g. levothyroxine)	Increased catabolism of clotting factors
Anti-thyroid agents (e.g. methimazole)	Decreased catabolism of clotting factors
Select herbals (e.g. danshen, garlic, ginger, gingko)	Antiplatelet
High vitamin K foods (e.g. spinach, greens, kale)	Increased production of vitamin k dependent clotting factors

Like aspirin, NSAIDs also inhibit the COX-1 enzyme and both interfere with platelet function and diminish the integrity of the GI mucosa [2]. GI erosions are dose-dependent and patients on anticoagulants are at a higher risk for NSAID-induced GI toxicity (odds ratio 12.7) [2, 5]. As such, GI protective therapy may be necessary if patients on warfarin remain on NSAID therapy [5].

Platelets have both serotonin receptors and a serotonin reuptake pump and selective-serotonin reuptake inhibitors (SSRIs) have the potential to increase bleeding risk through decreased platelet function [1]. The clinical significance is unclear and while case reports of bleeding have been reported, a population-based, nested, case-control study did not show an increase in risk of hospitalization for upper GI bleed for patients on warfarin initiated on an SSRI [8]. Of note, some SSRIs may inhibit CYP 2C9 and thus pose a pharmacokinetic interaction by decreasing the metabolism of warfarin.

What Clinical Aspects Should Be Considered When Evaluating Pharmacodynamic Drug-Drug Interactions?

The clinician must consider the risk-benefit of each drug presenting with a pharmacodynamic interaction with warfarin by considering the need for the interacting drug, the dose and alternatives (Table 30.2). In this case, it is necessary to continue anticoagulation for treatment of her recent DVT and other alternatives to ibuprofen are available to manage this patient's post-exercise lower back pain. In addition to non-pharmacologic measures to control pain, occasional acetaminophen (<2 g/day) may be an acceptable alternative. This patient has a clinical need to treat depression and continuating the SSRI and monitoring for bleeding is reasonable. Alternative SSRIs would not have a lower risk of bleeding and in fact some may also have a pharmacokinetic interaction with warfarin so the clinician should not consider switching to an alternative SSRI. Finally, this patient does not have a clinical indication for aspirin. She has no history of atherosclerotic cardiovascular disease (e.g. history of myocardial infarction or ischemic stroke) and started taking aspirin on her own presumably for primary prevention of atherosclerotic cardiovascular disease (ASCVD). Current recommendations from the American Diabetes Association are to consider aspirin therapy (75–16 mg/day) as primary prevention in patients with diabetes at increased risk of ASCVD (10-year risk >10%) [9]. She is currently at low risk

Table 30.2 Clinical risk-benefit considerations for pharmacodynamic interacting drug with an anticoagulant

(a) Is the **drug** necessary? (e.g. is there a specific indication)
(b) Is this **dose** of the drug necessary? (e.g. can the dose be lowered to minimize the potential impact)
(c) Are there clinically viable **alternatives**?

for ASCVD since she is less than 50 years old and has no major ASCVD risk factors (e.g. family history of ASCVD, hypertension, smoking, dyslipidemia or albuminuria). The risk of bleeding, especially given concurrent therapy with warfarin, would offset any potential benefit from aspirin. Therefore, it would be acceptable to discontinue aspirin in this patient. If she had a higher ASCVD risk, then the clinician may want to consider reducing the dose to 75–162 mg/day to be in line with recommended doses in clinical practice guidelines and minimize the risk of bleeding. The consideration of adding antiplatelet agents that increase bleeding risk to warfarin should be individualized considering the risk and benefits of each drug.

Would Switching to a Non-oral Vitamin K Anticoagulant (DOAC) Resolve the Pharmacodynamic Drug-Drug Interactions?

While DOACs are a therapeutic option for management of her DVT, these drugs also pose a risk of bleeding and similar pharmacodynamic interactions exist. Since these agents are newer, there are less data regarding the bleeding risk associated with these interactions. Nonetheless, the same theoretical interactions increasing the risk of bleeding exist. She is already managed on warfarin and there are no other clinical factors indicating a switch to a DOAC is necessary.

Key Points

- There are several possible mechanisms of pharmacodynamic interactions with anticoagulants.
    - Antiplatelet effect (e.g. aspirin, selective serotonin reuptake inhibitors, non-steroidal anti-inflammatory agents)
    - Injury to the gastrointestinal mucosa (e.g. aspirin, non-steroidal anti-inflammatory agents)
- The risk-benefit of concurrent therapy should be considered on an individualized basis.
- The clinician should consider if the interacting drug is necessary (e.g. is there a clinical indication), if the dose of the drug is necessary (e.g. can the dose be lowered) and/or if alternative non-interacting drugs may be suitable.
- It may not be possible to avoid all pharmacodynamic interactions and clinical monitoring (e.g. signs of bleeding) may be the best individualized approach.

Self-Assessment Questions

1. The mechanism(s) of the pharmacodynamic interaction between non-steroidal anti-inflammatory agents (NSAIDs) and warfarin include(s) that ibuprofen: SELECT ALL THAT APPLY.

    (a) Inhibits COX-1 for an antiplatelet effect to increase bleeding risk.
    (b) Inhibits of CYP 2C9 leading to an increased INR and bleeding risk.
    (c) Modulates serotonin and decreases platelet function and increases bleeding risk.
    (d) Decreases the integrity of the GI mucosa and increases GI bleeding risk.

Answers: A and D. NSAIDs inhibit the COX-1 enzyme and both interfere with platelet function and diminish the integrity of the GI mucosa. These actions increase bleeding risk. Answer B is incorrect as NSAIDs are not inhibitors of CYP 2C9 and this is also not an example of a pharmacodynamic interaction but instead a pharmacokinetic interaction. Answer C is incorrect as NSAIDs do not change serotonin activity; instead, SSRIs have the potential for antiplatelet function.

2. What impact does low-dose aspirin have on the INR when initiated in a patient stable on warfarin?

    (a) Increases the INR
    (b) Decreases the INR
    (c) No clinically significant impact on the INR

Answer: C. Low dose aspirin may increase the bleeding risk of a patient on warfarin through an antiplatelet effect but it does not significantly impact the INR. Therefore, both answers A and B are incorrect.

References

1. Hersh EV, Pinto A, Moore PA. Adverse drug interactions involving common prescription and over-the-counter analgesic agents. Clin Ther. 2007;29:2477–97.
2. Juurlink DN. Drug interactions with warfarin: what clinicians need to know. CMAJ. 2007;177(4):369–71.
3. Nutescu EA, Shapiro NL, Ibrahim S, West P. Warfarin and its interactions with foods, herbs and other dietary supplements. Expert Opin Drug Saf. 2006;5:433–51.
4. Mega JL, Simon T. Pharmacology of antithrombotic drugs: an assessment of oral antiplatelet and anticoagulant treatments. Lancet. 2015;386:281–91.
5. Lanza FL, Chan FKL, Quigley EMM, The Practice Parameters Committee of the American College of Gastroenterology. Guidelines for the prevention of NSAID-related ulcer complications. Am J Gastroenterol. 2009;104:728–38.
6. Delaney JA, Opatrny L, Brophy JM, Suissa S. Drug-drug interactions between antithrombotic medications and the risk of gastrointestinal bleeding. CMAJ. 2007;177(4):347–51.

7. O'Gara PT. American College of Cardiology for CAD, what is the recommended dose of aspirin and why? 2016. https://acc.org/latest-in-cardiology/articles/2016/03/29/10/08/for-cad-what-is-the-recommended-dose-of-aspirin-and-why. Accessed 13 July 2016.
8. Kurdyak PA, Juurlink DN, Kopp A, Hermann N, Mamdani MM. Antidepressants, warfarin, and the risk of hemorrhage. J Clin Psychopharmacol. 2005;25:561–4.
9. American Diabetes Association. Cardiovascular disease and risk management. Diabetes Care. 2016;39(Suppl 1):S60–71.

Chapter 31
Management of Direct Oral Anticoagulants with Mixed P-gp/3A4 Drug-Drug Interactions

Kathryn Wdowiarz

Abstract Direct oral anticoagulants (DOACs) interact with mixed P-gp/3A4 inhibitors and inducers to varying degrees. The degree of inhibition or induction of the interacting medication, as well as a patient's renal function, are important to assess when selecting a DOAC and an appropriate dose.

Keywords Direct oral anticoagulants (DOAC) • Drug interaction • Mixed P-gp/3A4 inhibitors • Renal function • Apixaban • Edoxaban • Dabigatran • Rivaroxaban

Case Introduction

A 70-year-old female presents to the emergency department with complaints of shortness of breath, palpitations, and dizziness. An EKG is obtained and reveals new onset atrial fibrillation. She has no history of arrhythmias. Her heart rate is 130 bpm and her blood pressure is 134/78. She weighs 160 lb and is 5′6″. Her past medical history includes hypertension, chronic kidney disease, gastroesophageal reflux disease, osteoarthritis of the knees, and a transient ischemic attack 2 months ago. Prior to admission, her home medication list included aspirin, lisinopril, ferrous sulfate, esomeprazole, atorvastatin, and acetaminophen. Baseline metabolic panel is within normal limits with the exception of a BUN of 30, a creatinine of 1.8 mg/dL, and a creatinine clearance of 33 mL/min.

She is initiated on a heparin infusion and a rate control strategy with diltiazem. When discussing options for chronic anticoagulation, she mentions that she would prefer to avoid frequent lab monitoring with warfarin therapy.

K. Wdowiarz, PharmD, BCPS
Midwestern University Chicago College of Pharmacy, 555 West 31st Street, Downers Grove, IL 60515, USA

Edward Elmhurst Healthcare, 801 South Washington Street, Naperville, IL 60540, USA
e-mail: kwdowi@midwestern.edu

Case Discussion

How Does the Presence of a Mixed P-gp/CYP3A4 Inhibitor like Diltiazem Affect the Choice of Treatment for this Patient? How Does the Patient's Renal Impairment Affect the Choice of Treatment?

Rivaroxaban and apixaban are both metabolized to varying degrees by the hepatic enzyme CYP3A4 while edoxaban and dabigatran are not substrates of CYP3A4 (see Fig. 22.1). All four of the direct oral anticoagulants (DOACs) are substrates of permeability-glycoprotein (P-gp) efflux transporter [1, 2]. If changing the rate control agent to a beta blocker such as metoprolol is an option, concern over drug-drug interactions with DOACs is no longer needed. In the setting where diltiazem is necessary, each of the four DOAC's drug-drug profile should be considered.

Rivaroxaban and Apixaban with Mixed P-gp/CYP3A4 Inhibitors

When assessing the appropriateness of initiating rivaroxaban or apixaban in patients currently taking a mixed P-gp/CYP3A4 inhibitor, it is necessary to be aware of the degree of inhibition of CYP3A4. Recommendations for use differ between strong and moderate CYP3A4 inhibition. While strong P-gp/CYP3A4 inhibitors are not recommended to be used with rivaroxaban, atrial fibrillation patients in the ROCKET AF trial were permitted to use moderate P-gp/CYP3A4 inhibitors with rivaroxaban without limitations [1–3]. However, it is expected that rivaroxaban exposure and anticoagulant effect are increased in the presence of P-gp/moderate CYP3A4 inhibitors [1]. The clinical significance of these increases is dependent on the patient's renal function and further studies are warranted. Because of the presence of impaired renal function in this patient, she should not receive rivaroxaban [1].

Apixiban is unique in that it is the only Xa inhibitor approved for use across the entire spectrum of renal impairment including hemodialysis. Data from patients on hemodialysis is based on a single dose study of 16 patients. It is important to recognize that the risk of accumulation with multiple doses of apixaban in hemodialysis has not been studied [4]. Renal impairment alone would not be a limiting factor when considering apixaban in this patient. When reviewing the drug interaction, diltiazem has been shown to increase apixaban exposure 1.3–1.4-fold when studied in healthy volunteers [1, 5]. Less is known about the drug interaction when combined with different severities of renal impairment. Experts suggest that apixaban can be used with caution with P-gp/moderate CYP3A4 inhibitors making it a possible choice for this patient [1, 5].

Edoxaban and Dabigatran with P-gp Inhibitors

Mixed P-gp/CYP3A4 inhibitors exert their effect of increased exposure of edoxaban primarily through P-gp inhibition. A wide variation of increased exposure exists between different P-gp inhibitors and edoxaban ranging from 12% with quinidine to 157% with dronedarone [6]. In the ENGAGE TIMI AF trial, 50% dose reductions were studied for patients on the strong P-gp inhibitors quinidine, verapamil, or dronaderone. Because blood levels of edoxaban were found to be lower in these patients compared to those on full dose edoxaban, current prescribing information does not recommend avoiding use or implementing dose adjustments for any of the P-gp inhibitors. However, it is important to note that the use of other P-gp inhibitors, such as cyclosporine and protease inhibitors, was not permitted in the ENGAGE TIMI AF trial. Therefore, combined use of P-gp inhibitors outside of those studied in ENGAGE TIMI AF should be avoided [2, 4]. Renal function is important to consider for edoxaban dosing as well because 50% of the medication is eliminated in the urine. Patients with creatinine clearances above 95 mL/min should not use edoxaban due to increased clearance of the medication [5]. Severe renal impairment prohibits use. Due to the degree of renal impairment for the patient above, and the unknown degree of increased edoxaban exposure with diltiazem, edoxaban should be avoided for this patient.

Similar to edoxaban, dabigatran is a P-gp substrate. Mixed P-gp/CYP3A4 inhibitors increase dabigatran exposure through the P-gp inhibition. Unique to dabigatran, recommendations for use with P-gp inhibitors is dependent upon the indication for treatment. The specific P-gp inhibitor is also a variable to be considered. In atrial fibrillation patients with impaired renal function between 30 and 50 mL/min, reduce the dose of dabigatran by 50% if patients use ketoconazole or dronedarone [1, 2]. Prescribing information does not provide recommendations for other P-gp inhibitors in patients with the same degree of renal impairment but does advise use with any P-gp inhibitor in patients <30 mL/min is not recommended. If a patient is using a P-gp inhibitor (other than ketoconazole and dronedarone), caution should be advised and dose reductions employed [4]. In this case scenario, the patient's renal function is severely impaired and near the cut-off for avoidance of use of dabigatran and P-gp inhibitors in combination. The risks of dabigatran accumulation and subsequent risk of bleeding likely outweigh the benefit of dabigatran.

Is Any Additional Monitoring Required When Adding a DOAC for this Patient?

The anticoagulant activity of the DOACs follows a predictable dose-response relationship [5]. This quality makes laboratory monitoring unnecessary in most scenarios, a main advantage of the DOACs when comparing them to warfarin.

However, there are some specific scenarios where the quantification of anticoagulant activity would be useful for the management of the patient. The need to identify if excessive levels of anticoagulation are present may be helpful in cases of hemorrhage, diminishing renal function, and drug interactions which may increase or decrease efficacy [5]. Utilizing an anti-Xa level in the setting of rivaroxaban, apixaban, and edoxaban use is preferred over PT or aPTT [7]. However, anti-Xa assays must be calibrated to the specific factor Xa inhibitor in order to assess the quantitative degree of anticoagulation [4]. Monitoring for excessive levels of dabigatran requires timely laboratory tests such as dilute thrombin time and ecarin clotting time [4, 7]. Because of the limited availability of these anticoagulant monitoring laboratory tests, application and widespread use is also limited.

Key Points

- The degree of inhibition of mixed P-gp/3A4 inhibitors is important in determining appropriate management of the interaction with the DOACs (see Tables 31.1 and 31.2).
- Renal function must be assessed as part of the drug interaction analysis with the DOACs.
- A majority of the guidance for use of mixed P-gp/CYP3A4 inhibitors combined with the DOACs is based on pharmacokinetic studies. Whether these interactions pose an increased risk of bleeding in actual patients remains unclear but caution is warranted.

Table 31.1 Mixed P-gp/CYP3A4 inhibitors and inducers [1, 4, 5]

Characteristic	Common medication examples[a]	
Strong mixed P-gp/CYP3A4 inhibitors	Clarithromycin	Nelfinavir
	Conivaptan	Posaconazole
	Indinavir	Ritonavir
	Intraconazole	Saquinavir
	Ketoconazole	Telithromycin
Moderate mixed P-gp/CYP3A4 inhibitors	Cyclosporine	Erythromycin
	Diltiazem	Tamoxifen
	Dronaderone	Verapamil
Strong mixed P-gp/CYP3A4 inducers	Carbamazepine	
	Phenytoin	
	Rifampin	
	St. John's wort	

[a]List is not exhaustive

31 Management of Direct Oral Anticoagulants with Mixed P-gp/3A4 Drug-Drug

Table 31.2 Drug interaction management [1, 4, 5]

Direct oral anticoagulant	Interacting medications	Management strategy
Apixaban	Strong mixed P-gp/CYP3A4 inhibitors	Reduce dose by 50% If on 2.5 mg BID, avoid combination
	Moderate mixed P-gp/CYP3A4 inhibitors	No dose adjustment required
	Strong mixed P-gp/CYP3A4 inducers	Avoid combination
Rivaroxaban	Strong mixed P-gp/CYP3A4 inhibitors	Avoid combination
	Moderate mixed P-gp/CYP3A4 inhibitors	Consider alternative if CrCl is <80 mL/min
	Strong mixed P-gp/CYP3A4 inducers	Avoid combination
Edoxaban	P-gp inhibitors	Afib: no dose adjustment required for quinidine, verapamil, or dronaderone. Avoid combination with other strong inhibitors[a] VTE: decrease dose from 60 to 30 mg daily
	P-gp inducers	Avoid combination[b]
Dabigatran	P-gp inhibitors	Afib: decrease dose from 150 to 75 mg BID if combined with dronaderone or ketoconazole when CrCl is 30–50 mL/min. If CrCl is <30 mL/min, avoid combination VTE treatment and prophylaxis after hip surgery: avoid combination if CrCl < 50 mL/min
	P-gp inducers	Avoid combination

[a]Recommendation based on expert opinion. CrCl = creatinine clearance
[b]Supporting data is with rifampin. Recommendation extrapolated to all strong P-gp inducers until more data is available

Self-Assessment Questions

1. A 68-year-old male presents to internal medicine clinic for his annual appointment. He has been taking rivaroxaban 20 mg daily for the past year for a history of atrial fibrillation. His other medical history includes hypertension, chronic kidney disease, and obesity. In addition to rivaroxaban, his medications include amlodipine, dronedarone, and losartan. Upon further review, you notice his renal function has steadily declined over the past year from a CrCl of 65 mL/min to a CrCl of 35 mL/min today. Which of the following is the most appropriate plan for his anticoagulation?

    (a) Continue rivaroxaban 20 mg daily
    (b) Continue rivaroxaban at a decreased dose of 15 mg daily
    (c) Stop rivaroxaban and initiate dabigatran 150 mg twice daily
    (d) Stop rivaroxaban and initiate warfarin titrated to an INR goal of 2–3

The correct answer is D. Although an interaction exists with dronedarone, the patient's INR can be monitored to prevent over-anticoagulation. Answer A and B are incorrect because the presence of renal impairment in combination with a moderate P-gp/CYP3A4 inhibitor is not recommended with rivaroxaban unless the benefits outweigh the risks. Answer C is incorrect because of dabigatran's interaction with P-gp inhibitors. In treatment of atrial fibrillation, dronaderone and dabigatran used in combination in patients with moderate renal failure (CrCl 30–50 mL/min) can increase dabigatran exposure to levels similar to those in severe renal failure. Therefore, the dose of dabigatran should be reduced to 75 mg twice daily.

2. Which of the following statements is true for a patient with normal renal function?

   (a) Rivaroxaban should be stopped if itraconazole is initiated
   (b) Apixaban should be stopped if itraconazole is initiated
   (c) Rivaroxaban should be stopped if verapamil is initiated
   (d) Apixaban should be stopped if verapamil is initiated

The correct answer is A. Rivaroxaban should be avoided when a strong P-gp/CYP3A4 inhibitor like itraconazole is initiated regardless of the patient's renal function. Apixaban can be continued in the presence of a strong P-gp/CYP3A4 inhibitor. A 50% dose reduction is warranted in this scenario. In the presence of verapamil, a moderate P-gp/CYP3A4 inhibitor, both rivaroxaban and apixaban can be continued when a patient's renal function is normal and therefore answer C and D are both incorrect choices.

References

1. Hellwig T, Gulseth M. Pharmacokinetic and pharmacodynamic drug interactions with new oral anticoagulants: what do they mean for patients with atrial fibrillation? Ann Pharmacother. 2013;47(11):1478–87.
2. Kovacs RJ, Flaker GC, Saxonhouse SJ, Doherty JU, Birtcher KK, Cuker A, Davidson BL, Giugliano RP, Granger CB, Jaffer AK, Mehta BH, Nutescu E, Williams KA. Practical management of anticoagulation in patients with atrial fibrillation. J Am Coll Cardiol. 2015;65(13):1340–60.
3. Patel MR, Mahaffey KW, Garg J, Pan G, Singer DE, Hacke W, Breithardt G, Halperin JL, Hankey GJ, Piccini JP, Becker RC, Nessel CC, Paolini JF, Berkowitz SD, Fox KA, Califf RM, The Rocket AF Steering Committee. Rivaroxaban versus warfarin in nonvalvular atrial fibrillation. N Engl J Med. 2011;365:883–91.
4. Nutescu EA, Burnett A, Fanikos J, Spinler S, Wittkowsky A. Pharmacology of anticoagulants used in the treatment of venous thromboembolism. J Thromb Thrombolysis. 2016;41: 15–31.
5. Burnett AE, Mahan CE, Vazquez SR, Oertel LB, Garcia DA, Ansell J. Guidance for the practical management of the direct oral anticoagulants (DOACs) in VTE treatment. J Thromb Thrombolysis. 2016;41:206–32.

6. Mendell J, Zahir H, Matsushima N, Noveck R, Lee F, Chen S, Zhang G, Shi M. Drug-drug interaction studies of cardiovascular drugs involving P-glycoprotein, an efflux transporter, on the pharmacokinetics of edoxaban, an oral factor Xa inhibitor. Am J Cardiovasc Drugs. 2013;13(5):331–42.
7. Cuker A, Siegal DM, Crowther MA, Garcia DA. Laboratory measurement of the anticoagulant activity of the non-vitamin K oral anticoagulants. J Am Coll Cardiol. 2014;64(11):1128–39.

Chapter 32
Pharmacokinetic Drug-Drug Interactions with Warfarin

Rachel C. Ieuter

Abstract Days since initiation of a drug, which has potential drug-drug interaction with warfarin, is an important factor to account for in determining anticipated clinical effect, timing of monitoring, and potential dose adjustments. It is important to understand how to assess approaches to warfarin management in the presence of pharmacokinetic interactions such as pre-emptive dose adjustments and "watch and wait" with additional monitoring.

Keywords Pharmacokinetic interactions • Phenytoin • Warfarin S-enantiomer • Warfarin R-enantiomer • Cytochrome P450 • Vitamin K oxide reductase • VKOR

Case Introduction

A 54-year-old woman receiving warfarin therapy for atrial fibrillation presents to the anticoagulation clinic on Monday for a 2-week follow up visit. The patient was diagnosed with atrial fibrillation 3 years ago and, presently, has remained therapeutic on warfarin 5 mg daily except 7.5 mg on Tuesday, Thursday, and Saturday. She reports that she was recently hospitalized for newly diagnosed seizure disorder and discharged on Friday with a prescription for phenytoin 100 mg three times daily. Prior to discharge her total phenytoin level was 12 mg/L, serum creatinine 0.9 mg/dL, serum albumin 4.2 g/dL, all other labs were within normal limits. Today her INR is 2.8. Since discharge she has resumed her home warfarin regimen and reports no side effects from phenytoin. Other medical problems include: hypertension and hyperlipidemia. Her only other medications are carvedilol, amlodipine, and atorvastatin—no additional new medications initiated since last anticoagulation visit.

R.C. Ieuter, PharmD, BCPS
Midwestern University Chicago College of Pharmacy, 555 31st Street, Downers Grove, IL 60515, USA

Loyola University Medical Center, 2160 S. First Avenue, Maywood, IL 60153, USA
e-mail: rieute@midwestern.edu

Case Discussion

What Factors Need to Be Considered When Assessing Potential Drug-Drug Interactions with Warfarin?

Several drug-drug interactions exist with warfarin, which are classified as either pharmacokinetic or pharmacodynamic drug-drug interactions. The focus of this case is pharmacokinetic interactions with warfarin; pharmacodynamic interactions are discussed elsewhere (see Chap. 30). Pharmacokinetics describes the movement of drug into, through, and out of the body [1]. More simply stated it is what the body does to the drug during the time that the drug is absorbed, distributed, metabolized, and excreted from the body. Briefly, warfarin is completely absorbed following oral administration with peak plasma concentrations within 4 h and is excreted mainly via urine and bile as inactive metabolites [2, 3]. Warfarin is highly protein bound to serum albumin, and therefore has a small volume of distribution with the drug largely remaining in the circulation. When there is competitive displacement of warfarin from its protein binding sites this leads to an increase in volume of distribution. As a result, there is an increased anticoagulant effect because more drug is free to inhibit the mechanism of action site, the Vitamin K Oxide Reductase. This enzyme plays a role in the production of vitamin K-dependent clotting factors [2, 3]. The most important enzyme system of phase I metabolism is cytochrome P450 (CYP450), because it is responsible for many drug-drug interactions in which one drug may enhance the toxicity or reduce the therapeutic effect of another drug [1]. Warfarin is metabolized via CYP2C9 (S enantiomer) and CYP1A2 and CYP3A4 (R enantiomer) [2, 3]. Thus, an understanding of how CYP inhibition or induction will effect warfarin dose requirements is important (see Table 32.1, Fig. 32.1).

Drug-Drug Interaction: Distribution

For patients newly initiated on phenytoin it is important to understand the bi-phasic drug-drug interaction with warfarin. Phenytoin and warfarin are both extensively protein bound at 90–95% and 99%, respectively. As a result, phenytoin displaces warfarin from its plasma protein binding sites which leads to a transient increase in its anticoagulant effects. This initial increase in INR occurs, typically, within 1–3 days [4]. This patient has been taking concomitant warfarin and phenytoin for more than 3 days and has likely experienced the transient increase in INR during hospitalization. We do not anticipate the patient's phenytoin dose to change in the immediate future based on the therapeutic total phenytoin level and no report of adverse drug events. Currently, it is not recommended to empirically dose adjust for this pharmacokinetic drug-drug interaction [5].

Table 32.1 Pharmacokinetic drug-drug interactions with warfarin

	Change in PK parameter	Expected change in INR	Drug interactions
Absorption	↓	↓ INR	Bile acid sequestrants
			Sucralfate
Distribution	↑	↑ INR	Metronidazole
			Phenytoin
			Salicylates (large doses)
			Sulfa (large doses)
Metabolism	↑	↓ INR	2C9:
			Carbamazepine
			Phenobarbital
			Phenytoin
			Rifampin
			3A4:
			Phenobarbital
			Phenytoin
			Rifampin
			St. John's wort
			1A2: tobacco smoke
	↓	↑ INR	2C9/19:
			Amiodarone
			Fluconazole
			Fluvastatin
			Metronidazole
			Propafenone
			Trimethoprim/sulfamethoxazole
			3A4:
			Cimetidine
			Clarithromycin
			Fluconazole
			Fluoxetine
			Gemfibrozil
			Ketoconazole
			Ritonavir

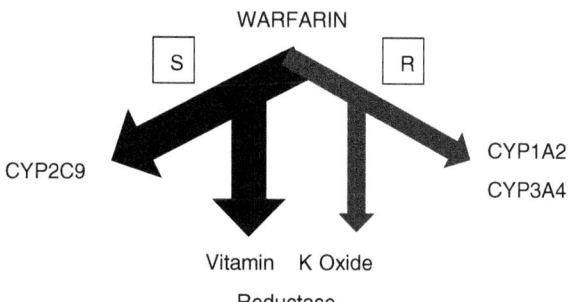

Fig. 32.1 Warfarin metabolism and relative potency

Drug-Drug Interaction: Metabolism

With long-term use of warfarin and phenytoin the drug-drug interaction transitions to induction of warfarin hepatic metabolism. This patient will be on lifelong anticoagulation for atrial fibrillation and, if otherwise tolerated, will remain on phenytoin long-term to control her seizure disorder. Therefore, it is important to understand the anticipated onset of induction in order to dose adjust warfarin appropriately. Warfarin is a racemic mixture consisting of an R-enantiomer and S-enantiomer [4]. Although it has a shorter half-life, the S-enantiomer is more pharmacologically active and impairs blood clotting 3–5 times more than the R-enantiomer. Each enantiomer is metabolized by different hepatic pathways. The S-enantiomer is predominantly hydroxylated via CYP2C9 enzymes whereas the R-enantiomer is metabolized via CYP3A4 and CYP1A2 enzymes (see Table 32.1) [4]. This is a key point given that phenytoin is a potent inducer of 2C9 and 3A4 [6]. Medications that preferentially induce metabolism of the more potent S-enantiomer increase its clearance and impair anticoagulation to a greater extent. This subsequent drug-drug interaction typically occurs within 1 week of concomitant therapy [7]. Although, the onset may demonstrate patient variability as there are case reports describing increased warfarin requirements after 2–4 weeks of concomitant therapy which may likely be due to continued induction of the CYP enzymes [5]. This patient will require close follow-up with weekly INR monitoring and warfarin dose increases as indicated to maintain therapeutic INR. Patient variability exists with warfarin dose adjustment ranging from 50–75% dose increase [8]. To add complexity to this drug-drug interaction continual assessment of the patient's overall status is important such as age, dietary vitamin K intake, hepatic dysfunction, renal dysfunction, and fluid overload state. Age: In the elderly, the half-life of some drugs may be remarkably long which results in increased therapeutic effects (i.e. phenytoin). Dietary vitamin K intake: Changes in the amount of vitamin K consumed can alter the metabolism of warfarin. For example, if a patient normally eats one serving per day of food high in vitamin K and suddenly increases to three servings per day there will be a subsequent decrease in INR. Therefore, a crucial counseling point for patients is to stress the importance of consistent vitamin K intake. Hepatic dysfunction: Due to decreased production of clotting factors, hepatic dysfunction may lead to a significantly elevated INR. This patient population will require decreased warfarin requirements. Renal dysfunction: Reduced renal function leads to the accumulation of renally excreted phenytoin. The resultant effect is increased serum levels of phenytoin and more potent CYP2C9 and CYP3A4-mediated induction of warfarin. Additionally, renal dysfunction is oftentimes associated with hypoalbuminemia. This is clinically significant because, as stated previously, warfarin and phenytoin are highly protein bound. Thus, hypoalbuminemia patients will require decreased warfarin requirements and close monitoring of total phenytoin levels to limit the risk of toxicity. Fluid overload state: In the presence of significant congestion warfarin is unable to reach its site of action, the liver, to be metabolized and exert its anticoagulant effects. This leads to increased warfarin requirements to maintain a therapeutic INR. Overall, it is important to continually weigh the risks and benefits of managing warfarin with certain drug-drug interactions as compared to switching anticoagulation therapy to a direct oral anticoagulant. These newer drugs are not without their own inherent interactions; therefore warfarin is commonly continued with more frequent monitoring.

Factors to Consider: Continuing Warfarin Versus Switching Anticoagulation Therapy

Ascertaining whether the patient can be initiated on alternative anticoagulation therapy, such as the direct oral anticoagulants, is challenging because phenytoin is also a potent CYP3A4 inducer [9]. The clinical implication is a decreased anticoagulation effect of the direct oral anticoagulants, thus increasing thrombotic risk. Additionally, the indication for anticoagulation should be considered since the direct oral anticoagulants do not have the same scope of FDA-approved indications as compared to warfarin. For example, the patient in our case has atrial fibrillation. It is important to assess the underlying etiology of her atrial fibrillation, valvular versus non-valvular. Adherence to warfarin is a crucial factor to assess if a patient is a candidate for warfarin therapy. Oftentimes patients' dose may vary from day-to-day (i.e. one-half tablet every other day) leading to a complex total weekly regimen. Furthermore, an understanding of dietary constraints and consistent vitamin K intake is another factor to assess in a patient who may have a history of labile INRs. Lastly, the percent time in therapeutic INR range should be assessed, especially in patients who require long-term anticoagulation. Usually, for those in the therapeutic INR range <60% of the time a direct oral anticoagulant would be a feasible option.

How Should the Patient's Situation Be Managed?

The patient should resume her current home warfarin regimen (5 mg daily except 7.5 mg on Tuesday, Thursday, and Saturday) given that she has been on concomitant warfarin and phenytoin for more than 3 days. The transient increase in INR due to displacement of warfarin from its protein binding sites is a less clinically significant drug interaction, and it is not recommended to empirically decrease the warfarin dose [5]. The patient should have more frequent clinic visits to monitor the INR trend. Ideally, repeat INR in 1 week (patient will be on phenytoin for 2 weeks at this point and more likely to see effects of metabolism induction) and adjust total weekly dose accordingly to maintain therapeutic INR.

Key Points

- Days since initiation of a medication, which has potential drug-drug interaction with warfarin, is an important factor to account for in determining anticipated clinical effect, timing of monitoring, and potential dose adjustments
- Assess approaches to warfarin management, such as pre-emptive dose adjustments as compared to "watch and wait" with additional monitoring
- For patients receiving warfarin the INR should be initially monitored more frequently when drug-drug interactions are introduced and appropriately adjust warfarin dose as necessary

Self-Assessment Questions

1. A 71-year-old man presents to the urgent care clinic complaining of prolonged bleeding from a cut on his cheek after shaving this morning. He is receiving warfarin 7.5 mg daily for atrial fibrillation. Other medical problems include: hypertension, type 2 diabetes, and hyperlipidemia. Labs including CBC are within normal limits. Today INR is 3.4. His vital signs are stable. Upon further questioning, the patient states that he quit smoking cigarettes 2 weeks ago cold turkey (30 pack year history). Which of the following is the correct drug-drug interaction between warfarin and cigarette smoke?

    (a) Cigarette smoke is a CYP1A2 inducer; therefore smoking cessation may result in an increase in warfarin total weekly dose.
    (b) Cigarette smoke is a CYP1A2 inhibitor; therefore smoking cessation may result in a decrease in warfarin total weekly dose.
    (c) Cigarette smoke is a CYP2C9 inducer; therefore smoking cessation may result in a decrease in warfarin total weekly dose.
    (d) Cigarette smoke is a CYP2C9 inhibitor; therefore smoking cessation may result in an increase in warfarin total weekly dose.

    Explanation: Correct answer is A. Cigarette smoke is a CYP1A2 inducer which leads to an increase in the metabolism of the R enantiomer of warfarin and thus may result in an increased warfarin total weekly dose. Therefore, upon cessation of tobacco products patients will require more frequent INR monitoring and, ultimately, may require a higher total weekly dose of warfarin.

2. A 59-year-old-woman receiving warfarin 4 mg daily for 2 months for an unprovoked PE was recently prescribed cholestyramine resin three times daily with meals for her difficult to control hypercholesterolemia. Which of the following is the best plan to manage this patient's new medication?

    (a) Take cholestyramine at least 30 min after warfarin dose in order to avoid decreased absorption of warfarin.

(b) Cholestyramine may cause an increase in INR via CYP3A4 inhibition; patient may require decrease in total weekly dose.
(c) Take cholestyramine at least 4 h after warfarin dose in order to avoid decreased absorption of warfarin.
(d) Cholestyramine may cause a decrease in INR via CYP2C9 induction; patient may require increase in total weekly dose.

Explanation: Correct answer is C. The drug-drug interaction between warfarin and cholestyramine is an absorption issue; it is not mediated by hepatic metabolism (answers B and D incorrect). Cholestyramine is a bile acid sequestrant that leads to decreased serum warfarin concentrations by ~50%. It mainly binds warfarin in the GI tract. Data demonstrates that following one dose administered 30 min after warfarin still decreased serum warfarin concentrations by 50% (answer A incorrect), therefore it is recommended to separate administration by at least 2 h, ideally would recommend to administer 4 h after.

References

1. Le J. Overview of pharmacokinetics. Merck Manuals. 2016. http://www.merckmanuals.com/professional/clinical-pharmacology/pharmacokinetics/overview-of-pharmacokinetics
2. Jacobs L. Warfarin pharmacology, clinical management, and evaluation of hemorrhagic risk for the elderly. Cardiol Clin. 2008;26:157–67.
3. Wells PS, Holbrook AM, Crowther NR, et al. Interactions of warfarin with drugs and food. Ann Intern Med. 1994;121(9):676–83.
4. Cropp JS, Bussey HI. A review of enzyme induction of warfarin metabolism with recommendations for patient management. Pharmacotherapy. 1997;17(5):917–28.
5. Bungard TJ, Yakiwchuk E, Foisy M, et al. Drug interactions involving warfarin: practice tool and practical management tips. CPJ. 2011;144(1):21–5.
6. Lexi-Comp online. Lexi-Interactions. Hudson, OH: Lexi-Comp, Inc.; 2015. https://online.lexi.com/lco/action/interact. Accessed 20 June 2016.
7. Levine M, Sheppard I. Biphasic interaction of phenytoin and warfarin. Clin Pharm. 1984;3(2):200–3.
8. Hansen JM, Siersbaek-Nielsen K, Kristensen M, et al. Effect of diphenylhydantoin on the metabolism of dicoumarol in man. Acta Med Scand. 1971;189:15.
9. Phenytoin. Lexi-Comp online. Lexi-Drugs. Hudson, OH: Lexi-Comp, Inc.; 2015. https://online.lexi.com/lco/action/doc/retrieve/docid/patch_f/7489. Accessed 20 June 2015.

Part VII
Special Populations

Chapter 33
Chronic Pain Management with Anticoagulation

Leah Sera

Abstract Many commonly used analgesics increase the risk of bleeding by various mechanisms. This case reviews this risk and how patients planning to undergo invasive procedures for chronic pain should discuss the risks and benefits of suspending anticoagulation with their care provider.

Keywords Chronic pain • Pain management • Interventional pain management NSAIDs • Gastrointestinal hemorrhage • Acetaminophen • Tramadol • Adjuvants Antidepressants

Case Introduction

OW is a 60-year old man with type 2 diabetes and persistent low back pain resulting from a motor vehicle accident for which he takes acetaminophen 650 mg every 4 h as needed (uses 2–3 doses per day). He is diagnosed with atrial fibrillation after presenting to the emergency department with shortness of breath and dizziness and was started on warfarin 5 mg daily. His other medications include gabapentin 300 mg three times daily for diabetic neuropathy, metformin, sitagliptin, and melatonin at night for insomnia. During a routine clinic visit 5 months later, he states that he has started seeing a pain specialist for his worsening back pain who has suggested an epidural steroid injection. He states that his current pain regimen includes naproxen 250 mg twice daily, oxycodone/acetaminophen 5 mg/325 mg two tablets every 4 h as needed (using 2–3 doses per day), and duloxetine 30 mg daily. His other medications have not changed.

L. Sera, PharmD, BCPS
Department of Pharmacy Practice and Science, University of Maryland School of Pharmacy, 9640 Gudelsky Dr., Building 1 Room 304, Rockville, MD 20850, USA
e-mail: lsera@rx.umaryland.edu

© Springer International Publishing AG 2017
K. Kiser (ed.), *Oral Anticoagulation Therapy*,
DOI 10.1007/978-3-319-54643-8_33

Case Discussion

Medical Management of Chronic Pain in Patients on Anticoagulants

How Do Different Classes of Pain Medications Interact with Anticoagulants?

Acetaminophen

Acetaminophen is considered the analgesic of choice for mild to moderate pain because of its relative safety compared to non-steroidal anti-inflammatory drugs (NSAIDs) [1]. The interaction between acetaminophen and warfarin leading to an increased risk of bleeding has long been recognized. Examples in the medical literature include case reports and prospective studies, many of which examine the association between acetaminophen use and elevated international normalized ratio (INR) [2]. While the mechanism underlying this interaction has yet to be fully elucidated, proposed mechanisms include the inhibition of warfarin metabolism or interference with the formation of clotting factors [3]. In prospective studies, doses between 2 and 4 g per day often resulted in increased INR measurements. This effect was reversed within days of discontinuing acetaminophen use [2]. The onset of this interaction generally occurred within 1–2 weeks [4]. Direct oral anticoagulants (DOACs) do not appear to interact with acetaminophen.

NSAIDs

The combination of NSAIDs and anticoagulants may increase the risk of gastrointestinal bleeding. NSAIDs cause gastrointestinal toxicity by both systemic and local mechanisms. NSAIDs inhibit cyclo-oxygenase (COX), an enzyme which is responsible for the generation of prostaglandins that protect the gastric and duodenal mucosa [5]. Additionally, NSAIDs, being acids, are not ionized in the acidic environment of the gastric lumen and may be absorbed across the gastric mucosa and cause cell damage [6]. NSAIDs also have antiplatelet activity due to the inhibition of COX-1 and consequently decreased production of thromboxane A2, which promotes platelet aggregation. The specific gastrointestinal risk varies between drugs and is dose-related [7]. In a prospective study of over 2000 patients undergoing colonoscopies, NSAIDs, warfarin, and low-dose aspirin were associated with acute lower gastrointestinal bleeding and diverticular bleeding, and increased the risk of clinically significant bleeding [8]. Another study of over 150,000 patients hospitalized with atrial fibrillation found that use of NSAIDs increased the risk of serious bleeding for patients on antithrombotic therapy, and even short term NSAID increased bleeding risk [9]. A similar result was seen in patients receiving antithrombotic therapy after myocardial infarction. The risk of bleeding was doubled if patients were taking NSAIDs in addition to antiplatelet agents or anticoagulants, and the increased risk occurred as early as 3 days after initiation of NSAID therapy [10]. According to the American College of Gastroenterology, patients taking NSAIDs along with anticoagulants, corticosteroids, or aspirin (even low-dose) are at moderate risk of GI bleed and should consider use of a COX-2 inhibitor or traditional non-selective NSAID plus misoprostol or a proton pump inhibitor (PPI) for gastroprotection [11]. Patients with additional risk factors, such as age greater than 65 or history of ulcer, should consider alternative therapy, or use of a COX-2 inhibitor plus misoprostol or high dose PPI if NSAID therapy is absolutely necessary [11].

Opioids

There are few clinically significant drug interactions between opioids and anticoagulants related to increased risk of bleeding or thrombosis, or interactions affecting the metabolism of anticoagulants. Three case reports have been published describing an interaction between tramadol and warfarin leading to supratherapeutic INR. A proposed mechanism of this interaction is competition for cytochrome P450 3A4 that increases R-warfarin levels [12]. In two case reports, INR returned to normal after discontinuation of tramadol [13, 14]. In the third case the patient INR was stabilized after dose adjustment of warfarin and tramadol was continued; in this case the authors recommended reducing the warfarin dose by 25% and monitoring INR closely if long-term tramadol therapy is being initiated [12]. This interaction has not been reported with DOACs. Although, sedation is a common adverse effect of opioids, likely related to their anticholinergic properties [15] a meta-analysis found that narcotic analgesics did not increase the risk of falls in the elderly [16]. Tolerance often develops to sedation and slow dose titration can help mitigate this adverse effect for patients requiring analgesics for severe pain [15].

Adjuvants

Antidepressants are frequently used in the treatment of neuropathic pain. Serotonergic drugs may increase the risk of gastrointestinal bleeding. The proposed mechanism impaired platelet aggregation resulting from decreased platelet serotonin [17]. A meta-analysis found that the use of SSRIs alone modestly increased the risk of gastrointestinal bleeding and this risk increased significantly when patients were also taking NSAIDs [18]. Several case reports describe episodes of bleeding with venlafaxine or duloxetine, which are serotonin-norepinephrine reuptake inhibitors (SNRIs). In two reports, bleeding associated with venlafaxine ceased approximately 1 week after discontinuation of the drug, a time course consistent with the platelet lifespan [19, 20].

Issues Related to Interventional Pain Management

When Should Anticoagulants Be Discontinued Prior to Interventional Pain Management Procedures?

Interventional pain management involves the use of invasive procedures for the management of chronic pain. Such procedures include targeted injection of drugs, nerve ablation, discectomy, and implantation of infusion pumps and spinal cord stimulators [21]. Decisions about discontinuation of antithrombotic therapy prior to a planned procedure depend on the patient's condition (i.e., risk of thrombosis) and the bleeding risk associated with the procedure [22]. Factors that increase the bleeding risk include larger needle size, close proximity to vascular or significant neurologic structures, and having the target in a confined space [22]. For high-risk or moderate-risk procedures, warfarin should be discontinued in time to achieve an INR less than 1.4 or 2.0, respectively. Dabigatran may be stopped between 1 and 4 days prior to a procedure in patients with normal renal function, depending on the associated bleeding risk (patients with impaired renal function should discontinue dabigatran at least 4–5 days prior to any procedure). Limited evidence suggests that rivaroxaban may be stopped for a day or longer prior to a planned procedure [22].

How Should this Patient Be Managed?

In order to optimize OW's pain management regimen while appropriately managing his atrial fibrillation with warfarin, his naproxen should be discontinued to decrease the risk of gastrointestinal bleeding. Continue the oxycodone/acetaminophen, but educate the patient that moderate to large daily doses of acetaminophen can affect INR. Duloxetine may also be continued, but it would be prudent to educate the patient regarding signs and symptoms of bleeding. Ask the patient to get more information about any planned invasive procedure with the interventional specialist so that a plan can be developed regarding temporary discontinuation of warfarin.

Key Points

- Acetaminophen, NSAIDs, tramadol, and antidepressants may all increase the risk of bleeding either by interfering with the metabolism of warfarin or by impairing the activity of platelets.
- The interaction between antithrombotic agents and NSAIDs is well-documented and leads to increased risk of gastrointestinal bleeding. Patients on antithrombotic therapy should utilize acetaminophen preferably to NSAIDs—despite the potential for acetaminophen to increase INR it is still considered the safer option for patients in need of an antipyretic or analgesic for mild to moderate pain.

- The decision to suspend anticoagulants prior to planned invasive procedures for chronic pain should be made with respect to the patient's condition and bleeding risk associated with the procedure.

Self-Assessment Questions

1. A 72-year old woman with a past medical history of atrial fibrillation on warfarin, hypertension, hyperlipidemia, and osteoarthritis presents for a routine clinic visit with an INR of 3.4. Her INRs have been therapeutic for the last several months without much fluctuation. She denies signs or symptoms of bleeding and the only change to her medications has been an increased use of acetaminophen (650 mg 4–5 times daily, pain is controlled). Up until 2 weeks ago when her pain worsened her pain was controlled with 1–2 doses of acetaminophen per day. Along with recommending workup for the new pain complaint with her primary care provide, what is the most reasonable course of action?
   (a) Adjust the warfarin dose and monitor INR more closely until stabilized.
   (b) Discontinue the acetaminophen and recommend tramadol 50 mg by mouth four times daily as needed
   (c) Decrease the acetaminophen to a maximum of two doses per day and recommend oxycodone 5 mg every 4 h as needed.
   (d) Continue the current plan of care and monitor INR more frequently.

   Rationale: A is the correct answer. Acetaminophen, although it may increase INR at doses >2 g per day, is preferred over NSAIDs for moderate pain. B is incorrect because tramadol may also increase the INR and therefore offers no individual benefit (and is less well tolerated than acetaminophen). C is not the best answer because her pain is controlled on acetaminophen and increasing pill burden is unnecessary when pain is not severe. D is not the best answer because continuing her current plan of care doesn't address the increased bleeding risk with a supratherapeutic INR.

2. A 68 year old man with a past medical history of hypothyroidism, depression, anxiety, hypertension, type 2 diabetes with peripheral neuropathy, and DVT is taking the following medications: rivaroxaban 20 mg daily, venlafaxine 75 mg daily, tramadol 50 mg every 6 h as needed (uses 1–2 doses per day), acetaminophen 650 mg every 4 h as needed for pain (uses occasionally), levothyroxine 50 mcg daily, lisinopril 10 mg daily, metformin 500 mg twice daily. Which of her medications (other than the rivaroxaban) is most likely to increase her risk of bleeding?

   (a) venlafaxine
   (b) tramadol
   (c) lisinopril
   (d) acetaminophen

Rationale: Venlafaxine is the correct answer due to its effect on platelet homeostasis. Tramadol and acetaminophen may increase the risk of bleeding by affecting warfarin metabolism, but this does not appear to be a problem with new oral anticoagulants. Lisinopril does not increase the risk of bleeding.

References

1. Shek KL, Chan L, Nutescu E. Wafarin-acetaminophen drug interaction revisited. Pharmacotherapy. 1999;19(10):1153–8.
2. Hughes GJ, Patel PN, Saxena N. Effect of acetaminophen on international normalized ratio in patients receiving warfarin therapy. Pharmacotherapy. 2011;31(6):591–7.
3. Mahe I, Bertrand N, Drouet L, Sollier C, Simoneau G, Mazoyer E, et al. Interaction between paracetamol and warfarin in patients: a double-blind, placebo-controlled, randomized study. Haematologica. 2006;91:1621–7.
4. Parra D, Beckey NP, Stevens GR. The effect of acetaminophen on the international normalized ratio in patients stabilized on warfarin therapy. Pharmacotherapy. 2007;27(5):675–83.
5. Cryer B, Feldman M. Cyclooxygenase-1 and cyclooxygenase-2 selectivity of widely used nonsteroidal anti-inflammatory drugs. Am J Med. 1998;104(5):413–21.
6. Flower RJ. The development of COX2 inhibitors. Nat Rev Drug Discov. 2003;2(3):179–91.
7. Moore N, Pollack C, Butkerait P. Adverse drug reactions and drug-drug interactions with over-the-counter NSAIDs. Ther Clin Risk Manag. 2015;11:1061–75.
8. Hreinsson JP, Palsdottir S, Bjornsson ES. The association of drugs with severity and specific causes of acute lower gastrointestinal bleeding: a prospective study. J Clin Gastroenterol. 2016;50:408–13.
9. Lamberts M, Lip GY, Hansen ML, Lindhardsen J, Oleson JB, Raunso J, et al. Relation of nonsteroidal anti-inflammatory drugs to serious bleeding and thromboembolism risk in patients with atrial fibrillation receiving antithrombotic therapy: a nationwide cohort study. Ann Intern Med. 2014;161(10):690–8.
10. Scherning Olsen AM, Gislason GH, McGettigan P, Fosbol E, Sorensen R, Hansen ML, et al. Association of NSAID use with risk of bleeding and cardiovascular events in patients receiving antithrombotic therapy after myocardial infarction. JAMA. 2015;313(8):805–14.
11. Lanza FL, Chan FK, Eamonn MM. Practice Parameters Committee of the American College of Gastroenterology. Prevention of NSAID-related ulcer complications. Am J Gastroenterol. 2009;104:728–38.
12. Dumo PA, Keilbasa LA. Successful anticoagulation and continuation of tramadol therapy in the setting of a tramadol-warfarin interaction. Pharmacotherapy. 2006;26(11):1654–7.
13. Sabbe JR, Sims PJ, Sims MH. Tramadol-warfarin interaction. Pharmacotherapy. 1998;18(4):871–3.
14. Scher ML, Huntington NH, Vitillo JA. Potential interaction between tramadol and warfarin (Letter). Ann Pharmacother. 1997;31:646–7.
15. Benyamin R, Trescotr AM, Datta S, et al. Opioid complications and side effects. Pain Physician. 2008;11(2 Suppl):S105–20.
16. Woolcott JC, Richardson KJ, Wiens MO, Patel B, Marin J, Khan KM, et al. Meta-analysis of the impact of 9 medication classes on falls in elderly persons. Arch Intern Med. 2009;169(21):1952–60.
17. Sereburany VL. Selective serotonin reuptake inhibitors and increased bleeding risk: are we missing something? Am J Med. 2006;119(2):113–6.
18. Anglin R, Yuan Y, Moayyedi P, Tse F, Armstrong D, Leontiadis GI. Risk of upper gastrointestinal bleeding with selective serotonin reuptake inhibitors with or without concurrent nonsteroidal anti-inflammatory use: a systemic review and meta-analysis. Am J Gastroenterol. 2014;109:811–9.

19. Linnebur SA, Saseen JJ, Pace WD. Venlafaxine-associated vaginal bleeding. Pharmacotherapy. 2002;22(5):652–5.
20. Yavasoglu I, Kadikoylu G, Bolaman Z. Gingival bleeding due to venlafaxine. Ann Pharmacother. 2008;42(1):144–5.
21. Manchikanti L, Falco FJ, Benyamin RM, et al. Assessment of bleeding risk of interventional techniques: a best evidence synthesis of practice patterns and perioperative management of anticoagulant and antithrombotic therapy. Pain Physician. 2013;16(2 Suppl):SE261–318.
22. Martinez Serrano B, Canser Cuenca E, Garcia Higuera E, et al. Anticoagulation and interventional pain management. Tech Reg Anesth Pain Manag. 2014;18:58–64.

Chapter 34
Anticoagulation Management in Atrial Fibrillation Catheter Ablation

Brian Cryder

Abstract Catheter ablation procedures carry both thrombotic and hemorrhagic risks that must be balanced in the periprocedural anticoagulant plan. Anticoagulation intensity should be reduced at the time of procedure, but maintained therapeutically before and after procedure to minimize risks.

Keywords Catheter ablation • Oral anticoagulants • Atrial fibrillation • Anticoagulation management • Periprocedural anticoagulation

Case Introduction

The patient is a 76 year old African American male patient who is taking warfarin due to a 2 year history of atrial fibrillation. His other past medical history includes heart failure (EF = 30%, which has worsened from 40% 1 year prior), CKD stage 3, hypertension, gout, and impaired fasting glucose. Current medications include: allopurinol, aspirin, atorvastatin, furosemide, lisinopril, metoprolol ER, pantoprazole, spironolactone, and warfarin 10 mg daily except 5 mg every Friday (65 mg weekly dose) with target INR 2–3. Current vitals include: BP 108/70, HR 72, RR 16, Wt 231 lb, BMI 36.2. Labs within normal limits except SCr 1.8 with GFR of 48. Last four INRs were 2.3, 2.5, 3.1 and 2.0. He has a family history of hypertension and stroke. All physical exam parameters were within normal limits at most recent physician visit. Most recent EKG: Atrial fibrillation with heart rate of 85 beats/min; Echocardiogram from last month: normal left ventricular size without hypertrophy, inferolateral hypokinesia present with decreased systolic function (EF 30%), abnormal left atrial volume, and normal right sided chamber dimensions. His cardiologist is recommending ablation to restore sinus rhythm due to his decline in systolic function.

B. Cryder, PharmD, BCACP
Midwestern University—Chicago College of Pharmacy, Downers Grove, IL 60515, USA

Advocate Medical Group, Chicago, IL 60625, USA
e-mail: bcryde@midwestern.edu

Case Discussion

Atrial fibrillation is among the most common arrhythmias and has links to several potential comorbidities. Cardiologists are more frequently recommending catheter ablation in symptomatic atrial fibrillation especially if the patient is refractory or intolerant of Class 1 or 3 antiarrhythmic medications [1]. In the past many held the popular belief that catheter ablation procedures would be corrective for atrial tachycardia thus eliminating the need for long term anticoagulation therapy. However, clinical experience with these procedures has shown that long term anticoagulation is still required in most cases despite initial sinus rhythm restoration.

When assessing anticoagulation therapy around the time of atrial fibrillation ablation, one must consider two major factors: (1) the change in thrombosis to hemorrhage risk balance before, during and after the procedure and (2) optimal anticoagulant medication selection [2].

Current guidelines recommend therapeutic anticoagulation a minimum of 4 weeks prior to ablation to minimize the risk of pre-existing thrombi dislodgement. Many clinicians will perform a pre-procedural transesophageal echocardiogram to ensure the lack of intracardiac thrombi, but recent research suggest that it may not be necessary in patients utilizing therapeutic warfarin or an oral Xa inhibitor [3, 4]. No data involving direct thrombin inhibitors and pre-procedure transesophageal echocardiogram is available at this time.

The procedure itself presents a complicated mix of thrombotic and hemorrhagic risks. The invasive nature of the catheterization usually would require full clearance or reversal of the anticoagulant, but the thrombotic risk triggered by the endothelial damage must be accounted for. Researchers have offered multiple anticoagulant strategies in the immediate days leading up to the ablation: (1) reverse or allow clearance of the chronic anticoagulant prior to ablation and "bridge" with low molecular weight heparin post-op if warfarin is the oral anticoagulant, or (2) do not interrupt the oral anticoagulant, but warfarin must be monitored closely to minimize hemorrhagic risk. Recent trends have favored continuous anticoagulation due to the associated lower bleeding risk with this method [1]. In our case scenario, warfarin was not interrupted, but a specific INR monitoring and dosing protocol is in place starting 2–3 days prior to the procedure to improve patient safety. While not formally addressed by the guidelines, a study by Kim and colleagues identified an INR target between 2.1 and 2.5 as the lowest hemorrhagic risk without compromising thromboembolic protection [5].

With all of the tight monitoring due to warfarin around the time of procedure, would it be preferable to utilize an oral direct thrombin or Xa inhibitor? Theoretically, the consistent therapeutic levels produced by the newer agents would provide a more predictable anticoagulant intensity with more room for lifestyle variation compared with warfarin. Most pre-procedural protocols request a 24–48 h window without dosing to allow clearance by the time of procedure. Recent data seems to imply that warfarin, apixaban, rivaroxaban, and dabigatran all have comparable

Table 34.1 Procedural considerations for anticoagulation for catheter ablation

	Pre-procedure (minimum 4 continuous weeks prior)	Peri-procedure	Post-procedure (minimum 2 continuous months after)
Warfarin	INR of at least 2.0	• Check INR 2–3 days prior to procedure • Ideal INR: 2.1–2.5 • If low: consider LMWH bridge • If high: reduce dose and monitor INR prior to procedure	INR of at least 2.0
DOAC	Ensure adherence with prescribed dose	• Last dose = 2 days prior to procedure • Restart at least 6 h after procedure completion	Ensure adherence with prescribed dose

safety data when used according to the appropriate drug specific protocols [6, 7]. Our case patient has been stable on warfarin chronically so there is no incentive at this time to alter medication selection, nor incentive to switch from a newer agent to warfarin if stable. Additionally, some cardiologists prefer warfarin due to its reversibility and amount of clinical experience with the drug.

Following the ablation, the patient remains at high thrombotic risk from the "stunning" of atrial tissue and direct endothelial injury induced by the procedure [1, 2]. Anticoagulants should be resumed within 6 h of vascular sheath removal and continued a minimum of 2 months [1]. Most patients will require long term anticoagulation regardless of cardiac rhythm if stroke risk is high as determined by the $CHADS_2$ or CHA_2DS_2-VASc scoring guidelines. In cases where low molecular weight heparins were used as a bridging agent, dosing should be continued until the warfarin has produced an INR ≥ 2.0. See Table 34.1 for a summary of catheter ablation procedure considerations around oral anticoagulants.

Key Points

- Catheter ablation procedures carry both thrombotic and hemorrhagic risks that must be balanced in the peri-procedural anticoagulant plan.
- Anticoagulation intensity should be reduced at the time of the procedure, with some preferring complete reversal and others advocating a lower, but still therapeutic level of intensity.
- All patients should receive therapeutically dosed anticoagulants for several weeks before and at least 2 months after ablation procedure.

- No current evidence suggests better outcomes with one specific oral anticoagulant medication over any other option.

Self-Assessment Questions

1. A common reason for catheter ablation is:
    (a) To eliminate the need for long term anticoagulants
    (b) To enhance the effectiveness of anticoagulant medications
    (c) To reduce patient symptoms associated with atrial fibrillation
    (d) To lower health related costs associated with atrial fibrillation

2. Thrombotic risk in catheter ablation is:
    (a) Only elevated if a thrombus is found in initial trans esophageal echocardiogram
    (b) Elevated due to the endothelial damage induced by the procedure
    (c) Elevated, but the hemorrhagic risk is significantly higher in priority
    (d) Only modestly elevated and does not require anticoagulant treatment in the several weeks surrounding the ablation procedure

3. Patients taking warfarin chronically prior to catheter ablation
    (a) Should have INR closely monitored, with pre-procedure target near 2.1–2.5
    (b) Should have INR closely monitored, with pre-procedure target near 1.4–1.9
    (c) Should have warfarin therapy interrupted with no additional heparin-based coverage
    (d) Should have warfarin switched to apixaban to further reduce periprocedural bleeding risk

Answers

1. C is correct; ablation does not eliminate anticoagulant need as risk of atrial fibrillation recurrence is high even if sinus rhythm is initially restored. There is no correlation between ablation and relative potency or effectiveness of anticoagulant medications. At this time there is no data suggesting health associated cost reduction from catheter ablation.
2. B is correct; thrombus identification does represent risk, but is not the only scenario in which the thrombotic risk is elevated. Both thrombotic and hemorrhagic risks are significant in catheter ablation, requiring careful modula-

tion of anticoagulant medication use in the immediate peri-procedural time period
3. A is correct; this INR intensity was shown to have the lowest risk compared to both lower and higher INR targets. Changing from warfarin to apixaban is not known to either increase or decrease hemorrhagic risk when either is used correctly in the setting of catheter ablation.

References

1. Calkins H, Kuck KH, Cappato R, et al. 2012 HRS/EHRA/ECAS Expert Consensus Statement on Catheter and Surgical Ablation of Atrial Fibrillation: recommendations for patient selection, procedural techniques, patient management and follow-up, definitions, endpoints, and research trial design. Heart Rhythm. 2012;9(4):632–717.
2. Weitz JI, Healey JS, Skanes AC, Verma A. Periprocedural management of new oral anticoagulants in patients undergoing atrial fibrillation ablation. Circulation. 2014;129:1688–94.
3. DiBiase L, Burkhardt JD, Santangeli P, et al. Periprocedural stroke and bleeding complications in patients undergoing catheter ablation of atrial fibrillation with different anticoagulation management. Circulation. 2014;129:2638–44.
4. DiBiase L, Briceno DF, Trivedi C, et al. Is transesophageal echocardiogram mandatory in patients undergoing ablation of atrial fibrillation with uninterrupted novel oral anticoagulants? Results from a prospective multicentre registry. Heart Rhythm. 2016;13(6):1197–202.
5. Kim JS, Jongnarangsin K, Latchamsetty R, et al. The optimal range of international normalized ratio for radiofrequency catheter ablation of atrial fibrillation during therapeutic anticoagulation with warfarin. Circ Arrhythm Electrophysiol. 2013;6:302–9.
6. Armbruster HL, Lindsley JP, Moranville MP, et al. Safety of novel oral anticoagulants compared with uninterrupted warfarin for catheter ablation of atrial fibrillation. Ann Pharmacother. 2015;49(3):278–84.
7. Rillig A, Lin T, Plesman J, et al. Apixaban, rivaroxaban, and dabigatran in patients undergoing atrial fibrillation ablation. J Cardiovasc Electrophysiol. 2016;27(2):147–53.

Chapter 35
Anticoagulation Management Considerations for Mechanical Valves

Denise M. Kolanczyk

Abstract All patients who receive mechanical valves should be anticoagulated with a vitamin K antagonist such as warfarin. The INR goal will be determined based on the type and location of the valve and patient-specific risk factors for thromboembolism.

Keywords Mechanical valves • On-X valves • Anticoagulation for mechanical valves • INR goal intensification • Valve thrombosis

Case Introduction

A 57-year-old Caucasian male is post-operative day #2 after undergoing a mechanical valve replacement for mitral stenosis. His past medical history includes hypertension, atrial fibrillation, and type 2 diabetes. He has had an uneventful post-operative course, and the cardiothoracic surgery team is ready to initiate warfarin for his mechanical valve. Prior to surgery, the patient was receiving rivaroxaban for stroke prevention in the setting of his atrial fibrillation. The patient has requested that he remain on rivaroxaban because he does not want to deal with the dietary restrictions and frequent INR monitoring appointments with warfarin.

D.M. Kolanczyk, PharmD, BCPS (AQ Cardiology)
Midwestern University Chicago College of Pharmacy, Downers Grove, IL 60515, USA

Loyola University Medical Center, Maywood, IL 60153, USA
e-mail: dkolan@midwestern.edu

Case Discussion

What Is the Appropriate Oral Anticoagulant to Use in the Setting of a Mechanical Valve?

All patients who undergo a mechanical valve replacement require lifelong anticoagulation with an oral vitamin K antagonist (i.e., warfarin) in order to prevent valve thrombosis and embolic events [1]. The prosthetic material increases the risk of thrombus formation and abnormal flow conditions can lead to platelet activation. Many studies have demonstrated warfarin's effectiveness at preventing valve thrombosis and thromboembolic events. In addition to warfarin, all patients should receive aspirin 75–100 mg daily.

Newer oral anticoagulants should be avoided in the presence of mechanical valves [1]. The RE-ALIGN trial, which was a phase 2 dose-validation study, evaluated the use of dabigatran compared to warfarin in patients with mechanical valves [2]. The trial was terminated early due to an excess of thromboembolic and bleeding events in the dabigatran group. Based on the results from RE-ALIGN, the FDA issued a boxed warning stating that dabigatran is contraindicated in patients with mechanical heart valves [3]. Due to the lack of safety and efficacy data with the oral anti-Xa agents (rivaroxaban, apixaban, and edoxaban), it is strongly advised that these agents also be avoided in patients with mechanical valves [1].

Additionally, one can argue that the patient described in the vignette should not have been prescribed rivaroxaban prior to surgery. These agents have only been approved for non-valvular atrial fibrillation, and the cause of this patient's atrial fibrillation may be a complication from mitral stenosis (i.e., valvular atrial fibrillation).

What Factors Should Be Considered When Determining an INR Goal for a Patient with a Mechanical Valve?

All mechanical valves generate flow patterns which differ from native valves [4]. High velocity and high shear can cause damage to circulating blood elements. This leads to activation of platelets, endothelial cells and coagulant proteins, further increasing the risk for thrombus formation. Localized regions of turbulent flow can further lead to stasis and thrombus formation [5].

The position and type of valve play a critical role in determining an INR goal [1]. The risk of valve thrombosis and thromboembolic events are higher in the mitral position than in the aortic position due to different flow conditions and hemodynamics across the valve itself [1]. Due to overall cardiac hemodynamics, low blood flow and/or reduced cardiac output increases the risk of thrombosis around the mitral valve [5]. During systole, blood is ejected through the aortic valve when the leaflets are widely separated [6]. This minimizes stasis, or contact time, between blood and the thrombogenic material of the mechanical valve. Mitral valve leaflets have more contact with blood in the left atria during diastole and in the left ventricle during systole since the leaflets are closed.

The different generations of mechanical valves vary from one another in terms of thrombogenicity. Caged-ball prostheses have the highest thrombogenic potential resulting from stagnant and circumferential blood flow [7]. Both single-leaflet (or tilting-disk) and bileaflet valves are enabled for central flow of blood, which decreases the thrombogenicity risk. Bileaflet valves have the lowest risk of embolic events [8]. See Fig. 35.1 for pictures of each type of valve (A—caged-ball; B/C—tilting disk; D—bileaflet).

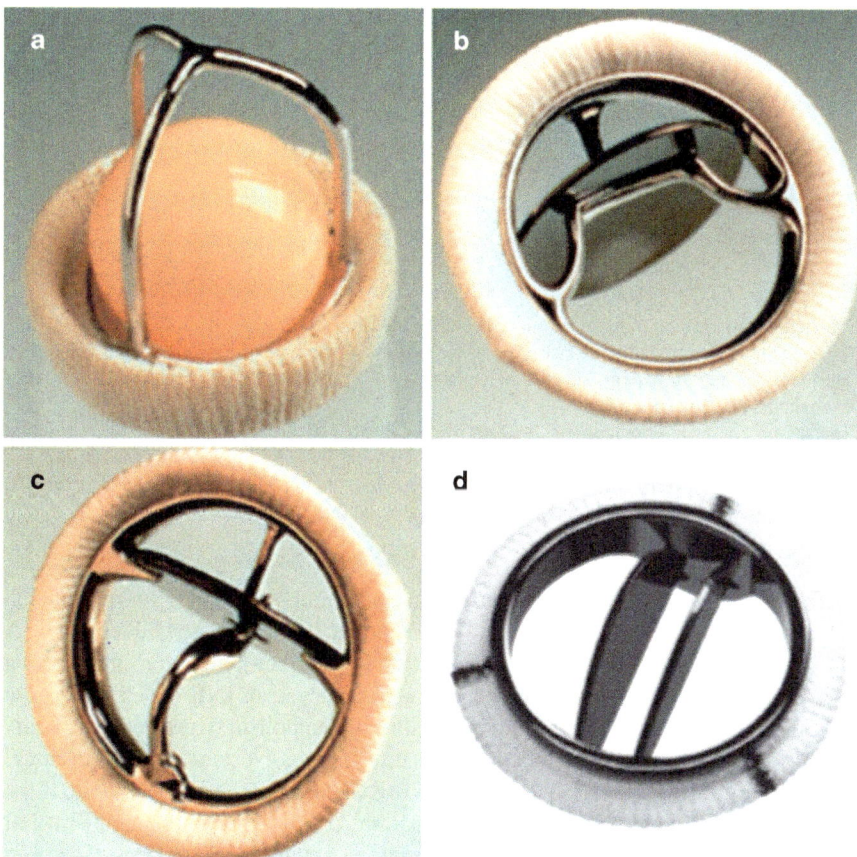

Fig. 35.1 Examples of mechanical heart valves. (**a**) Starr-Edwards caged-ball valve which is associated with the highest thrombogenicity. (**b**) Bjork-Shiley tilting-disk valve is an example of a tilting-disk valve which has intermediate risk of thrombogenicity. (**c**) Medtronic Hall tilting-disk valve. (**d**) St. Jude Medical Regent is an example of a bileaflet valve which has the lowest risk of thrombogenicity. Reprinted with permission from Lancet. 2009;374:565–76

Table 35.1 Antithrombotic recommendations for mechanical heart valves based on the 2014 AHA/ACC valvular heart disease guidelines [1, 10]

Valve type	Description	Trade names	Valve position	INR goal	INR goal with risk factors[a]
1st generation	Caged-ball	Starr-Edwards [DSC]	Aortic	2.5–3.5	
			Mitral	2.5–3.5	
2nd generation	Single-tilting disk	Omnicarbon [DSC]	Aortic	2.0–3.0	2.5–3.5
			Mitral	2.5–3.5	
		Bjork-Shiley [DSC]	Aortic	2.0–3.0	2.5–3.5
			Mitral	2.5–3.5	
		Medtronic Hall	Aortic	2.0–3.0	2.5–3.5
			Mitral	2.5–3.5	
3rd generation	Bileaflet tilting disk	Edwards-Duromedis [DSC]	Aortic	2.0–3.0	2.5–3.5
			Mitral	2.5–3.5	
		St. Jude	Aortic	2.0–3.0	2.5–3.5
			Mitral	2.5–3.5	
		Carbomedic	Aortic	2.0–3.0	2.5–3.5
			Mitral	2.5–3.5	
		Open pivot	Aortic	2.0–3.0	2.5–3.5
			Mitral	2.5–3.5	
4th generation	Bileaflet tilting disk (silicon free)	On-X	Aortic	2.0–3.0 (1.5–2.0)[b]	

In patients who have an older generation mechanical AVR such as caged-ball, the goal is 2.5–3.5, independent of thromboembolic risk factors. Regardless of the type of valve and its position, it is recommended that all patients receive an aspirin dosed 75–100 mg daily for additional thromboprophylaxis. *DSC* discontinued

[a]Risk factors for thromboembolism: atrial fibrillation, history of thromboembolism, left ventricular dysfunction, or known hypercoagulable conditions

[b]The INR goal for an On-X mechanical aortic valve is recommended to be 2.0–3.0 during the first three months. Afterwards, it is recommended to lower the INR goal to 1.5–2.0

Table 35.1 provides recommendations to antithrombotic therapy for mechanical heart valves based on the 2014 AHA/ACC Valvular Heart Disease Guideline [1]. A mechanical valve in the aortic position (bileaflet or current-generation single tilting disc) should have optimal anticoagulation that achieves an INR of 2.5 (INR goal 2.0–3.0) in patients with no risk factors for thromboembolism. However, if a patient has other risk factors for thromboembolism, more aggressive anticoagulation should be considered. Achieving an INR of 3.0 (INR goal 2.5–3.5) may be warranted if the following risk factors such as atrial fibrillation, previous thromboembolism, left ventricular dysfunction, and/or hypercoagulable conditions are present. However, there is a lack of data to support the recommendation of routinely targeting higher INR goals in patients with additional risk factors. Decisions on whether to intensify INR goals should be based on individual patient risk assessments for thrombosis and bleeding. Older-generation mechanical valves (i.e., caged-ball) in the aortic position are also recommended to achieve an INR of 3.0 (INR goal 2.5–3.5) due to higher risk of thromboembolic complications, regardless if risk factors are present or not.

One study found that rates of thromboembolism in patients with mechanical mitral valves were lower in patients with higher INR goals compared to those with lower INR goals [9]. In patients with mechanical valves in the mitral position, anticoagulation with warfarin is recommended to achieve an INR of 3.0 (INR goal 2.5–3.5) [1]. In patients who have mechanical valves in both the mitral and aortic positions, anticoagulation with warfarin should achieve an INR of 3.0 (INR goal 2.5–3.5).

Newer valves, such as the On-X aortic mechanical valve, may allow patients to be managed with a lower INR goal. The On-X valve is made entirely out of carbon and is free of silicone, which reduces the risk of blood damage [10]. Initially, patients are anticoagulated with an INR goal of 2.0–3.0. After three months, the INR goal is reduced to 1.5–2.0. The PROACT trial demonstrated that reducing the intensification of anticoagulation not only reduced bleed rates, but there was also no change in the rate of stroke [11].

What Diagnostic or Surgical Procedures Require a Temporary Interruption in Oral Anticoagulation?

Any patient who is anticoagulated and requires a procedure should have the risk of increased bleeding weighed against the increased risk of thromboembolism. Anticoagulation should not be stopped for procedures where bleeding is not likely or very low [1]. Examples of these include surgery on the skin, dental cleaning, and eye surgeries for cataracts or glaucoma.

Patients with a bileaflet mechanical aortic valve and have no risk factors for thromboembolism are generally considered to be low-risk [1]. Depending on the procedure, bridging anticoagulation could be avoided. Patients who are at higher risk of thromboembolism (presence of risk factors described above plus all patients with mechanical valves in the mitral position) that require interruption of warfarin should be bridged with an agent that can easily be stopped before the procedure and restarted afterwards when appropriate.

Patients who require interruption of warfarin therapy are recommended to be "bridged" with either intravenous unfractionated heparin (UFH) or subcutaneous low molecular weight heparin (LMWH) such as enoxaparin [1].

If Embolic Events Occur Despite Therapeutic INRs, What Is the Approach to Antithrombotic Therapy?

In the event that a patient experiences a thromboembolic event on therapeutic anticoagulation, intensification of the INR goal can be considered [1]. For example, if valve thrombosis occurs in a patient with an aortic mechanical valve that has been anticoagulated and managed with an INR goal of 2.0–3.0, it is recommended to change the INR goal to 2.5–3.5. The INR goal may be changed from 2.5–3.5 to 3.0–4.0 in patients with mechanical mitral valves who experience an embolic event. Aspirin 75–100 mg daily is also recommended to minimize thromboembolic events. Clinicians should consider patient preferences and their bleed risk when deciding if intensification is appropriate.

As previously mentioned, direct oral anticoagulants should be avoided in patients who continue to have recurrent embolic events despite therapeutic INRs. Other agents such LMWH should be used with caution in patients with recurrent embolic events. LMWHs, such as enoxaparin, have insufficient data to support long-term use for thromboprophylaxis [12]. The current AHA/ACC valvular heart disease guidelines do not mention the use of LMWH in non-pregnant patients [1]. If a patient has a history of recurrent embolic events despite therapeutic INRs and wishes to start enoxaparin, providers should discuss the benefits and risks of switching and the lack of evidence to support its long-term use. Anti-Xa levels should be strongly considered for monitoring. Due to the lack of evidence, optimal peak ranges to prevent valve thrombosis are unknown in non-pregnant patients. In pregnant patients with mechanical valves, anti-Xa levels are measured 4–6 h after injection, and suggested peaks range from 0.8 to 1.2 units/mL.

Key Points

- Warfarin is the only recommended oral anticoagulant to prevent cardioembolic events in a patient with a mechanical valve. Aspirin 75–100 mg daily is also recommended to minimize these thrombotic events in all patients with mechanical valves.
- The INR goal should be based on the type and location of the valve and patient-specific risk factors for thromboembolism.
- Temporary interruption of oral anticoagulation should be based on the type of procedure, risk factors, and the type, location, and number of heart valve prosthesis(es). Bridging anticoagulation with unfractionated heparin or low molecular weight heparin is recommended during these times.
- Intensifying INR goals and ensuring a daily aspirin (75–100 mg) is on board is a practical approach to a patient who has suffered an embolic event in the setting of therapeutic INRs. Patient preferences and bleed risk should also be considered.

Self-Assessment Questions

1. A 64-year-old woman has a history of hypertension, atrial fibrillation, type 2 diabetes, peptic ulcer disease, and severe symptomatic aortic stenosis. She undergoes surgery and a St. Jude mechanical valve is placed in the aortic position.

On post-operative day #3, hers labs are within normal limits, and her vitals are stable. The team is planning on initiating warfarin therapy today. Which of the following is the best INR goal range for this patient?

(a) 1.5–2.0
(b) 2.0–3.0
(c) 2.0–3.0 for 3 months, then decrease to 1.5–2.0
(d) 2.5–3.5
(e) 2.5–3.5 for 3 months, then decrease to 2.0–3.0

The correct answer is B. Mechanical valves in the aortic position are recommended to achieve an INR goal of 2.5 (INR goal 2.0–3.0). The On-X mechanical valve is the only mechanical valve that can be anticoagulated with a lower INR goal after three months of anticoagulation targeting a goal of 2.0–3.0. Her history of atrial fibrillation does increase her risk for thromboembolism, but due to her history of peptic ulcer disease and a lack of evidence to support a more aggressive anticoagulation plan, the higher goal of 2.5–3.5 may put her at more risk for bleeding. The AREVA trial demonstrated that moderate anticoagulation (INR goal 2.0–3.0) was as effective as conventional anticoagulation (INR goal 3.0–4.0) in patients with mechanical aortic valves [13]. Moderate anticoagulation also reduced the risk of bleeding events. Patients with risk factors for thromboembolism were excluded in this study which makes it hard to extrapolate in this patient vignette. In clinical practice, providers should carefully weigh a patient's thrombosis and bleed risk, and discuss this with the patient. Some patients may be willing to accept a higher bleed risk to avoid cardioembolic events. Incorporation of a validated scoring system such as HAS-BLED may assist in clinical decision-making when determining this patient's risk. Caution should be applied using this scoring system outside the nonvalvular atrial fibrillation population. It should not be used as an excuse to target a lower goal of 2.0–3.0, but to highlight patients that warrant additional monitoring. If this patient did not have peptic ulcer disease, a goal of 2.5–3.5 would be appropriate due to the additional thrombosis risk.

2. A 62-year-old male with a history of hypertension, hyperlipidemia, and history of recurrent VTE is admitted for a mechanical mitral valve replacement. Prior to surgery, the patient was taking apixaban for his history of VTE. The surgery is successful, and once the patient is hemodynamically stable, the team would like to resume apixaban. Which of the following is the best plan to recommend?

(a) Resume apixaban
(b) Transition to dabigatran
(c) Transition to warfarin, INR goal 2.0–3.0
(d) Transition to warfarin, INR goal 2.5–3.5

The correct answer is D. Regardless of the patient's VTE history, a mechanical valve in the mitral position has the highest thrombogenic risk, and requires a more aggressive INR goal of 2.5–3.5. Resuming apixaban or transitioning to any other anti-Xa agent, such as rivaroxaban or edoxaban, is not recommended due to the lack of data supporting their use. Dabigatran has a boxed warning to avoid use in patients with mechanical valves based on results from the RE-ALIGN study.

References

1. Nishimura RA, Otto CM, Bonow RO, Carabello BA, Erwin III JP, Guyton RA, O'Gara PT, Ruiz CE, Skubas NJ, Sorajja P, Sundt III TM, Thomas JD. 2014 AHA/ACC guideline for the management of patients with valvular heart disease: a report of the American College of Cardiology/American Heart Association Task Force on practice guidelines. J Am Coll Cardiol. 2014;63:e57–185.
2. Eikelboom JW, Connolly SJ, Brueckmann M, et al. Dabigatran versus warfarin in patients with mechanical heart valves. N Engl J Med. 2013;369:1206–14.
3. Food and Drug Administration. FDA Drug Safety Communication: Pradaxa (dabigatran etexilate mesylate) should not be used in patients with mechanical prosthetic heart valves. 2012. Web. 10 June 2016.
4. Yoganathan AP, Chandran KB, Sotiropoulos F. Flow in prosthetic heart valves: state-of-the-art and future directions. Ann Biomed Eng. 2005;33(12):1689–94.
5. Roudaut R, Serri K, Lafitte S. Thrombosis of prosthetic heart valves: diagnosis and therapeutic considerations. Heart. 2007;93:137–42.
6. Schoen FJ. Evolving concepts of cardiac valve dynamics: the continuum of development, functional service, pathobiology, and tissue engineering. Circulation. 2008;118:1864–80.
7. Sun J, Davidson MJ, Lamy A, Eikelboom JW. Antithrombotic management of patients with prosthetic heart valves: current evidence and future trends. Lancet. 2009;374(9689):565–76.
8. Vongpatanasin W, Hillis LD, Lange RA. Prosthetic heart valves. N Engl J Med. 1996;335(6):407–16.
9. Horstkotte D, Bergemann R, Althaus U, et al. German experience with low intensity anticoagulation (GELIA): protocol of a multi-center randomized, prospective study with the St. Jude Medical valve. J Heart Valve Dis. 1993;2(4):411–9.
10. On-X Life Technoligies, Inc. On-X prosthetic heart valve design and features. Web. 10 June 2016.
11. Puskas J, Gerdisch M, Nichols D, et al. Reduced anticoagulation after mechanical aortic valve replacement: interim results from the prospective randomized on-X valve anticoagulation clinical trial randomized Food and Drug Administration investigational device exemption trial. J Thorac Cardiovasc Surg. 2014;147(4):1202–10.
12. Seshadri N, Goldhaber SZ, Elkayam U, et al. The clinical challenge of bridging anticoagulation with low-molecular-weight heparin in patients with mechanical prosthetic heart valves: an evidence-based comparative review focusing on anticoagulation options in pregnant and non-pregnant patients. Am Heart J. 2005;150:27–34.
13. Acar J, Lung B, Boissel JP. AREVA: multicenter randomized comparison of low-dose versus standard-dose anticoagulation in patients with mechanical prosthetic heart valves. Circulation. 1996;94(9):2107–12.

Chapter 36
Management of Antiphospholipid Antibody Syndrome

Margaret A. Felczak

Abstract The gold standard of treatment for antiphospholipid antibody syndrome (APS) remains VKAs (goal INR 2.0–3.0). The gold standard for monitoring of patients with APS remains INR testing, although chromogenic Factor Xa assays may be considered for certain individuals.

Keywords Thrombophilias • Antiphospholipid antibody syndrome (APS) • Hypercoagulable states • Chromogenic factor X levels • Thrombocytopenia

Case Introduction

A 78-year-old female presents to your anticoagulation clinic for follow up. She has been taking warfarin since 2000 to prevent recurrent thrombotic events due to antiphospholipid antibody syndrome. Past medical history includes systemic lupus erythematosus (SLE), hypothyroidism, coronary artery disease, dyslipidemia, hypertension, depression, and new onset dementia. Previous events include myocardial infarction in 2010 and multiple transient ischemic attacks (2006, 2013). In addition, patient has history of venous thromboembolism (LLE DVT 2000, PE 2010). Current medications include hydroxychloroquine, levothyroxine, metoprolol succinate, lisinopril, atorvastatin, amlodipine, paroxetine, donepezil, aspirin, and warfarin 4 mg tablets—as directed by anticoagulation clinic. Patient presents with daughter to visit today with concerns about patient not being able to do her ADL's. The patient's dementia is progressing and she is no longer able to drive herself to appointments. The daughter would like to know if there are any other anticoagulants the patient may take due to difficulty with transportation and frequency of visits.

M.A. Felczak, PharmD, BCPS
Midwestern University Chicago College of Pharmacy, 555 31st Street,
Downers Grove, IL 60515, USA
e-mail: mfelcz@midwestern.edu

Case Discussion

What Is Antiphospholipid Antibody Syndrome (APS) and How Is it Diagnosed?

Antiphospholipid antibody syndrome is a condition characterized by venous or arterial thrombosis and pregnancy loss. Antiphospholipid (aPL) antibodies are a group of autoantibodies directed against phospholipid-binding proteins. The diagnosis of APS is made upon detection of circulating aPL antibodies, namely lupus anticoagulant (LA), anticardiolipin (aCL) antibodies, and anti beta$_2$-glycoprotein 1. When the syndrome occurs alone, it is termed primary APS. However, when it occurs in the presence of other conditions, such as SLE, it is called secondary APS [1, 2]. In 2006, there was an update to the diagnosis of APS, which are now called the Sydney criteria for APS. APS diagnosis requires the combination of at least one clinical and one laboratory criterion. The laboratory criterion must be repeated at least 12 weeks apart from initial testing to confirm the diagnosis [3]. One reason testing for aPL is problematic is due to lack of laboratory standardization. It has been reported that up to 10% of healthy individuals will test positive for aPL, while up to 30–50% of patients with SLE will have a positive assay [1].

What Are Other Common Thrombophilias Encountered in Clinical Practice?

Thrombophilias are either inherited or acquired hypercoagulable states. Recently, a guidance document was published strongly recommending against the routine testing for hypercoagulable states in patients with unprovoked VTE [4]. Therefore, thrombophilia testing should be limited to very rare instances, such as certain females with family history of thrombophilia contemplating pregnancy [4]. Common thrombophilias along with their respective risk for thrombosis are listed in the Table 36.1.

How Is APS Treated?

APS patients are treated with VKAs, such as warfarin, which reduces the risk of recurrent venous and arterial thrombosis. Current CHEST guidelines recommend VKAs with a moderate intensity INR range (2.0–3.0) [6]. Due to the recurrent nature of arterial and venous episodes, researchers explored a higher intensity anticoagulation strategy to see if secondary thrombosis could be prevented. However, in a prospective, randomized trial by Crowther et al., researchers found that 10.7% of patients in the high-intensity warfarin group (INR goal 3.1–4.0) vs. 3.4% of patients

Table 36.1 Common thrombophilias and risk of thrombosis [5]

Hypercoagulable state	Prevalence (%)	Risk for thrombosis
Activated protein C resistance (Factor V Leiden mutation)	5–15	3.8-fold increase for heterozygotes[a] 18-fold increase for homozygotes[b]
Prothrombin G20210A	2–6	2–3-fold increase
Elevated factor VIII levels	10	>150 IU/dL increases risk by 4.8-fold compared to <100 IU/dL
Antithrombin deficiency	<1	8.1-fold increase 1% annual risk
Protein C deficiency	0.2	25–50-fold increase 1% annual risk
Protein S deficiency	<1	10–15-fold increase 1% annual risk
Antiphospholipid antibody syndrome	2–4	5.5% annual risk
Hyperhomocysteinemia	5–10	2.6-fold increase

in the moderate-intensity warfarin group (INR goal 2.0–3.0) reached the primary endpoint of recurrent thrombotic event over 2.7 years (hazard ratio 3.1, 95% CI 0.6-15, $p = 0.15$). The authors concluded that for prevention of recurrent thrombosis in patients with aPL, moderate intensity was appropriate [7]. At this time, there is no recommendation to add antiplatelet therapy to VKA for secondary thrombosis prevention.

Since management of VKAs may be problematic due to numerous drug-drug interactions, drug-food interactions, need for frequent monitoring, and unreliability of INR as a coagulation test (see below), the use of DOACs in this patient population is being explored. Currently, two prospective randomized controlled trials are underway exploring the potential for using rivaroxaban or apixaban in APS patients [8, 9]. However, at this time DOACs should be used with caution in aPL as they have not yet been well studied in this population. Therefore, above patient should remain on VKA until further studies are available.

What Considerations for Monitoring APS Patients Should Be Examined?

aPL antibodies may differentially affect thromboplastin reagents, potentially affecting the international normalized ratio (INR) [10]. This could render the INR test unreliable in certain APS patients by falsely elevating the INR. Alternative monitoring strategies include chromogenic Factor X assays, which has its own disadvantages, such as lab availability and cost. General cost for venipuncture INR is about $10 versus point of care INRs $15–20 versus venipuncture chromogenic Factor X level $440. Furthermore, chromogenic Factor X levels would likely need to be sent to an outside lab, with results taking 24–72 hours, delaying warfarin management in the patient. Notwithstanding, in the majority of APS patients, INR measurements should be reliable. In select lupus anticoagulant patients in whom Factor X levels would be beneficial, it is recommended to work with a hematologist to determine appropriate anticoagulation intensity [11, 12].

What Considerations for Bleeding Should Be Addressed in APS?

Some things to consider in an APS patient that may affect bleeding include higher rates of thrombocytopenia. As the risk of bleeding in patients with thrombocytopenia is closely associated with the platelet count, platelet counts may need to be monitored more closely. Furthermore, due to a high baseline risk of thrombosis, the management of major bleeding in APS patients will present a challenge. If anticoagulation therapy is to be withheld, it should be re-instated as soon as possible once bleeding has ceased and hemostasis is restored [13].

Key Points

- APS diagnosis requires the combination of at least one clinical and one laboratory criterion. The laboratory criterion must be repeated at least 12 weeks apart from initial testing to confirm the diagnosis.
- The gold standard of treatment for APS remains VKAs (goal INR 2.0–3.0)
- The gold standard for monitoring of patients with APS remains INR testing, although chromogenic Factor X assays may be considered for certain individuals.
- Factor V Leiden mutation is one of the most common thrombophilias.
- Testing for thrombophilias is NOT recommended in most patients due to cost, inappropriate timing of testing, and misinterpretation of results.

Self-Assessment Questions

1. A 69-year-old was seen by hematology for consult after myocardial infarction and recent silent stroke. Patient has a remote history for a left lower extremity DVT (2005). Patient was placed on aspirin 81 mg daily and clopidogrel 75 mg daily by her cardiologist, however, her primary care physician is concerned whether she is on appropriate therapy. The hematologist places the following lab orders: lupus anticoagulant, beta 2 glycoprotein panel, and anticardiolipin panel. Labs are repeated in 16 weeks and patient meets the criteria for APS. Which of the following is appropriate anticoagulation for this patient?

(a) continue aspirin and clopidogrel.
(b) switch to warfarin; goal INR 2.0–3.0.
(c) switch to warfarin; goal INR 2.5–3.5.
(d) switch to rivaroxaban 20 mg daily.

Correct answer is B. The appropriate INR range for patients with APS is 2.0–3.0. Low intensity warfarin was not associated with increased bleeding risk or a difference in thrombotic outcomes, thus low intensity is recommended. Answer A is incorrect since the diagnosis of APS was confirmed. Answer D is incorrect since rivaroxaban is still being studied as a treatment for APS in a prospective trial—results still unknown.

2. A 56-year-old male with APS presents to your anticoagulation clinic for follow up. Last four INR's have been stable (2.0, 2.4, 2.6, 2.1). At today's visit, patient reports no missed/extra doses, no changes in vitamin K consumption, no recent illness, no medication changes, denies EtOH, no illness. His INR today is 4.0 with no known etiology. Which of the following statements is false?

(a) High titers of aPL may be interfering with phospholipid component of thromboplastin reagent, resulting in falsely elevated INR.
(b) Chromogenic factor X assays may be used in APS patients as an alternative to INR testing.
(c) Chromogenic factor X assays are readily available at most laboratories.
(d) Chromogenic factor X assays are less costly than INR tests.

Correct answer is C. All of the other options are correct. Chromogenic factor X assays may not be available at all lab facilities.

References

1. Lim W, Crowther MA, Eikelboom JW. Management of antiphospholipid antibody syndrome. JAMA. 2006;295(9):1050–7.
2. Pengo V, Banzato A, Bison E, et al. Laboratory testing for antiphosholipid antibody syndrome. Int J Lab Hematol. 2016;38(Suppl 1):27–31. doi:10.1111/ijlh.12507.
3. Miyakis S, Lockshin MD, Atsumi T, et al. International consensus statement on an update of the classification criteria for definite antiphospholipid syndrome (APS). J Thromb Haemost. 2006;4:295–306.
4. Stevens SM, Woller SC, Bauer KA, et al. Guidance for evaluation and treatment of hereditary and acquired thrombophilia. J Thromb Thrombolysis. 2016;41:154–64.
5. Michaud J. Hypercoagulability testing. In: Dager WE, Gulseth M, Nutescu E, editors. Anticoagulation therapy: a point-of-care guide. Bethesda, MD: American Society of Health-System Pharmacists; 2011. p. 427–55.
6. Holbrook A, Schulman S, Witt DM, et al. Evidence-based management of anticoagulant therapy: antithrombotic therapy and prevention of thrombosis, 9th ed: American College of Chest Physicians evidence-based clinical practice guidelines. Chest. 2012;141:e152S–84S.
7. Crowther MA, Ginsberg JS, Julian J, et al. A comparison of two intensities of warfarin for the prevention of recurrent thrombosis in patients with the antiphospholipid antibody syndrome. N Engl J Med. 2003;349:1133–8.

8. Pengo V, Banzato A, Bison E, et al. Efficacy and safety of rivaroxaban vs warfarin in high-risk patients with antiphospholipid syndrome: rationale and design of the Trial on Rivaroxaban in Anti Phospholipid Syndrome (TRAPS) trial. Lupus. 2016;25:301–6.
9. Woller SC, Stevens SM, Kaplan DA, et al. Apixaban for the secondary prevention of thrombosis among patients with antiphospholipid syndrome: study rationale and design (ASTRO-APS). Clin Appl Thromb Hemost. 2016;22(3):239–47.
10. Chaturvedi S, McCrae KF. The antiphopholipid syndrome: still an enigma. Hematology Am Soc Hematol Educ Program. 2015;2015:56–60.
11. Crowl A, Schullo-Feulner A, Moon JY. Warfarin monitoring in antiphospholipid syndrome and lupus anticoagulant. Ann Pharmacother. 2014;48(11):1479–83.
12. Isert M, Miesbach W, Schuttfort G, et al. Monitoring anticoagulant therapy with vitamin K antagonists in patients antiphospholipid syndrome. Ann Hematol. 2015;94(8):1291–9.
13. Pazzola G, Zuily S, Erkan D. The challenge of bleeding in antiphosholipid antibody-positive patients. Curr Rheumatol Rep. 2015;17(2):7. doi:10.1007/s11926-014-0481-0.

Chapter 37
Venous Thromboembolism and Pregnancy

Erika L. Hellenbart

Abstract Pregnancy is associated with a significant increase in risk of venous thromboembolism compared to that of non-pregnant patients of comparable age. Anticoagulation therapy is challenging as guideline recommendations are largely based on observational studies and extrapolations from non-pregnant patients. Low molecular weight heparin is the therapy of choice in these patients, but treatment plans including dosing, peripartum plans, and length of therapy must be individualized based on risk assessment and patient characteristics.

Keywords Pregnancy-associated venous thromboembolism • Pregnancy • Venous thromboembolism • Low-molecular weight heparin • Adjusted-dose low molecular weight heparin • Enoxaparin • Anti-Factor Xa levels

Introduction

VR is a 33 year old Hispanic female who presents to your anticoagulation clinic on warfarin for history of recurrent DVTs (2009 and 2012) and PE (2012) as well as heterozygous factor V Leiden mutation (FVL) and history of late miscarriage at 20 weeks gestation in 2009. During the patient interview, she states she is pregnant based on a home testing kit. You send the patient to the lab to confirm pregnancy by laboratory testing. VR's weight is 103 kg and her CrCl is 98.2 mL/min. Knowing warfarin crosses the placental barrier and fatal hemorrhage to the fetus and other teratogenic effects have been well-documented, you assist with transitioning VR to an alternative anticoagulant.

E.L. Hellenbart, PharmD, BCPS
University of Illinois at Chicago College of Pharmacy, University of Illinois Hospital and Health Sciences System, 833 South Wood Street, Suite 164, Chicago, IL 60612, USA
e-mail: ehellen@uic.edu

What is the Risk of Venous Thromboembolism During Pregnancy and the Post-Partum Period?

Anticoagulation therapy for the treatment or prevention of VTE during pregnancy is challenging due to the need for considerations of fetal complications such as loss of pregnancy and congenital malformations, as well as maternal complications. This is accompanied by the fact that guideline recommendations are largely based on observational studies and extrapolations from non-pregnant patients [1]. Pregnancy is associated with a four to fivefold increased risk in venous thromboembolism (VTE), including deep vein thrombosis (DVT) and pulmonary embolism (PE), compared to that of non-pregnant women of comparable age [2]. This risk is further increased during the first 6 weeks post-partum [1–3]. Reported incidence of VTE ranges from 0.6 to 1.7 episodes per 1000 deliveries [3]. Considering the post-partum period is significantly shorter than the ante-partum period, the daily risk of VTE is increased 15–35-fold during this time compared with non-pregnant patients of similar age [1]. In developed countries, thromboembolism is one of the leading causes of maternal death [2].

Which Agents are Available for Use During Pregnancy and When Should They Be Initiated?

Both unfractionated heparin (UFH) and low molecular weight heparin (LMWH) do not cross the placenta and are safe for use during pregnancy. However, LMWH is recommended over UFH due to a more predictable therapeutic response as well as decreased rates of bleeding, heparin induced thrombocytopenia (HIT), and heparin-associated osteoporosis [1–3]. UFH is preferred in patients with renal dysfunction (CrCl < 30 mL/min) but requires aPTT monitoring, which can be less reliable during pregnancy [1]. Pregnant women were excluded in clinical trials evaluating direct oral anticoagulants (DOACs) including dabigatran, rivaroxaban, apixaban, and edoxaban. The package inserts of dabigatran and rivaroxaban report pregnancy loss and fetal harm in animals but reproductive risk in humans is unknown for all DOACs and is therefore, not recommended at this time. Similar to warfarin, as soon as a patient on a DOAC is confirmed pregnant, transition to LMWH is recommended [1, 4]. It is, however, recommended to continue oral anticoagulants until pregnancy is confirmed rather than initiating LMWH if a patient expresses a desire to become pregnant due to the burden of daily injections as well as the cost of LMWH [1].

Which Agent Should Be Recommended for VR? How Should She Be Monitored?

Table 37.1 lists the treatment recommendations and dosing by the American College of Chest Physicians (ACCP) for various clinical scenarios. Our patient, VR, is currently receiving long-term vitamin K antagonist (VKA) therapy and would thus require either adjusted dose LMWH or 75% of therapeutic dose. Current guidelines do not make recommendations regarding one LMWH over another and can be based on patient preference or insurance formularies. However, one key feature of enoxaparin over dalteparin is the calibrated syringes, allowing for necessary dose adjustments without having to use (and pay for) new syringe strengths. This is especially helpful when monitoring anti-Xa levels.

Based on VR's weight and renal function, an appropriate recommendation would be enoxaparin 100 mg q12 h. Some recommend twice-daily dosing to compensate for increases in renal clearance of LMWH during pregnancy, however in non-pregnant patients, once daily dosing has been proven as safe and effective at treating acute VTE. It has also been suggested that the increased renal clearance of LMWH during pregnancy may require routine monitoring of anti-Xa levels to measure the efficacy of the LMWH, however this remains controversial. Previous iterations of the ACCP guidelines suggested targeting a prophylactic peak (3–5 h post-dose) anti-Xa level of 0.2–0.6 units/mL as well as a therapeutic peak anti-Xa level of 0.6–1.0 units/mL for twice daily regimens and recommend slightly higher ranges if once-daily regimens are chosen [5, 6]. However, current guidelines do not mandate the routine monitoring of LMWH with anti-Xa levels, reiterating the cost and inconvenience of testing as well as the uncertainty for appropriate target ranges and low frequency with which dose adjustments are required [3]. Despite this, the American College of Obstetricians and Gynecologists (ACOG) recommend targeting a peak anti-Xa level of 0.6–1 units/mL for twice daily regimens in patients receiving adjusted dose LMWH and note that slightly higher anti-Xa levels may be needed for once-daily regimens [2]. One single-centered retrospective study showed that dose changes for LMWH throughout pregnancy based on anti-Xa levels were common, especially dose increases in those receiving prophylactic doses, prompting this health-center to begin monitoring anti-Xa levels routinely [7].

Similar to non-pregnant patients, anti-Xa levels may be helpful in patients with renal impairment or extremes of body weight [1]. It is therefore reasonable to weigh all factors when considering whether or not to routinely monitor anti-Xa levels in high-risk pregnant patients. If a center has the ability to run the laboratory test on-site with relatively quick turnaround time and it is covered by insurance, it may be prudent to monitor. It is important to note that various LMWHs have different factor Xa/IIa activity and the laboratory test should be calibrated for the drug in use [8].

Table 37.1 Clinical considerations for VTE prophylaxis and treatment during and after pregnancy [5]

Clinical scenario	Antepartum	Postpartum
Prophylaxis: No prior VTE		
Homo-FVL or prothrombin mutation		
FH VTE	Prophylactic or immediate dose LMWH	Prophylaxis for 6 weeks post-partum with prophylactic or immediate dose LMWH or VKA (INR 2–3) over no prophylaxis
No FH for VTE	Clinical vigilance	Prophylaxis for 6 weeks post-partum with prophylactic or immediate dose LMWH or VKA (INR 2–3) over routine care
All other thrombophilias		
FH VTE	Clinical vigilance	Prophylactic or immediate dose LMWH or VKA (INR 2–3; if not protein C or S deficient) over routine care
No FH for VTE	Clinical vigilance	Clinical vigilance
Prophylaxis: Prior VTE		
Low risk: Single episode of VTE with transient risk factor not related to pregnancy or use of estrogen	Clinical vigilance	Prophylaxis for 6 weeks post-partum with prophylactic or immediate dose LMWH or VKA (INR 2–3) over no prophylaxis
Moderate to high risk: Single unprovoked VTE, pregnancy- or estrogen-related VTE, multiple prior unprovoked VTE not receiving long-term anticoagulation	Prophylactic or intermediate dose LMWH rather than clinical vigilance or routine care	Prophylaxis for 6 weeks post-partum with prophylactic or immediate dose LMWH or VKA (INR 2–3) over no prophylaxis
Moderate to high risk: Receiving long-term VKA	Adjusted dose LMWH or 75% of therapeutic dose	Resumption of long-term anticoagulation
Treatment	Adjusted dose LMWH over adjusted dose UFH or VKA	Anticoagulants continued for at least 6 weeks post-partum (minimum of 3 months total duration)

FH, family history (first-degree relative); *Homo-FVL*, Homozygous factor V Leiden mutation; *VKA*, vitamin K antagonist

Clinical vigilance: alertness of patient and provider to signs and symptoms of VTE and awareness of need for timely and appropriate objective investigation and diagnosis

Adjusted-dose UFH: UFH SC q12 h in doses adjusted to target a mid-interval aPTT in the therapeutic range

Prophylactic LMWH: dalteparin 5000 units SC q24 h; tinzaparin 4500 SC q24 h; enoxaparin 40 mg SC q24 h (dose modifications may be required at extremes of body weight)

Intermediate-dose LMWH: dalteparin 5000 units SC q12 h; enoxaparin 40 mg SC q12 h

Adjusted-dose LMWH: weight-adjusted or full-treatment doses of LMWH, given once daily or BID; dalteparin 200 units/kg daily; tinzaparin 175 units/kg daily; dalteparin 100 units/kg q12 h; enoxaparin 1 mg/kg q12 h

Table 37.2 Sample nomogram for therapeutic dosing of LMWH based on peak anti-Xa levels [9]

Peak anti-Xa level[a] (units/mL)	Dose adjustment[b]
< 0.35	↑ by 25%
0.35–0.49	↑ by 10%
0.5–1	No dose adjustment
1.1–1.5	Once daily: No dose adjustment Twice daily: ↓ by 20%
1.6–2	Once daily: No dose adjustment Twice daily: ↓ by 30%
> 2	HOLD 1–2 doses then ↓ by 40%

[a]Peak anti-Xa levels are 3–5 h post dose administration once steady-state is reached
[b]Frequency of subsequent anti-Xa levels are dependent on the clinical scenario; ideally once new dose reaches steady state. Levels within goal ranges are considered "therapeutic" and can be monitored less frequently (ex. monthly)

Table 37.2 includes recommended dose adjustments based on a 4-h peak anti-Xa level once at steady-state, initially developed for pediatric patients but is widely accepted in the pregnant population [9]. It is important to confirm the patient has not missed at least any of the previous three doses prior to checking an anti-Xa level to ensure steady state has been achieved. The frequency of subsequent levels is patient specific. Typically, repeat levels should be checked after dose adjustments, then monthly once levels are within the target range. Patients on prophylactic doses of LMWH may be monitored less frequently once "therapeutic", at least once each trimester. In addition to anti-Xa levels, it is also wise to monitor for changes in renal function, especially if dysfunction is present at baseline, as well as platelets to assess for any evidence of HIT.

What Does VR Need to be Aware of as Her Due Date Approaches?

All pregnant women should have an individualized peripartum plan. Due to a very high risk of recurrent VTE close to the expected due date, planned deliveries by induction or cesarean section may be beneficial to minimize the duration of time a patient is without anticoagulation. If the delivery is planned, adjusted-dose UFH or LMWH should be discontinued at least 24 h before expected time of delivery or epidural analgesia. If once-daily LMWH is being used, patients should only take 50% of the dose 24 h prior to delivery. Alternatively, high risk patients can be switched to IV UFH, which can be discontinued 4–6 h prior to epidural analgesia [1, 3, 10]. Patients can also be switched to a comparable dose of subcutaneous UFH at approximately 36 weeks of gestation to improve the likelihood of epidural anesthesia use [10]. Of note, multi-dose vials of UFH and LMWH contain benzyl alcohol, with which cases of fetal gasping syndrome in neonates have been reported. Preservative-free vials or single-dose syringes should always be used [11]. All pregnant women should be advised to discontinue anticoagulants immediately upon the onset of spontaneous labor. Heparin levels can be checked if possible or time since last injection can be considered to determine if epidural analgesia can be used [1, 3, 10]. Epidural analgesia should not be used with prophylactic doses administered within 12 h or therapeutic doses within 24 h [10].

What are VR's Options During the Post-partum Period?

Patients who are receiving long-term anticoagulation should continue anticoagulation following pregnancy as suggested by ACCP and ACOG guidelines (Table 37.1) [2, 3]. Warfarin is not detected in breast milk and is safe to resume following pregnancy. LMWH has been detected in small quantities in breast milk however, given the low bioavailability, clinically relevant amounts are unlikely and deemed safe to use by the ACCP and ACOG. Breast-feeding women were excluded from all DOAC trials so these should be avoided in these women [2, 3]. The patient in this case, VR, should continue long-term anticoagulation by either switching back to warfarin or continuing LMWH. Should she return to warfarin, bridging with LMWH until the INR is therapeutic should be considered due to high risk of post-partum VTE [2]. This may require frequent INR monitoring; depending on how well-controlled the patient's INRs were prior to pregnancy. Patients who are on prophylactic anticoagulation should remain on anticoagulation for 6 weeks post-partum and may consider continuing LMWH to avoid frequent visits for INR monitoring, especially with the demands of a newborn. Similarly, VR may decide to continue LMWH for 6 weeks and then resume warfarin. Patients with a newly diagnosed VTE during pregnancy should continue anticoagulation for at least a total of 3 months or 6 weeks post-partum, whichever is longer to ensure the VTE is adequately treated. The decision to continue anticoagulation past 3 months would be based on the same risk factors and considerations as non-pregnant patients [3].

Key Points

- Pregnancy is associated with a four to fivefold increased risk of VTE, including DVT and PE, compared to that of non-pregnant women of comparable age. Considering the post-partum period is significantly shorter than the ante-partum period, the daily risk of VTE is increased 15–35-fold during this time compared with non-pregnant patients of similar age.
- The determination of appropriate dose of LMWH is based on individual risk assessment and monitoring of anti-Xa levels should be considered if available and feasible. If anti-Xa levels are monitored, the level should be drawn approximately 3–5 h after injection once steady state has been reached. Subsequent levels should

be tested until "therapeutic" levels have been reached, followed by monthly testing during pregnancy.
- Enoxaparin pre-filled syringes are calibrated, making dose adjustments easier than with dalteparin. Multi-dose vials of LMWH and UFH contain benzyl alcohol and should be avoided. Preservative-free vials are available if use is necessary.
- All pregnant women should have an individualized peripartum plan. For epidural analgesia to be used safely, planned delivery is preferred. Otherwise, patients should discontinue anticoagulants immediately at onset of labor. Epidural analgesia should not be used within 12 h of prophylactic doses or 24 h of therapeutic doses.
- Warfarin and LMWH are both safe during breast-feeding. All DOACs should be avoided.
- Patients with a newly diagnosed VTE during pregnancy should remain on anticoagulation for 6 weeks post-partum or at least 3 months, whichever is longer to ensure the VTE is adequately treated

Self-Assessment Questions

1. MJ is a 31 yo AAF who is 22 weeks pregnant and has just been diagnosed with a right femoral vein DVT. MJ weighs 123 kg and her CrCl is 87 mL/min. Which is the best treatment option for MJ?

    (a) Warfarin daily (INR 2–3)
    (b) Enoxaparin 120 mg daily
    (c) Dalteparin 12,500 units q12 h
    (d) Adjusted dose UFH q12 h

    Based on the options provided, dalteparin 12,500 units q12 h is the best option for MJ because the guidelines recommend adjusted-dose LMWH over adjusted dose UFH or VKA therapy (Table 37.1). LMWH is usually recommend over UFH due to having a more predictable therapeutic response and decreased rates of bleeding, heparin induced thrombocytopenia, and heparin-associated osteoporosis. Warfarin can technically be used after the first trimester of pregnancy but is typically only reserved for the highest risk patients such as mechanical mitral valve replacements. Enoxaparin can be preferred over dalteparin if anti-Xa levels will be monitored because the prefilled syringes are calibrated making dose adjustments easier. However, 1 mg/kg q12 h is the dose that is recommended and 1 mg/kg daily is what is listed above. Once daily enoxaparin has been suggested to be safe but should be dosed at 1.5 mg/kg daily, similar to non-pregnant patients. Adjusted-dose dalteparin is the other option for LMWH and can be dosed at either 200 units/kg/day or 100 units/kg q12 h. Dalteparin 100 units/kg would equate to 12,300 units q12 h so based on available syringe strengths, dalteparin 12,500 units q12 h would, therefore, be the best option of the above choices.

2. RL is a 23 yo Caucasian female with PMH significant for heterozygous FVL and multiple DVT/PE, receiving long-term anticoagulation. Pt is now 12 weeks pregnant on adjusted-dose enoxaparin 80 mg q12 h since becoming pregnant. RL has a peak anti-Xa level of 0.37 units/mL, which is to be managed by your anticoagulation clinic. Of the following options, which should be completed at RL's visit with the pharmacist? Please select all that apply.

   (a) **Ensuring RL has not missed any recent doses**
   (b) **Confirming time of last injection**
   (c) Assessing any changes in vitamin K diet
   (d) Continue RL on enoxaparin 80 mg q12 h
   (e) **Increase enoxaparin to 90 mg q12 h**

   When monitoring peak anti-Xa levels, confirming the time of the last injection is important to ensure the level was drawn within 3–5 h to be an accurate peak level. It is also imperative to ensure that the patient has been taking the current dose for long enough to have reached steady-state. RL has been taking this dose since becoming pregnant but it is important to ask if the patient has missed any of at least the past three doses, making the patient no longer at steady-state. Assessing for changes in vitamin K diet is only necessary while a patient is taking a vitamin K antagonist and does not interfere with the efficacy of LMWH. Once you have confirmed that the available anti-Xa level is an accurate peak, you can decide if any dose adjustments are necessary. When taking adjusted-dose LMWH twice daily, the goal peak anti-Xa level is suggested as 0.6–1.0 units/mL per ACOG guidelines and has been suggested as 0.5–1.0 units/mL in other literature [2, 9]. Table 37.2 includes a sample nomogram for the therapeutic dosing of LMWH and suggests that with a level of 0.37 units/mL, RL's dose should be increased by 10%. Therefore, continuing RL on this dose would be incorrect. In the scenario where RL had missed a dose the day prior, continuing the current dose and rechecking an anti-Xa level within the next week would also be appropriate. However, if RL has not missed any doses and the timing of the lab is appropriate, her dose should be increased to 88 mg q12 h. Enoxaparin is available in 80 and 100 mg calibrated pre-filled syringes. The 100 mg syringes are calibrated per 1 mL or 10 mg so the best recommendation would be to have the patient inject 90 mg of enoxaparin twice daily using 100 mg syringes and repeat a peak anti-Xa level once the new steady state has been achieved.

References

1. Bates SM, Middeldorp S, Rodger M, et al. Guidance for the treatment and prevention of obstetric-associated venous thromboembolism. J Thromb Thrombolysis. 2016;41:92–128.
2. American College of Obstetricians and Gynecologists Women's Health Care Physicians. Practice bulletin no. 123: thromboembolism in pregnancy. Obstet Gynecol. 2011;118(3): 718–29.
3. Bates SM, Greer IA, Middeldorp S, et al. Venous thromboembolism, thrombophilia, antithrombotic therapy, and pregnancy: antithrombotic therapy and prevention of thrombosis, 9th

ed: American College of Chest Physicians evidence-based clinical practice guidelines. Chest. 2012;141(2 Suppl):e691S–736S.
4. Burnett AE, Mahan CE, Vazquez SR, et al. Guidance for the practical management of the direct oral anticoagulants (DOACs) in VTE treatment. J Thromb Thrombolysis. 2016;41: 206–32.
5. Bates SM, Greer IA, Hirsh J, et al. Use of antithrombotic agents during pregnancy. The seventh ACCP conference on antithrombotic and thrombolytic therapy. Chest. 2004;126:627S–44S.
6. Bates SM, Gree IA, Pabinger I, et al. Venous thromboembolism, thrombophilia, antithrombotic therapy, and pregnancy: American College of Chest Physicians evidence-based clinical practice guidelines (8th edition). Chest. 2008;133:844S–86S.
7. Shapiro NL, Kominiarek MA, Nutescu EA, et al. Dosing and monitoring of low-molecular-weight heparin in high-risk pregnancy: single-center experience. Pharmacotherapy. 2011; 31(7):678–85.
8. Duhl AJ, Paidas MJ, Ural SH, et al. Antithrombotic therapy and pregnancy: consensus report and recommendations for prevention and treatment of venous thromboembolism and adverse pregnancy outcomes. Am J Obstet Gynecol. 2007;197:457.e1–e21.
9. Ohler KH. Pediatrics. Anticoagulation therapy: a point-of-care guide. Bethesda, MD: American Society of Health-System Pharmacists; 2011. p. 369–88.
10. American College of Obstetricians and Gynecologists Women's Health Care Physicians. Practice bulletin no. 138: inherited thrombophilias in pregnancy. Obstet Gynecol. 2013; 122(3):706–17.
11. Shapiro NL. Pregnancy. Anticoagulation therapy: a point-of-care guide. Bethesda, MD: American Society of Health-System Pharmacists; 2011. p. 343–67.

Chapter 38
Venous Thromboembolism in Active Malignancy

Margaret A. Felczak

Abstract Selection of cancer-associated venous thromboembolism treatment is influenced by several patient specific factors. In most cases, LMWH for 3–6 months is the treatment of choice.

Keywords Malignancy • Dalteparin • Chemotherapy • Malnutrition • Duration • Cancer-associated venous thromboembolism

Case Introduction

A 65-year-old man with stage IV colon cancer, in addition to pulmonary and liver metastases, is receiving palliative chemotherapy with oxaliplatin, leucovorin, fluorouracil, and bevacizumab. He presents to the emergency room with shortness of breath. CT of the chest reveals a right-sided pulmonary embolism. Venous dopplers performed on the lower extremities are positive for DVT in the left femoral vein. Patient is started on heparin drip in the emergency room. Patient denies any chest pain, cough, or hemoptysis. Also denies abdominal pain, melena, and hematemesis. Patient's PMH includes systolic heart failure (compensated), chronic kidney disease stage III, and chronic anemia. Patient reports no known drug allergies. Patient's height = 5'9". Patient's weight = 180 lbs. Laboratory data includes Sodium 142, potassium 3.7, BUN 13, creatinine 1.4. LFTs wnl. Troponin negative. WBC 4, hemoglobin 10, platelets 161 K, D-dimer is 17, BNP 110. A 2D echocardiogram showed ejection fraction of 20–25%.

M.A. Felczak, PharmD, BCPS
Midwestern University Chicago College of Pharmacy, 555 31st Street, Downers Grove, IL 60515, USA
e-mail: mfelcz@midwestern.edu

Case Discussion

What Treatment Strategies Are Recommended for Cancer-Associated Venous Thromboembolism?

Current CHEST guidelines, as well as international guidelines, suggest low molecular weight heparin (LMWH) as the treatment of choice for the first 3–6 months of anticoagulation, with unfractionated heparin (UFH) as the alternative [1–4]. If an oral treatment is preferred, vitamin K antagonists (VKA) are preferred over dabigatran, rivaroxaban, apixaban, and edoxaban for long-term treatment [1, 2]. This recommendation is based on limited evidence of efficacy and safety of direct oral anticoagulants (DOACs) in the setting of cancer. After initial therapy with the preferred agent (LMWH) of 3–6 months, switching to an oral agent such as VKA may be considered. However, preference should be given to continuing the first selected agent (LMWH). Consideration for LMWH over VKA should be given in the following clinical scenarios: newly diagnosed cancer, extensive VTE and/or very symptomatic, metastatic cancer, vomiting, and in patients receiving chemotherapy [2].

Currently, a randomized controlled trial to compare edoxaban with dalteparin for the treatment of venous thromboembolism in patients with cancer is underway (NCT02073682) and will shed some light on this topic. In a single center registry of patients at the Mayo Clinic with venous thromboembolism (VTE) and active malignancy, 118 patients out of 296 VTE patients received rivaroxaban for at least 3 months and had a confirmed malignancy (vs. 178 who had no cancer). No difference was found between the groups with respect to VTE recurrence (3.3% vs. 2.8%, $p = 0.533$). In terms of safety, borderline higher rates of major bleeding ($p = 0.06$) vs. non-major clinically relevant bleeding ($p = 0.08$) were seen in the patients with cancer [5].

What Is the Optimal Duration of Treatment?

The recommendation of 3–6 months is based on randomized controlled trials in which patients were treated for a maximum of 6 months. The 2016 Chest VTE disease guideline update favors extended therapy over discontinuing anticoagulation in 3 months, if patient is not at high bleeding risk. Thus, in most cases, patients should be considered for long-term treatment if their cancer is still active. It is also recommended to have ongoing re-evaluation of bleeding risks at least annually [2].

What Are the Advantages of LMWH Over VKA?

LMWH is preferred both for efficacy and safety, when compared with VKA. In a study by Prandoni et al., VKA was less effective than LMWH and was associated with a 1 year VTE recurrence rate over 20% versus 6.8% in patients with cancer (hazard ratio 3.2). In addition, VKA were associated with more than a doubling of the rate of major bleeding, despite well-controlled INR's [6].

What Patient Specific Factors Need to Be Considered?

The patient's specific chemotherapy regimen will need to be assessed for drug-drug interactions with the chosen anticoagulant (see Table 38.1). If needed, possible modification to chemotherapy regimen could be considered. In addition, degree of patient's anemia and chronic kidney disease need to be closely monitored. Furthermore, patient's tolerability for daily injections, cost of medication, and need for laboratory monitoring should also be considered.

Table 38.1 Chemotherapy agents with possible interactions with warfarin [7]

Chemotherapy agent	Effect on INR	Proposed mechanism
Androgens/antiandrogens	Increase	Unknown
Bevacizumab	None	Increased bleeding risk
Capecitabine	Increase	Down-regulation of CYP2C9
Carboplatin	Increase	Unknown
Cyclophosphamide	Increase/decrease	Unknown
Doxorubicin	Increase	Unknown
Erlotinib	Increase	Unknown
Estrogens	Decrease	Increased synthesis of clotting factors
Etoposide	Increase	Unknown
Fluorouracil	Increase	Inhibition of CYP2C9
Gefitinib	Increase	Unknown
Ifosfamide/mesna	Increase	Unknown
Imatinib	Increase	Inhibition of CYP2C9, CYP3A4, CYP2D6
Mechlorethamine	Increase	Unknown
Mercaptopurine	Decrease	Unknown
Methotrexate	Increase	Unknown
Nilotinib	Increase	Inhibition of CYP2C9 and CYP3A4
Paclitaxel	Increase	Change in protein binding
Procarbazine	Increase	Unknown
Sorafenib	Increase	Unknown
Tamoxifen	Increase	Inhibition of CYP2C9
Thalidomide/lenalidomide + dexamethasone	None	Increase rate of VTE, up to 20%
Toremifene	Increase	Unknown
Trastuzumab	Increase	Unknown
Vincristine	Increase	Unknown
Vindesine	Increase	Unknown
Vorinostat	Increase	Unknown

In general, treatment of the cancer patient requires special attention to drug-drug interactions, malnutrition, vomiting, liver dysfunction, potential need for invasive procedures (quick on/off anticoagulant preferred), and monitoring for chemotherapy-induced pancytopenia [8]. For example, LMWH is more reliable in patients who may be having significant vomiting with chemotherapy. Gastrointestinal absorption of oral medications may be impaired with repeated vomiting. Also, nutrition may be affected due to fluctuations in appetite due to chosen chemotherapy. Thus, patients on oral VKA may not be able to be consistent with vitamin K consumption.

Despite all of this, there may be circumstances in which VKA therapy may need to be used over LMWH. Some of the reasons include inability to afford the cost of LMWH and/or not qualifying for any patient assistance programs, patients who refuse to self-administer injections, and patients with severe renal dysfunction or fluctuating renal function.

VKA management during cancer chemotherapy may present a challenge for maintaining INR at goal for several reasons. Several studies have shown that patients with cancer have lower time-in-therapeutic range than patients without cancer. Patients need more INR visits than patients without cancer due to possible malnutrition due to age/vomiting due to cancer chemotherapy, changes in renal/liver function (including liver metastases) and anemia monitoring, as well as close monitoring is needed due to drug-drug interactions with chemotherapy or antimicrobials used during treatment of cancer.

In Which Situations, If Any, Is Primary Thromboprophylaxis Recommended in Cancer Patients?

Primary thromboprophylaxis is recommended in cancer patients, in absence of contraindication, and is summarized in Table 38.2 [9].

Table 38.2 VTE prophylaxis recommendations based on setting [9]

Inpatient setting	Outpatient setting

• Hospitalized cancer patients with acute medication illness
• All patients undergoing major surgical intervention
  – Preferred agent is LMWH
  – Prophylaxis should be started before surgery or as soon as possible post-op
	• Patients diagnosed with multiple myeloma receiving treatment with thalidomide or lenalidomide plus chemotherapy or dexamethasone
	  – LMWH is preferred for high-risk patients
	  – Aspirin may be used for low-risk patients
	• Primary thromboprophylaxis is generally not recommended in ambulatory patients receiving chemotherapy
	  – It may be considered in patients with advanced pancreatic cancer or with Khorana score ≥ 3*, and low bleeding risk
	• Primary thromboprophylaxis is also not recommended in cancer patients with central venous catheters (CVC)

Khorana score is a predictive model for chemotherapy-associated VTE [10]. Total possible score of 7. See Table 38.3 for determining Khorana score

38 Venous Thromboembolism in Active Malignancy

Table 38.3 Predictive model for chemotherapy-associated VTE (Khorana score)

Patient characteristic	Risk score
Site of cancer	
– Very high risk (stomach, pancreas)	2
– High risk (lung, lymphoma, gynecologic, bladder, testicular)	1
Pre-chemotherapy platelet count 350×10^9/L or more	1
Hemoglobin level less than 100 g/L or use of red cell growth factors	1
Pre-chemotherapy leukocyte count more than 11×10^9/L	1
BMI 35 kg/m^2 or more	1

What Are Treatment Strategies for Management of Recurrent Venous Thromboembolism in Cancer Patients?

Despite adequate anticoagulation for VTE disease in the cancer patient, patients may have a recurrent VTE while on anticoagulant therapy. Depending on initial choice of anticoagulant, there are some options for "treatment failure" while on anticoagulation in the cancer patient.

An international consensus working group suggests three options [11]

- Switching from VKA to LMWH in patients treated with VKA as initial anticoagulant
- Increasing LMWH dose in patients treated with LMWH
- Inserting a vena cava filter

There is currently no literature to support the use of DOAC in this clinical scenario.

What Are Your Final Recommendations for Anticoagulation? Provide Drug Name, Dose, Route, Frequency and Duration

The guidelines do not specify which LMWH agent is preferred. Interestingly, dalteparin is the only LMWH with a FDA approved indication for cancer associated VTE [12]. However, typically it is necessary to check a patient's formulary to see which LMWH is covered. Furthermore, injectable medications are usually set at a higher copay. AWP of a 30 day supply of enoxaparin 100 mg subcutaneously BID would be approximately $5358 [13]. Generally, a prior authorization would need to be submitted to patient's third party prescription plan to determine eligibility of coverage. Despite dalteparin's indication in VTE, the most common encountered LMWH in clinical practice is enoxaparin. Enoxaparin dosing for VTE is 1 mg/kg subcutaneously every 12 h, given CrCL is >30 mL/min. The patient's dose for enoxaparin would be 80 mg subcutaneously every 12 h for a minimum of 3–6 months. At that time, may consider switching to VKA if injections are no longer favorable and/or cost issues.

Key Points

- LMWH is the preferred agent in the treatment of cancer-associated VTE.
- Duration of treatment is usually 3–6 months, and then re-evaluate cancer status and risk of recurrent VTE for long-term treatment.
- Primary prophylaxis of the cancer patient is only indicated in a few situations, usually in the hospital setting.
- There is a limited proven role for primary prophylaxis in the ambulatory patient.

Self-Assessment Questions

1. A 69-year old woman presents to the ER with left upper extremity swelling. Her PMH includes breast cancer, currently being treated with trastuzumab, type 2 diabetes, osteopenia, and GERD. Her medications include metformin 1000 mg po BID, Lantus Solostar 20 units subcutaneously daily, alendronate 35 mg po weekly, and omeprazole 20 mg po daily. Venous dopplers of upper extremity reveal deep venous thrombosis in the left axillary and proximal brachial veins. Which of the following long-term anticoagulant strategies is best for this patient?
    (a) VKA with target INR 2.0–3.0.
    (b) rivaroxaban 15 mg po BID for 3 weeks, then 20 mg po daily.
    (c) refer to interventional radiology for insertion of vena cava filter.
    (d) enoxaparin 1 mg/kg subcutaneously every 12 h.

The correct answer is D. According to current guidelines, LMWH is the preferred agent in the setting of cancer-associated VTE. Patient is currently undergoing chemotherapy, thus, not yet in remission, and we are uncertain of the length of chemotherapy treatment at this time. Patient should be treated with LMWH for 3–6 months and then treatment should be re-evaluated for further need for anticoagulation. Answer A is incorrect since proven inferior to LMWH. Answer B is incorrect since DOACs have not yet been compared head-to-head with gold standard of LMWH to prove non-inferiority. Studies are currently underway to determine DOACs role as a treatment option in cancer patients. Answer C is incorrect at this time since this is not a recurrent VTE event, thus, vena cava filters should not be considered at this time.

2. A 75-year-old presents to your anticoagulation clinic as a new referral. Her PMH includes hypertension, hyperlipidemia, osteoarthritis, and newly diagnosed multiple myeloma. Her oncologist has recommended starting thalidomide with dexamethasone, plus chemotherapy. She is considered high risk for VTE due to her chemotherapeutic regimen. Which of the following recommendations is correct?

    (a) Primary thromboprophylaxis is not indicated since patient is ambulatory.
    (b) Primary thromboprophylaxis is indicated due to type of cancer and treatment patient is receiving.
    (c) Wait until patient develops a DVT to provide LMWH therapy.
    (d) Insert a vena cava filter as prophylaxis for DVT.

The correct answer is B. Multiple myeloma patients who are receiving thalidomide and dexamethasone, plus chemotherapy should receive primary thromboprophylaxis with either LMWH (high risk) or aspirin (low risk). In this situation, would recommend LMWH since presenting as high risk patient as determined by oncology. Answer A is incorrect. Answer C is incorrect due to high risk of DVT in this setting and primary thromboprophylaxis is indicated. Answer D is incorrect as vena cava filter insertions are only indicated when contraindications to anticoagulation exist.

References

1. Kearon C, Akl EA, Comerota AJ, et al. Antithrombotic therapy for VTE disease: antithrombotic therapy and prevention of thrombosis, 9th ed: American College of Chest Physicians evidence-based clinical practice guidelines. Chest. 2012;141:e419S–94S.
2. Kearon C, Akl EA, Ornelas J, et al. Antithrombotic therapy for VTE disease: CHEST guideline and expert panel report. Chest. 2016;149(2):315–52.
3. Imberti D, Di Nisio M, Donati MB, et al. Treatment of venous thromboembolism in patients with cancer: guidelines of the Italian Society for Haemostasis and Thrombosis (SISET). Thromb Res. 2009;124:e32–40.
4. Farge D, Debourdeau P, Beckers M, et al. International clinical practice guidelines for the treatment and prophylaxis of venous thromboembolism in patients with cancer. J Thromb Haemost. 2013;11:56–70.
5. Bott-Kitslaar DM, Saadiq RA, McBane RD, et al. Efficacy and safety of rivaroxaban in patients with venous thromboembolism and active malignancy: a single-center registry. Am J Med. 2016;129(6):615–9.
6. Prandoni P, Lensing AW, Piccioli A, et al. Recurrent venous thromboembolism and bleeding complications during anticoagulant treatment in patients with cancer and venous thrombosis. Blood. 2002;100(10):3484–8.
7. Lohr L. Warfarin drug interactions can affect INR values. HemOnc Today 2008. Accessed 28 July 2016.
8. Bauersachs R. LMWH in cancer patients with renal impairment—better than warfarin? Thromb Res. 2016;140(S1):S160–4.
9. Garcia Escobar I, Antonio Rebollo M, Garcia Adrian S, et al. Safety and efficacy of primary thromboprophylaxis in cancer patients. Clin Transl Oncol. 2017;19(1):1–11.

10. Khorana AA, Kuderer NM, Culakova E, Lyman GH, Francis CW. Development and validation of a predictive model for chemotherapy-associated thrombosis. Blood. 2008;111(10):4902–7.
11. Romualdi E, Ageno W. Management of recurrent venous thromboembolism in cancer patients. Thromb Res. 2016;140(S1):S128–31.
12. Eisai. Fragmin [package insert]. Woodcliff Lake, NJ: Eisai; 2015.
13. Redbook Online [online database]. Greenwood Village, CO: Truven Health Analytics. Accessed 28 July 2016.

Chapter 39
Anticoagulation Management in Patients Undergoing Gastric Bypass Procedures

Brian Cryder

Abstract Patients undergoing gastric bypass surgery are at high risk for venous thromboembolic events, especially those with a history of prior events. Limited clinical studies are available to evaluate safe anticoagulant use in the periprocedural time period so close monitoring is essential.

Keywords Gastric bypass • Bariatric surgery • Oral anticoagulants • Venous thromboembolism • Periprocedural anticoagulation • Inferior vena cava filter

Case Introduction

A 57 year old female patient taking warfarin due to a history of recurrent pulmonary emboli was identified as a candidate for gastric bypass surgery. Other past medical history includes protein C deficiency, hypertension, GERD, sleep apnea, osteoarthritis of the knees, and vitamin D deficiency. She has family history of hypertension and coronary artery disease. Current vitals include BP 138/88, HR 88, RR 20, O2 sat 100%, weight 275 lb, height 66 in., BMI 44.4. All labs and physical exam parameters are within normal limits at the time of pre-operative clearance examination. SCr 0.9 mg/dL. She is highly motivated to receive the surgery as her efforts from diet and exercise alone have provided only modest improvements. The surgeon would like to perform a gastric sleeve procedure, but needs appropriate peri-procedural anticoagulation management to be arranged.

B. Cryder, PharmD, BCACP
Midwestern University—Chicago College of Pharmacy, Downers Grove, IL, USA

Advocate Medical Group, Chicago, IL, USA
e-mail: bcryde@midwestern.edu

Case Discussion

What Are the Pre-procedural Anticoagulation Consideration for this Patient?

In preparing for surgery, the anticoagulation provider will need to assess the hemorrhagic and thrombotic risks involved. Due to its invasive nature, gastric bypass surgery requires full anticoagulation interruption (timing dependent on anticoagulant medication and renal function). Thrombotic risk will be high for most chronically anticoagulated patients with few exceptions. The American Society for Metabolic and Bariatric Surgery Clinical Issues Committee considers every gastric bypass patient either moderate or high risk for venous thromboembolism, with all patients with prior thromboembolism fitting into the latter category [1]. Other conditions that would justify high risk include, advanced age, immobility, known thrombophilia condition, obesity, hypoventilation syndrome, pulmonary hypertension, venous stasis disease, hormonal therapy, expected long operative time, open surgical approach and male gender [1]. Likewise, CHEST guidelines would rate this patient has high risk for thromboembolism due to her protein C deficiency [2].

Due to her high risk status, low molecular weight heparin bridging utilizing therapeutic weight-based dosing would be indicated peri-procedurally while warfarin is temporarily discontinued. It is well documented that low molecular weight heparin dosing may not be as reliable in the morbidly obese population, with limited safety and efficacy evidence beyond 144, 190, and 165 kg for enoxaparin, dalteparin and tinzaparin respectively [3]. Some have proposed anti-Xa level monitoring, but this may not be readily available at all clinical sites in the timeline needed. Our patient's weight of 125 kg remains within the acceptable dosing limits, but this does present a problem for many other morbidly obese patients.

Based on limited cohort study data [4, 5], many surgeons have implemented the practice of inserting inferior vena cava filters (IVC) prior to surgery as added layer of pulmonary embolism prophylaxis. Many surgeons insist on their use in patients with prior thromboembolic events despite no randomized controlled studies and a systematic review that labeled the results "highly heterogeneous" among the 18 included studies [6]. CHEST guidelines do not address the use of IVC filters as a preventative measure, and broadly discourage their use in a secondary prevention role [7]. Retrievable filters are frequently chosen in an effort to limit filter related complications long term. In this case, the patient would be considered high risk due to both her protein C deficiency and recurrent venous thromboembolism, thus potentially prompting surgeon recommendations for IVC filter placement on the preceding day to the gastric sleeve surgery, with filter removal 2–3 months after surgery.

Pre-operative dietary changes specific to gastric bypass procedures must also be taken into account for certain anticoagulants. The final 1–2 weeks before surgery patients are required to limit oral intake to non-caffeinated, non-carbonated, sugar free beverages and liquid protein meal replacement shakes; in some cases small amounts of lean meat or vegetables are permitted. For patients taking warfarin, this may significantly change their routine dietary vitamin K consumption so dosing accommodations are to be expected. Planning and close INR monitoring during this time will be helpful to avoid unanticipated INR elevations.

What Are the Post-procedural Anticoagulation Considerations?

After surgery in the general population, not specific to those with prior embolic history since this data is not available, the post-operative venous thromboembolism rates have been cited at 1–2% at 30 days despite unfractionated heparin prophylaxis and external pneumatic compression [8, 9]. This rate is comparable to thromboembolic rates after knee arthroplasty so appropriate anticoagulation management, including medication selection and intensity, in this time period is important.

Our case patient would be recommended to resume warfarin in addition to therapeutic weight-adjusted dose low molecular weight heparin post-operatively until therapeutic INR levels are achieved. The warfarin dose requirement after surgery is frequently lower than their pre-surgery maintenance dose. It is likely that malabsorptive surgeries such as roux-en-Y or gastric sleeve have more significant dose changes than restrictive surgeries such as gastric banding [10]. Theories have focused on changes in vitamin K absorption or intake, altered warfarin absorption, changes in gut bacterial flora, and other peri-operative metabolic changes related to weight loss, but no consensus etiology has been agreed upon [10–12]. Some reports even note that the warfarin dose frequently regresses back toward pre-surgical amounts over time [10].

So with All of These Complicating Factors with Warfarin, Would it Be More Useful to Choose an Alternate Agent Such as an Oral Xa or IIa Inhibitor?

This is a difficult comparison as data with these anticoagulants are very limited in the gastric bypass population. All of the oral Xa and IIa inhibitors are substrates for p-glycoprotein efflux channels in the GI tract, thus reducing the functional intestine length and potentially altering the efflux-reabsorption pattern. Additionally, the prodrug dabigatran etexilate starts the bioconversion process to its active form of dabigatran in the intestinal tract, introducing another potential source of variability. Clinical accounts of pharmacokinetic alterations among these medications are limited to a few case reports. One case report identified potential malabsorption issues with dabigatran resulting in an on-treatment pulmonary embolism [13] while another case report showed no absorption limitations with rivaroxaban [14]. Recognizing this gap in research, a clinical study is planned to evaluate apixaban in the post-gastric bypass population [15].

Without more extensive clinical information, the use of Xa and IIa inhibitors should be with caution following gastric bypass surgery. In light of the limited data some practitioners advocate for closely monitored warfarin over alternative oral anticoagulants until more is known [16].

Key Points

- Patients undergoing gastric bypass surgery are at high risk for venous thromboembolic events, especially with a history of prior events.
- Inferior vena cava filters are frequently used in patients with a prior history of venous thromboembolism, despite limited support from clinical studies and practice guidelines.
- Warfarin dosing often requires significant reduction following malabsorptive gastric bypass procedures, prompting frequent INR monitoring in the periprocedural time period.
- Limited evidence is available in the medical literature to evaluate the appropriate role of oral Xa and IIa inhibitors in patients following gastric bypass surgery.

Self-Assessment Questions

1. Post-operative warfarin doses are expected to change the least following type of gastric bypass procedure?

    (a) Roux-en-Y
    (b) Gastric banding
    (c) Gastric sleeve
    (d) All procedures impact warfarin dosing equally

    B is the correct answer; Malabsorptive surgeries such as Roux-en-Y and gastric sleeve seem to have greater impact on warfarin dosing post-operatively than restrictive surgeries such as gastric banding.

2. In patients taking rivaroxaban prior to gastric bypass surgery

    (a) Rivaroxaban should be switched to enoxaparin to avoid malabsorptive changes post-operatively
    (b) Rivaroxaban should be switched to dabigatran due to lower risk of gastrointestinal hemorrhage
    (c) Rivaroxaban should be switched to apixaban because apixaban can be crushed and administered with liquid diet restrictions around time of surgery
    (d) Not enough information is available yet to fully assess the safety and efficacy of rivaroxaban in these patients

    D is the correct answer; A is not ideal due to the fact that enoxaparin dosing is not well established in morbidly obese patients; B is incorrect as there is no evidence to suggest that rivaroxaban has a higher GI hemorrhage risk than dabigatran in any patient population; C is incorrect as either medication may be crushed for administration.

References

1. The American Society of Metabolic and Bariatric Surgery Clinical Issues Committee. ASMBS updated position statement on prophylactic measures to reduce the risk of venous thromboembolism in bariatric surgery patients. Surg Obes Relat Dis. 2013;9:493–7.
2. Douketis JD, Spyropoulos AC, Spencer FA, et al. Perioperative management of antithrombotic therapy: antithrombotic therapy and prevention of thrombosis, 9th ed: American College of Chest Physicians evidence-based clinical practice guidelines. Chest. 2012;141(2 Suppl):e326S–50S.
3. Garcia DA, Baglin TP, Weitz JI, Samama MM. Parenteral anticoagulants: antithrombotic therapy and prevention of thrombosis, 9th ed: American College of Chest Physicians evidence-based clinical practice guidelines. Chest. 2012;141(2 Suppl):e24S–43S.
4. Vaziri K, Bhanot P, Hungness ES, Morasch MD, Prystowsky JB, Nagle AP. Retrievable inferior vena cava filters in high-risk patients undergoing bariatric surgery. Surg Endosc. 2009;23(10):2203–7.
5. Vaziri K, Devin-Watson J, Harper AP, et al. Prophylactic inferior vena cava filters in high-risk bariatric surgery. Obes Surg. 2011;21:1580–4.
6. Rowland SP, Dharmarajah B, Moore HM, et al. Inferior vena cava filters for prevention of venous thromboembolism in obese patients undergoing bariatric surgery: a systematic review. Ann Surg. 2015;261:35–45.
7. Kearon C, Akl EA, Ornelas J, et al. Antithrombotic therapy for VTE disease: CHEST guideline and expert panel report. Chest. 2016;149(2):315–52.
8. Prystowsky JB, Morasch MD, Eskandari MK, Hungness ES, Nagle AP. Prospective analysis of the incidence of deep venous thrombosis in bariatric surgery patients. Surgery. 2005;138:759–65.
9. Froehling DA, Daniels PR, Mauck KF, Collazo-Clavell ML, Ashrani AA, Sarr MG, Petterson TM, Bailey KR, Heit JA. Incidence of venous thromboembolism after bariatric surgery: a population-based cohort study. Obes Surg. 2013;23(11):1874–9.
10. Irwin AN, McCool KH, Delate T, Witt DM. Assessment of warfarin dosing requirements after bariatric surgery in patients requiring long-term warfarin therapy. Pharmacotherapy. 2013;33(11):1175–83.
11. Chan LN. Warfarin dosing changes after bariatric surgery: implications on the mechanism for altered dose requirements and safety concerns—an alternate viewpoint. Pharmacotherapy. 2014;34(4):e26–9.
12. Steffen KJ, Wonderlich JA, Erickson AL, Strawsell H, Mitchell JE, Crosby RD. Comparison of warfarin dosages and international normalized ratios before and after roux-en-y gastric bypass surgery. Pharmacotherapy. 2015;35(9):876–80.
13. Lachant DJ, Uraizee I, Gupta R, Pedulla R. Novel oral anticoagulants after gastric bypass surgery: caveat emptor. Int J Case Rep Imag. 2013;4(11):663–5.
14. Mahlmann A, Gehrisch S, Beyer-Westendorf J. Pharmacokinetics of rivaroxaban after bariatric surgery: a case report. J Thromb Thrombolysis. 2013;36(4):533–5.
15. APB study: Apixaban pharmacokinetics in bariatric patients. https://clinicaltrials.gov/ct2/show/NCT02406885. Accessed 4 Apr 2016.
16. Domienik-Karlowicz J, Pruszczyk P. The use of anticoagulants in morbidly obese patients. Cardiol J. 2016;23(1):12–6.

Chapter 40
Patient Presenting with Minor Bleeding

Daniel M. Witt

Abstract When patients receiving anticoagulation therapy present with minor bleeding, bleeding severity and hemodynamic stability should be assessed in a timely manner. The need to reverse anticoagulation should be individualized based on bleeding severity, hemodynamic stability, underlying thromboembolic risk, and degree of INR elevation (for patients receiving warfarin).

Keywords Hemorrhage • Anticoagulation • Warfarin • Minor bleeding • Rectal bleeding • Mechanical heart valve • Therapeutic management

Case Introduction

A 67-year-old man receiving warfarin therapy for an On-X mechanical aortic valve prosthesis presents to urgent care complaining of rectal bleeding. His blood pressure is 126/84 mmHg, pulse 78 bpm, and O_2 saturation is 100% on room air. He reports that he has been seeing blood streaks on the toilet paper following bowel movements off and on for several months. Today following a difficult to evacuate bowel movement he noticed about two teaspoonsful of bright red blood in the toilet bowl and on the stool surface. There was a significant amount of blood on the toilet paper with wiping but after about 10 min this bleeding was controlled. His INR today is 2.9. Two years ago a colonoscopy revealed no polyps or other abnormalities. He takes aspirin 81 mg daily. His only other medication is Vicodin taken as needed for chronic back pain. He reports that he has been taking Vicodin twice daily pretty regularly for about the past week. He has no other medical problems.

D.M. Witt, PharmD, FCCP, BCPS
University of Utah College of Pharmacy, 30 South 2000 East,
Salt Lake City, UT 84112, USA
e-mail: dan.witt@pharm.utah.edu

Case Discussion

What Factors Need to Be Considered When Developing a Plan to Manage this Patients Bleeding Episode?

Bleeding Severity and Hemodynamic Stability

For patients presenting with anticoagulation-related bleeding it is important to assess extent of blood loss and impact on hemodynamic stability. Several bleeding severity categorization schemes have been developed but in general major bleeds are those that result in death, are life-threatening, cause chronic sequelae or consume major healthcare resources [1]. Most other bleeding events are categorized as minor (Table 40.1). Clinically relevant non-major bleeding is a term used in research studies but has limited utility in real-world clinical management [2]. This patient is not hypotensive, has a non-elevated pulse, and adequate O_2 saturation. A complete blood count including platelets could be measured to detect potential anemia related to blood loss. Bleeding into critical sites (e.g., the central nervous system, pericardial space, retroperitoneal space) can be life threatening even in the absence of hemodynamic instability [1]. The characteristics of this patient's bleeding are consistent with minor bleeding associated with hemorrhoids (pending definitive diagnosis) and are not life-threatening.

Risk for Ongoing and/or Further Bleeding

Ascertaining whether bleeding is ongoing is critical to determine whether interventions to reverse anticoagulation and control bleeding will be urgently required [3]. Our patient is current not experiencing ongoing bleeding and does not need urgent intervention. However, the use of aspirin therapy and his history indicates that further bleeding is likely unless the bleeding source can be identified and corrected.

Underlying Thromboembolic Risk

Weighing the patient-specific thromboembolic risk against bleeding severity helps determine how aggressively anticoagulation should be reversed [3, 4]. This patient has relatively low underlying thromboembolic risk based on the type (On-X—target

Table 40.1 Common types of minor bleeding

Gingival bleeding
Epistaxis
Bruising
Heavier than normal menstrual bleeding
Bleeding from minor cuts or scrapes
Hemorrhoidal bleeding

INR range 1.5–2.0 after the first 3 months provided aspirin is co-administered) and position (aortic) of his mechanical valve [5].

Need for Invasive Diagnostic/Interventional Procedure

At some point the source of this patient's bleeding should be identified and corrected if possible. This should occur non-urgently sometime in the near future [3].

Should this Patient Receive Vitamin K to Reverse Warfarin Therapy?

Factors arguing against administering oral vitamin K in this patient include the following:

- INR is only slightly elevated.
- Is not currently experiencing bleeding symptoms [4].
- Vitamin K administration increases the potential for INR overcorrection [6, 7].
- The target INR for patients with On-X aortic valves is lower than other valve types (i.e. 1.5–2.0 provided the valve was placed at least 3 months previously and the patient is co-administering aspirin) [5].

How Should this Patient's Situation Be Managed (See Fig. 40.1)?

The next dose of warfarin should probably be skipped [3]. Potential causes for the slightly elevated INR such as interacting drugs, changes in dietary vitamin K intake, ethanol consumption, and illness should be investigated. This patient has been taking increased amounts of a narcotic pain reliever that contains acetaminophen. Evidence indicates that sustained increases in acetaminophen intake (2 g per day or more) is associated with increased risk for elevated INRs [8]. If ongoing acetaminophen use is anticipated, the weekly warfarin dose should be decreased by 10–20%. A repeat INR should be checked within the next 5–7 days (sooner if bleeding symptoms return). Ideally the dose of warfarin should be titrated to keep the patient's INR toward the lower end of the target INR range. Measures aimed at managing constipation and hemorrhoids such as increasing fluid, fiber, and physical activity are relatively benign and should be instituted while a work up to identify the bleeding source is occurring. Since this patient's constipation is likely associated with narcotic analgesic use, a stimulant laxative may be necessary to relieve constipation. If needed, measures to definitively control the source of bleeding (e.g., hemorrhoid surgery) should occur as soon as possible.

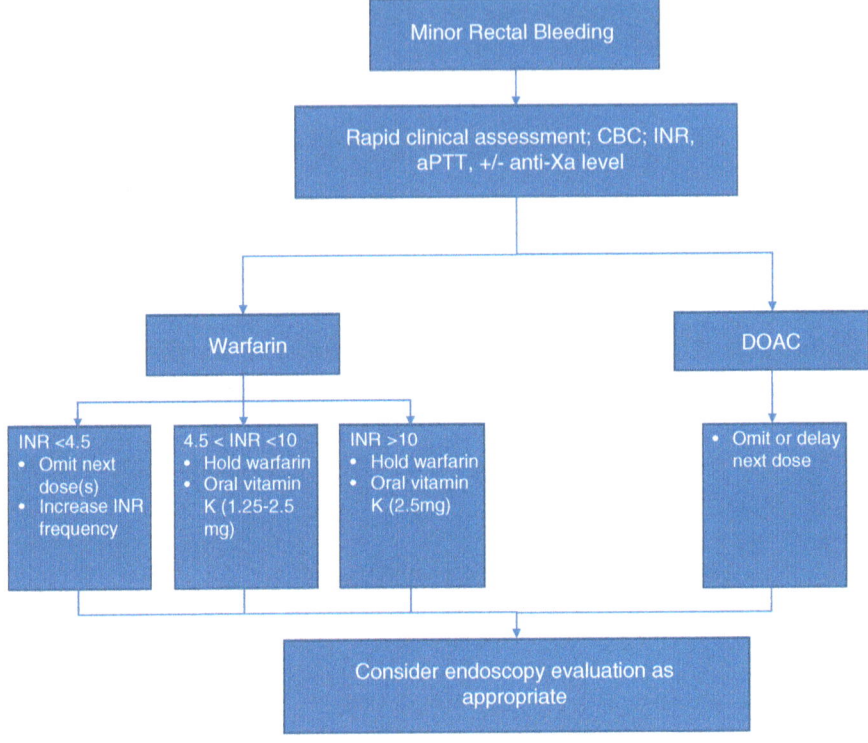

Fig. 40.1 Clinical decision chart for management of oral anticoagulant with minor rectal bleeding

Key Points

- Bleeding severity and hemodynamic stability should be assessed in a timely manner.
- Underlying thromboembolic risk should be determined.
- For patients receiving warfarin the INR should be measured.
- Need to reverse anticoagulation should be individualized based on bleeding severity, hemodynamic stability, underlying thromboembolic risk, and degree of INR elevation.
- The underlying cause of bleeding should be identified and corrected if possible.

Self-Assessment Questions

1. A 74-year-old woman presents to the urgent care clinic complaining of prolonged bleeding (oozing) from a tooth extraction site. She is receiving warfarin for atrial fibrillation and has mechanical aortic and mitral valves. Other medical

problems include hypertension, heart failure, and history of cardioembolic stroke. Labs including CBC are within normal limits. INR is 2.1. Blood pressure is 125/82 mmHg and pulse is 78 bpm. A lower molar was extracted yesterday as has been oozing blood since the patient returned home from the dentist's office. The patient skipped warfarin on the day prior to the extraction and also skipped last night's dose due to the persistent oozing. Which of the following is the best plan for managing this patient's situation?

(a) Resume usual dose of warfarin and attempt to control bleeding with local measures (e.g., direct pressure using a moistened tea bag or transexamic acid solution).
(b) Continue to hold warfarin and administer oral vitamin K 2.5 mg.
(c) Continue to hold warfarin and attempt to control bleeding with local measures (e.g., direct pressure using a moistened tea bag or transexamic acid solution).
(d) Continue to hold warfarin and administer 10 mg intravenous vitamin K.

The correct answer is A. This patient's underlying thromboembolic risk is very high (mechanical valves in the aortic and mitral position, prior history of stroke and several additional stroke risk factors). Subtherapeutic INRs should be avoided in this patient and local measures are likely to be sufficient to control the type of bleeding this patient is experiencing. Based on the current INR (probably already below target INR range of 2.5–3.5) and underlying thrombembolic risk answers B and D are incorrect because she is experiencing minor bleeding and is currently hemodynamically stable and further lowering of the INR with vitamin K places the patient at risk for thromboembolism and most guidelines recommend against holding warfarin doses for tooth extraction. Answer C is incorrect because the patient has already skipped two doses of warfarin resulting in further decline of the INR and increased thromboembolic risk.

2. A 62-year-old man has been taking rivaroxaban 20 mg daily for the past 4 months for a DVT that occurred following a total knee replacement. His creatinine clearance is 40 mL/min. Today he complains of a nosebleed that took nearly 30 min to control. He has been having frequent nosebleeds for the past several days. Which of the following represents the best plan to manage this patient's situation?

(a) Skip the next rivaroxaban dose and then resume anticoagulation if no further nosebleeds occur.
(b) Skip the next two rivaroxaban doses and then resume anticoagulation if no further nosebleeds occur.
(c) Discontinue rivaroxaban and follow up with patient in a few days to see if nosebleeds have improved.
(d) Refer the patient to the nearest emergency department for management of his recurrent nosebleeds.

Because this patient's DVT was associated with a transient risk factor (knee replacement surgery) 3 months of anticoagulation therapy is sufficient. Therefore, the correct answer is C because the risk of bleeding now outweighs the risk of recurrent

DVT. Answers A and B are incorrect because anticoagulation therapy is no longer indicated for the aforementioned reasons. Answer D is incorrect because this patient's bleeding is not severe enough to warrant going to the emergency department.

References

1. Schulman S, Kearon C on behalf of the Subcommittee on Control of Anticoagulation of the Scientific and Standardization Committee of the International Society on Thrombosis and Haemostasis. Definition of major bleeding in clinical investigations of antihemostatic medicinal products in non-surgical patients. Scientific and Standardization Committee Communication. J Thromb Haemost. 2005;3:692–4.
2. Kaatz S, Ahmad D, Spyropoulos AC, Schulman S, for the Subcommittee on Control of Anticoagulation. Definition of clinically relevant non-major bleeding in studies of anticoagulants in atrial fibrillation and venous thromboembolic disease in non-surgical patients: communication from the SSC of the ISTH. J Thromb Haemost. 2015;13:2119–26.
3. Radaelli F, Dentali F, Repici A, et al. Management of anticoagulation in patients with acute gastrointestinal bleeding. Dig Liver Dis. 2015;47:621–7.
4. Holbrook A, Schulman S, Witt DM, et al. Evidence-based management of anticoagulant therapy: antithrombotic therapy and prevention of thrombosis, 9th ed: American College of Chest Physicians evidence-based clinical practice guidelines. Chest. 2012;141(2 Suppl):e152S–84S.
5. Puskas J, Gerdisch M, Nichols D, et al. Reduced anticoagulation after mechanical aortic valve replacement: interim results from the prospective randomized on-X valve anticoagulation clinical trial randomized Food and Drug Administration investigational device exemption trial. J Thorac Cardiovasc Surg. 2014;147:1202–11.
6. Crowther MA, Ageno W, Garcia D, et al. Oral vitamin K versus placebo to correct excessive anticoagulation in patients receiving warfarin. Ann Intern Med. 2009;150:293–300.
7. Patel RJ, Witt DM, Saseen JJ, Tillman DJ, Wilkinson DS. Randomized, placebo-controlled trial of oral phytonadione for excessive anticoagulation. Pharmacotherapy. 2000;20:1159–66.
8. Lopes RD, Horowitz JD, Garcia DA, Crowther MA, Hylek EM. Warfarin and acetaminophen interaction: a summary of the evidence and biologic plausibility. Blood. 2011;118:6269–73.

Chapter 41
Patient Presenting with Major, Life-Threatening Bleeding

Daniel M. Witt

Abstract Initial management of anticoagulation-related major bleeding should involve stopping the anticoagulant, starting general supportive measures, measuring coagulation status, and locating and treating the source of bleeding if possible. Anticoagulation reversal strategies are specific to anticoagulation therapy type (warfarin vs. DOACs). The default strategy for most patients should be to resume anticoagulation therapy following resolution of bleeding.

Keywords Hemorrhage • Major bleeding • Life-threatening bleeding • Dabigatran Idarucizumab • Direct oral anticoagulant • Warfarin • Therapeutic management • Intracranial hemorrhage

Case Introduction

A 77-year-old man is brought to the emergency department by ambulance after being found unresponsive in his apartment by his daughter. He is taking dabigatan 150 mg orally twice daily to prevent stroke associated with paroxysmal non-valvular atrial fibrillation. His last known dabigatran dose was taken approximately 24 h ago (yesterday morning)—it is unclear whether he took last night's dose. He has a history of type 2 diabetes, congestive heart failure, poorly controlled hypertension, and chronic kidney disease (estimated creatinine clearance is 36 mL/min). He switched from warfarin to dabigatran 2 months ago after suffering a cardioembolic stroke when his INR was 2.3. He has fully recovered from that event without residual deficits. His other medications include lisinpril, HCTZ, metformin, furosemide, and amiodarone. Upon emergency department arrival the following were noted: T-98.6°, P-61 bpm, BP-201/96 mm Hg; Pupils-equal, sluggish, reactive; CV-NSR, no

---

D.M. Witt, PharmD, FCCP, BCPS
University of Utah College of Pharmacy,
30 South 2000 East, Salt Lake City, UT 84112, USA
e-mail: dan.witt@pharm.utah.edu

murmur; Skin-Bruise on hip; no gag reflex present, withdraws from pain, and has a Glasgow Coma Score of 4. CT scan reveals a large basal ganglia hematoma. Labs include an aPTT of 85 s (>2× the upper limit of normal). Neurosurgery would like to proceed with craniotomy as soon as possible.

Case Discussion

What Are the Initial Priorities for this Patient?

In addition to general supportive care (IV access, maintaining diuresis, hemodynamic support, etc.) key priorities include blood pressure management and anticoagulant reversal. Interventions to lower SBP >180 mmHg are warranted for patients presenting with intracranial hemorrhage (ICH) [1]. Achieving a SBP between 140 and 160 mmHg within 4 h of presentation has been associated with lower rates of hematoma enlargement [1].

How Should Anticoagulation Be Reversed?

Efforts to reverse dabigatran should be guided by the likelihood that anticoagulant effect is present. Knowing when the last dose of dabigatran was taken and estimating renal function will allow clinicians to reasonably predict whether anticoagulant effect is present [2]. Since the patient's family last saw him well yesterday, it should be assumed that he took a dose dabigatran last night (approximately 12 h ago). Based on this assumption, dabigatran's half-life in a patient with a creatinine clearance between 30–50 mL/min (estimated time to normalized hemostasis 96 h) (Table 41.1), and coadministration of the P-gp inhibitor amiodarone (further delay to normalized hemostasis), it is reasonable to assume that dabigatran anticoagulant effect is present. Although the aPTT cannot quantify the degree of anticoagulation, a value >2× after at least 12 h since the last dose indicates high bleeding risk [3]. The presence of life-threatening bleeding and the need for urgent surgical intervention are strong arguments for rapid dabigatran reversal using idarucizumab, which is FDA approved for these indications after demonstrating near complete reversal of

Table 41.1 Time to normalized hemostasis following DOAC cessation [2]

Creatinine clearance	Approximate time to normalized hemostasis	
	Dabigatran	Apixaban, rivaroxaban, edoxaban
>80 mL/min	24–48 h	24–48 h
50–80 mL/min	48–72 h	24–48 h
30–50 mL/min	72–96 h	24–48 h
15–30 mL/min	Not recommended	36–48 h
<15 mL/min	Not recommended	Not recommended

anticoagulation within minutes of administration [4]. The idarucizumab dose should be 5 g administered IV [4].

How Can the Effect of Idarucizumab Be Assessed?

Hemostatic efficacy of idarucizumab can be assessed by monitoring the patient for further signs of clinical deterioration and also by repeat CT scanning to detect hematoma enlargement. A normal aPTT may provide reassurance that the patient can be taken to surgery [2]. A normal thrombin time (TT) or dilute thrombin time (dTT) can also be used as qualitative evidence that dabigatran's anticoagulant effect has been reversed [2]. Repeat aPTT/TT/dTT testing may be needed during the hospitalization to detect re-emergence of dabigitran's anticoagulant effect as idarucizumab's effect wears off. A dTT >65 s indicates high bleeding risk [3].

What if Idarucizumab Is Not Available?

If idarucizumab is unavailable the administration of prothrombin complex concentrate (PCC) can be considered but reductions in blood loss and improved outcomes have not been demonstrated in actively bleeding patients and the potential prothrombotic effects must be considered [2]. The role of recombinant factor VIIa is poorly understood and not recommended by most experts [2]. Dabigatran can be removed by hemodialysis and this modality can be tried as a last resort [3].

If the Patient Survives to Hospital Discharge, Should Anticoagulation Therapy Be Resumed?

The answer to this question is multifactorial and depends on factors such as the location of the bleed (lobar or deep), the underlying thromboembolic risk, the patient's prognosis, and anticipated quality of life [5]. Compared to bleeds occurring in the deep structures of the brain, recurrent ICH is more common following lobar bleeds [5]. Resuming anticoagulation therapy should be more strongly considered in patients with high underlying thromboembolic risk [5]. This patient suffered a deep ICH and has many stroke risks including heart failure, hypertension, prior stroke history, and diabetes. These considerations argue in favor of resuming anticoagulation provided the patient's prognosis and anticipated quality of life are reasonably favourable [5]. High quality evidence to inform the optimal timing of anticoagulation therapy resumption and the choice of anticoagulant are not currently available. Given this patient's renal function and the presence of interacting amiodarone therapy resuming therapy with warfarin is worth considering. However, DOACs like dabigatran are associated with lower risk of ICH although patients with recent ICH were likely excluded from DOAC clinical trials.

Key Points

- Initial management of anticoagulation-related major bleeding should involve stopping the anticoagulant, starting general supportive measures, measuring coagulation status (aPTT, INR, TT, dTT, anti-Xa level depending on the type of anticoagulant), and locating and treating the source of bleeding if possible.
- For DOACs, determining when the last dose was administered, estimating renal function, and documenting whether interacting drugs are present, the severity of bleeding, and need for invasive interventions are helpful to assess whether reversal strategies (idarucizumab for dabigatran, PCCs for rivaroxaban, apixaban, and edoxaban) will be needed (see Table 41.2).
- For warfarin, elevated INRs should be reversed with vitamin K (IV for severe or life threatening bleeding, oral otherwise). The severity of bleeding and need for invasive interventions are helpful to assess whether PCC or FFP will be needed (PCC preferred over FFP due to ease of administration and more rapid reversal) (see Table 41.2).
- The default strategy should be to resume anticoagulation therapy following resolution of bleeding. Patient-specific factors such as low underlying thromboembolic risk, very high risk for recurrent bleeding, or patient preference should dictate whether the default strategy should be abandoned.

Self-Assessment Questions

1. A 75-year-old man is seen in the emergency department complaining of a three-day history of black, tarry stool, syncope, and fatigue. He is taking warfarin for a DVT that occurred 6 months ago following hip replacement surgery. His hemoglobin is 9 g/dL and his INR is 6.2. He has been taking ibuprofen 800 mg

Table 41.2 Anticoagulant reversal strategies for patients with major bleeding

Anticoagulant	Reversal strategy
Warfarin	Non-life-threatening: Oral vitamin K 2.5–5 mg Life-threatening or need for urgent invasive intervention: IV vitamin K 5–10 mg plus PCC or FFP (PCC preferred over FFP due to ease of administration and more rapid reversal)
Dabigatran	Life-threatening or need for urgent invasive intervention: IV idarucizumab 5 g
Apixaban Rivaroxaban Edoxaban	Life-threatening or need for urgent invasive intervention: 4-factor PCC or IV andexanet (approval pending)

three times daily for about a week for lower back pain. An NSAID-induced upper GI tract bleed is suspected and the medical team would like to perform endoscopy as soon as possible. In addition to stopping warfarin and general supportive measures, which of the following is the best management plan for this patient?

(a) 2.5 mg oral vitamin K
(b) 5 mg IV vitamin K plus PCC 50 units/kg
(c) PCC 50 units/kg
(d) 5 mg oral vitamin K plus 2 units of FFP

Because the INR is elevated and an urgent invasive procedure is needed the correct answer is B. A and D are incorrect because oral vitamin K and FFP will not correct the INR rapidly enough to facilitate urgent endoscopy. Oral vitamin K won't correct the INR for about 24 h and FFP must be thawed prior to infusion and requires prolonged infusion time. C is incorrect because without vitamin K administration to support production of functional clotting factors, once PCCs wear off, the INR will become elevated again putting the patient at risk for further bleeding complications.

2. It has been 2 weeks since the patient from the previous question was discharged from the hospital following treatment of his GI tract bleed. He has stopped using ibuprofen and is taking omeprazole 20 mg daily to facilitate healing of a gastric ulcer. His physician would like a recommendation from you regarding whether his warfarin therapy should be resumed. Which of the following represents the best plan for this patient?

(a) This patient should not resume warfarin therapy
(b) This patient should resume anticoagulation therapy with apixaban, which has a lower risk of GI tract bleeding
(c) This patient should resume warfarin therapy to prevent further VTE
(d) This patient should be switched to low-dose daily aspirin

This patient had a provoked DVT and should have stopped warfarin therapy 3 months ago. Therefore, the correct answer is A. B, C and D are incorrect because the underlying risk of thromboembolism is not high enough to outweigh bleeding risk. Furthermore, aspirin increases the risk for GI tract bleeding and should be avoided unless there is a compelling indication, which is not the case for this patient.

References

1. Kuramatsu JB, Gerner ST, Schellinger PD, et al. Anticoagulant reversal, blood pressure levels, and anticoagulant resumption in patients with anticoagulation-related intracerebral haemorrhage. JAMA. 2015;313:824–36.
2. Heidbuchel H, Verhamme P, Alings M, et al. Updated European Heart Rhythm Association practical guide on the use of non-vitamin K antagonist anticoagulants in patients with non-valvular atrial fibrillation. Europace. 2015;17:1467–507.

3. Weitz JI, Pollack CV. Practical management of bleeding in patients receiving non-vitamin K oral anticoagulants. Thromb Haemost. 2015;114:1113–26.
4. Pollack CV, Reilly PA, Eikelboom J, et al. Idarucizumab for dabigatran reversal. N Engl J Med. 2015;373:511–20.
5. Goldstein JN, Greenberg SM. Should anticoagulation be resumed after intracerebral hemorrhage? Cleve Clin J Med. 2010;77:791–9.

Chapter 42
Overdose of Dabigatran

Alicia Potter DeFalco

Abstract With the limited availability of reversal agents, it may be difficult to treat a patient who has overdosed on a direct oral anticoagulant (DOAC). Treatment of these patients may be guided by time elapsed since ingestion, laboratory values, and overall clinical stability.

Keywords Anticoagulant reversal agents • Direct oral anticoagulants • Idarucizumab (Praxbind®) • Andexanet alfa • Ciraparantag • Dabigatran overdose • Laboratory monitoring

Case Introduction

A 57 year-old-female receiving dabigatran for treatment of deep vein thrombosis at home presents to the emergency department after intentional ingestion of ten 150 mg dabigatran capsules approximately 90 min ago. Her current blood pressure is 132/88 mmHg, heart rate is 76 beats per minute, respiratory rate is 18 per minute, and oxygen saturation is 100% on room air. The patient is conscious and following commands. She denies any signs or symptoms of bleeding, and her physical exam is negative for evidence of bleeding. Pertinent labs are as follows: hemoglobin (hgb) is 13.1, hematocrit (hct) is 38.2%, platelets (plt) are 180×10^9/L, prothrombin time (PT) is 22, international normalized ratio (INR) is 2.8, and activated partial thromboplastin time (aPTT) is 42 s. Her estimated creatinine clearance is 88 mL/min. The patient is also taking lisinopril 20 mg by mouth daily at home.

A.P. DeFalco, PharmD, BCPS
South College School of Pharmacy, 400 Goody's Lane, Knoxville, TN 37922, USA
e-mail: apotter@southcollegetn.edu

Case Discussion

What Factors Should Be Considered When Developing a Plan for Treatment of an Anticoagulant Overdose?

Time Since Ingestion

Time elapsed since ingestion of an anticoagulant is helpful in assessing the potential for anticoagulant absorption, and thus can provide guidance in management of the overdose. For patients who present within a few hours of ingestion, administration of activated charcoal may be beneficial in preventing further absorption of the anticoagulant [1]. Due to the rapid absorption of dabigatran, activated charcoal would provide the greatest benefit if administered within 2 h of ingestion [2]. For patients who present with massive overdoses of dabigatran or if several hours have passed since ingestion of dabigatran, hemodiaylsis has been shown to remove up to 2/3 of the drug within 2 h due to the low protein binding exhibited by dabigatran. However, the highly protein bound factor Xa inhibitors and warfarin are unable to be sufficiently removed by hemodialysis. Emergency access to hemodialysis may be limited, making the recently approved idarucizumab a potentially favorable treatment option in the setting of dabigatran overdose [3].

Hemodynamic Stability and Bleeding Complications

In a patient experiencing direct oral anticoagulant (DOAC) or warfarin overdose, hemodynamic stability and bleeding complications including bleeding site, blood volume lost, and severity of bleed must be assessed [4]. If evidence of bleeding is absent, as the case here describes, clearance of the anticoagulant and maintaining hemodynamic stability are the mainstays of care. Supportive care measures include fluid administration and maintaining adequate renal perfusion. Due to the short half-lives of DOACs, supportive care in patients with normal renal function is typically sufficient for removal of the agent in the absence of bleeding complications [1].

Lab Monitoring

There are several laboratory measurements and coagulation assays being investigated to evaluate direct oral anticoagulant (DOAC) concentrations, however, their limited availability and the lack of FDA approved reference levels and assays restrict their utility in clinical practice [4]. See Table 42.1 for a summary of coagulation assay monitoring. Prothrombin time and INR results are unreliable in assessing anticoagulation activity of DOACs. INR lacks sensitivity to dabigatran related anticoagulation, causing relatively normal INR values at therapeutic dabigatran levels, and slight increases at higher dabigatran concentrations [6]. The PT/INR results will differ across laboratories secondary to the differences in the sensitivities of reagents to the

Table 42.1 Oral anticoagulants and coagulation assay monitoring [3, 5]

Drug	Coagulation assay	Sensitivity	Utility
Dabigatran	TT	Very sensitive—Detects lower levels of dabigatran but maximum TT levels may result before achieving therapeutic concentration of dabigatran	Sensitivity limits utility in quantifying anticoagulation; helpful at low levels of dabigatran but value is lost at higher concentrations
	PT/INR	Insensitive	Elevated values may indicate presence of drug, but may not correlate anticoagulation effects
	aPTT	More sensitive than PT/INR	Cannot be used to measure concentration of dabigatran. Readily available assay
	dTT	Sensitive	Quantifies serum concentration. Limited availability. Not FDA approved
	ECT	Sensitive	Quantifies serum concentration. Limited availability. Not FDA approved
Rivaroxaban Apixaban Edoxaban	Chromogenic Factor Xa	Sensitive and accurate	Limited availability. Not FDA approved
	PT/INR	Rivaroxaban and apixaban—More sensitive at higher concentrations. Edoxaban—More sensitive than aPTT, insensitive at low levels	May suggest high drug concentrations if significantly elevated
	aPTT	Low sensitivity	Readily available assay. Not ideal
Warfarin	PT/INR	Sensitive	May not show significant elevations for 24–48 h post ingestion
	aPTT	Low sensitivity	Not ideal, value increases with warfarin ingestion

effects of dabigatran [2]. Thrombin time (TT) is a sensitive assay that may provide information regarding the anticoagulation activity of dabigatran, however, due to the sensitivity of the assay, maximum TT levels may result before achieving therapeutic levels of dabigatran. A diluted thrombin time (dTT) and an ecarin clotting time (ECT) can both provide a quantitative measurement of dabigatran, however availability of these assays is limited and their efficacy in monitoring dabigatran anticoagulant activity has not been established by the Food and Drug Administration (FDA) [7]. In the RE-LY study, patients receiving dabigatran 150 mg twice daily yielded median trough concentrations of 93 ng/mL and median peak concentrations of 184 ng/mL. Anticoagulant effects of dabigatran are not expected at plasma concentrations below 20 ng/mL [8]. Activated partial thromboplastin time (aPTT) may be utilized to confirm that a patient is anticoagulated with dabigatran, as aPTT will be prolonged in a dose-dependent response to dabigatran. The aPTT may be prolonged for 8–12 h, and in some patients, aPTT elevations may be observed as long as 24 h after dabigatran ingestion. Evidence suggests that aPTT will peak 2 h after ingestion of dabigatran [2]. While aPTT elevation may be associated with the presence of dabigatran, these elevations do not quantify the dabigatran plasma concentration [3].

Factor Xa inhibitors, such as rivaroxaban, apixaban, and edoxaban, do not effect TT or ECT and produce changes in PT/INR and aPTT values that are unreliable in evaluating drug levels. Prothrombin time prolongation is typically more significant with higher concentrations of factor Xa inhibitors, which may provide further confirmation of an overdose. Chromogenic anti-factor Xa assays have been evaluated in the measurement of heparin and enoxaparin as well as the oral factor Xa inhibitors. The chromogenic anti-factor Xa assay must be calibrated for each specific factor Xa inhibitor to be utilized in assessing plasma concentrations of specific factor Xa inhibitors. When measuring levels of factor Xa inhibitors, chromogenic anti-factor Xa assays are more accurate than PT, INR, and aPTT [3], however, at this time, specific chromogenic anti-factor Xa assays for DOACs are not available worldwide [6].

Additionally, complete blood count (CBC) and renal function should be monitored to assess for bleeding complications and clearance of the medication, respectively.

Reversal Agents Available

Management of direct oral anticoagulant (DOAC) overdose can typically be managed by temporary removal of the anticoagulant and supportive care. If urgent reversal is warranted, the addition of clotting factor supplements may be indicated. Supportive care may include hemodynamic support to promote removal of the anticoagulant, and if bleeding is evident, volume replacement, blood transfusion, and bleeding site control may be beneficial [4].

Idarucizumab (Praxbind®) is a humanized monoclonal antibody fragment approved for reversal of the anticoagulant properties of dabigatran in the setting of emergency surgery, urgent procedures, or in life-threatening or uncontrolled bleeding [8]. Data is lacking on the utility of idarucizumab in the treatment of dabigatran overdose in the absence of bleeding or the need for emergent surgery or urgent procedures but case reports suggest benefit. In one case report, aPTT and PT values normalized quickly and remained normalized for 24 h in a patient who was treated with idarucizumab after intentional ingestion of 125 capsules of dabigatran 150 mg [9].

To date, there are no antidotes approved for the reversal of the oral factor Xa inhibitors, rivaroxaban, apixaban, and edoxaban. Of note, there are two reversal agents, andexanet alfa and ciraparantag, in clinical trials that have been granted expedited reviews by the FDA [3]. Andexanet alfa is being evaluated for the reversal of oral factor Xa inhibitors, low molecular weight heparin, and fondaparinux, while ciraparantag is being evaluated for the reversal of oral direct thrombin inhibitors and heparin in addition to oral factor Xa inhibitors, low molecular weight heparin, and fondaparinux. There are reports to support prothrombin complex concentrates

(PCCs) and activated prothrombin complex concentrates (aPCCs) in treatment of bleeding complications associated with DOACs, however, data to support their use in overdose patients without evidence of bleeding is limited. A disadvantage of using prothrombin complex concentrates includes the risk of thrombosis which may occur as a result of pre-existing risk factors for thrombosis and the introduction of additional clotting factors into a patient in effort to reverse anticoagulation in a patient predisposed to thrombosis [3]. See Table 42.2 for a summary of oral anticoagulant reversal options.

Table 42.2 Oral anticoagulants and reversal agents [1, 5, 10]

Reversal option	Dabigatran	Rivaroxaban, apixaban, edoxaban	Warfarin
Activated charcoal	Within 2 h of ingestion—may reduce absorption	Within 2 h of ingestion—may reduce absorption	Within 2 h of ingestion—may reduce absorption
Hemodialysis	Removes approximately 80% of drug	Not effective	Not effective
Phytonadione	Not effective	Not effective	**INR 4.5–10, no bleed**: not indicated **INR > 10, no bleed**: 5 mg PO × 1 **Serious, life threatening bleed at any INR***: 10 mg IV × 1 *May also require prothrombin complex concentrate and/ or fresh frozen plasma in addition to phytonadione
Activated factor VIIa [Novoseven RT]	If serious, life-threatening bleeding or emergent reversal indicated, may combine with 3-factor PCC; would be less preferred option	If serious, life-threatening bleeding or emergent reversal indicated, may combine with 3-factor PCC; would be less preferred option	If serious, life-threatening bleeding or emergent reversal indicated, may be administered with or without 3-factor PCC
3-factor PCC [Profilnine]	Limited evidence; If serious, life-threatening bleeding or emergent reversal indicated, recommended in combination with activated factor VIIa (Novoseven®); avoid as monotherapy for dabigatran reversal if possible	Limited evidence; If serious, life-threatening bleeding or emergent reversal indicated, recommended in combination with activated factor VIIa (Novoseven®); avoid as monotherapy for factor Xa-inhibitor reversal if possible	If serious, life-threatening bleeding or emergent reversal indicated, may be administered

(continued)

Table 42.2 (continued)

Reversal option	Dabigatran	Rivaroxaban, apixaban, edoxaban	Warfarin
4-factor PCC [Kcentra]	May consider as alternative to aPCC	If serious, life-threatening bleeding or emergent reversal indicated, may be administered	Preferred PCC for warfarin associated serious, life-threatening bleeding or emergent reversal
Activated 4-factor PCC (aPCC) [Feiba]	Recommended by dabigatran manufacturer for serious, life-threatening bleeding or emergent reversal	If serious, life-threatening bleeding or emergent reversal indicated, may be administered	May consider as alternative to Kcentra
Idarucizumab [Praxbind®]	Known overdose, no bleed, aPTT or dTT/ECT significantly elevated: May consider 5 g IV × 1 Moderate—serious bleeding: 5 g IV × 1	Not effective	Not effective
Andexanet alfa	Not effective	Potential benefit—not yet approved	Not effective
Ciraparantag	Potential benefit—not yet approved	Potential benefit—not yet approved	Not effective

Table 42.3 DOAC half-life based on renal function [5, 11]

Renal function	Half-life (hours) based on renal function			
	Dabigatran	Rivaroxaban	Apixaban	Edoxaban
CrCl >80 mL/min	14	8	15	14
CrCl 50–79 mL/min	17	9	15	18
CrCl 30–49 mL/min	19	9	18	24
CrCl <30 mL/min	28	10	17	24

How should this patient be managed?

This patient is currently hemodynamically stable without evidence of bleeding complications. She ingested a supratherapeutic dose of dabigatran less than 2 h ago. The most appropriate first line therapy would be activated charcoal to prevent further absorption of the medication.

Administer fluids to maintain perfusion and monitor hemodynamic stability throughout the encounter. Her current estimated creatinine clearance is 88 mL/min. It is crucial to maintain adequate renal perfusion to ensure clearance of the absorbed medication. See Table 42.3 for a summary of DOAC half-lives based on renal clearance. If the patient requires hospitalization, a serum creatinine should be obtained daily and creatinine clearance calculated utilizing the Crockcoft-Gault equation.

Her PT, INR, and aPTT are all elevated. Ideally, a dTT and/or ECT would be ordered to quantify the serum concentration of the dabigatran; however, these assays are not widely available in emergency situations. If dTT and ECT are unavailable, aPTT may provide guidance regarding the anticoagulant effect of dabigatran, although the aPTT does not quantify the serum concentration of dabigatran. At a minimum, the aPTT should be drawn at baseline, at 2 h post exposure, and every 12 h until aPTT returns to normal [2].

Is idarucizumab indicated for this patient?

At this time, it would not be necessary to administer idarucizumab. The patient is showing no symptomatic or clinical signs of bleeding and her CBC is within normal limits. While her aPTT is elevated, it would be more appropriate to continue to monitor the patient and obtain an aPTT post activated charcoal administration prior to making the decision to administer idarucizumab. If the patient presented several hours post ingestion and was showing significantly prolonged aPTT values (or elevated dTT, ECT, if available), or if the same patient presented similarly, but with signs of bleeding, idarucizumab may be indicated.

Key Points

- In evaluating an overdose patient, time elapsed since ingestion is crucial in developing a treatment plan.
- In the absence of bleeding, many patients who have overdosed on a DOAC may be managed by limiting absorption of the DOAC, maintaining hemodynamic stability, and facilitating clearance of the DOAC.
- There are no reversal agents approved for the oral factor Xa inhibitors. Idarucizumab is the only approved reversal agent for dabigatran.
- Patients who have overdosed on a DOAC require monitoring of CBC and renal function. Other potential labs that may be helpful in assessing a patient who has overdosed on dabigatran are aPTT, dTT, and ECT. Chromogenic antiXa assays, if available, can be helpful in assessing a patient who has overdosed with a factor Xa inhibitor.

Self-Assessment Questions

1. A 61 year-old-female who is on dabigatran 150 mg twice daily for atrial fibrillation presents to the emergency department via ambulance. The patient's sister found her at home with a suicide note. The patient reports taking 60 dabigatran 150 mg capsules approximately 5 h ago. She is also on metoprolol succinate 100 mg once daily at home. Her current blood pressure is 150/92 mmHg, heart rate is 80 beats per minute, respiratory rate is 18 per minute, and oxygen saturation is 98% on room air. The patient is conscious and following commands. She denies

any signs or symptoms of bleeding, and her physical exam is negative for evidence of bleeding. Pertinent labs are as follows: hemoglobin (hgb) is 12.8, hematocrit (hct) is 36.0%, platelets (plt) are 160×10^9/L, prothrombin time (PT) is 34, international normalized ratio (INR) is 4.0, and activated partial thromboplastin time (aPTT) is 76 s. Additionally, a dTT reveals a dabigatran serum concentration of 680 ng/mL. Her estimated creatinine clearance is 96 mL/min. What is the most appropriate treatment option for this patient at this time?

(a) Activated charcoal
(b) Fluids
(c) Hemodialysis
(d) Idarucizumab

Correct answer: D. idarucizumab.

Rational: The patient ingested the dabigatran approximately 5 h ago. Due to the time elapsed since ingestion, activated charcoal will be ineffective. The patient's labs suggest a great deal of the medication has been absorbed (PT 28, INR 4.0, aPTT 76, and dabigatran concentration 680 ng/mL). The patient requires more than fluid resuscitation for treatment of this overdose. While there is no evidence of bleeding, the aPTT and dabigatran are significantly elevated and warrant reversal of dabigatran. Hemodialysis is less readily available and more invasive than administering a reversal agent. Idarucizumab will neutralize the circulating dabigatran.

2. A 56 year-old-male who is on rivaroxaban 20 mg daily for deep vein thrombosis at home presents to the emergency department after an intentional overdose of 15 rivaroxaban 20 mg tablets. The patient reports ingesting all 15 tablets approximately 60 min ago. The patient is also on sertraline 100 mg daily and alprazolam 0.5 mg three times daily as needed for anxiety. His current blood pressure is 146/92 mmHg, heart rate is 62 beats per minute, respiratory rate is 16 per minute, and oxygen saturation is 100% on room air. The patient is conscious and following commands. He denies any signs or symptoms of bleeding, and his physical exam is negative for evidence of bleeding. Pertinent labs are as follows: hemoglobin (hgb) is 14.1, hematocrit (hct) is 38.0%, platelets (plt) are 162×10^9/L, prothrombin time (PT) is 24, international normalized ratio (INR) is 1.8, and activated partial thromboplastin time (aPTT) is 36 s. Chromogenic antiXa assay for rivaroxaban is unavailable at your institution's laboratory. His estimated creatinine clearance is 100 mL/min. What is the most appropriate treatment option for this patient at this time?

(a) Activated charcoal
(b) Andexanet alfa
(c) Idarucizumab
(d) Prothrombin complex concentrate

Correct answer: A. activated charcoal.

The patient presents within 2 h of ingestion, therefore activated charcoal may be administered to limit the absorption of tablets ingested. Andexanet alfa is not yet approved, therefore would not be an available or appropriate selection. Idarucizumab is specific for dabigatran and will be ineffective for reversal of other medications. The patient is not bleeding and aPTT, PT, and INR are not critically elevated, therefore, the risk of thrombosis associated with administration of prothrombin complex concentrate outweighs any potential benefit at this time.

References

1. Kaatz S, et al. Guidance on the emergent reversal of oral thrombin and factor Xz inhibitors. Am J Hematol. 2012;87:S141–5.
2. Alikhan R, et al. The acute management of haemorrhage, surgery and overdose in patients receiving dabigatran. Emerg Med J. 2014;31:163–8.
3. Dager W, Hellwig T. Current knowledge on assessing the effects of and managing bleeding and urgent procedures with direct oral anticoagulants. Am J Health Syst Pharm. 2016;73(Suppl 2):S14–26.
4. Gulseth MP. Overview of direct oral anticoagulant therapy reversal. Am J Healh Syst Pharm. 2016;73(Suppl 2):S5–13.
5. Nutescu EA, et al. Management of bleeding and reversal strategies for oral anticoagulants: clinical practice considerations. Am J Health Syst Pharm. 2013;70:1914–29.
6. Tummala R, Kavtaradze A, Gupta A, Ghosh RK. Specific antidotes against direct oral anticoagulants: a comprehensive review of clinical trials data. Int J Cardiol. 2016;214:292–8.
7. Thakkar A. Reversal of dabigatran etexilate: current strategies and the RE-VERSE AD trial. 2015. http://www.acc.org/latest-in-cardiology/articles/2015/09/25/09/51/reversal-of-dabigatran-etexilate
8. Praxbind® [package insert]. Ridgefield, CT: Boehringer Ingelheim Pharmaceuticals, Inc.; 2015.
9. Peetermans M, et al. Idarucizumab for dabigatran overdose. Clin Toxicol. 2016;54(8):644–6. doi:10.1080/15563650.2016.1187737.
10. Guyatt GH, et al. Executive summary: antithrombotic therapy and prevention of thrombosis, 9th ed: American College of Chest Physicians evidence-based clinical practice guidelines. Chest. 2012;141(2 Suppl):7S–47S.
11. Savaysa® [package insert]. Tokyo, Japan: Daiichi Sankyo Co., Ltd; 2015.

Index

A
Acetaminophen, 19, 93, 121, 209, 213, 231, 232, 234–236, 285
ACS. *See* Acute coronary syndrome (ACS)
Activated partial thromboplastin time (aPTT)
  dabigatran, 297–298
  idarucizumab, 291
Activated prothrombin complex concentrates (aPCCs), 298–299
Acute coronary syndrome (ACS)
  apixaban, 171, 172
  bleeding avoidance, 170
  CABG
    bridging therapy, 188
    DOACs interruptions, 189
    elective, 188
    heart valves, 188
    idarucizumab, 190, 191
    patient history, 187
    urgent/emergent, 189–191
    warfarin, 188, 189, 191, 192
  catheterization, 171
  DOACs, 169
  PCI, 168–170
  post PCI
    bleeding risk, 174
    DAPT duration, 175
    double *vs.* triple therapy, 175
    ischemic risk, 174
    patient history, 173
    pharmacotherapy regimen, 174–175
    STEMI, 181–184
    triple therapy, 174–178
    warfarin, 174–176, 178
  VKA management, 169
  warfarin, 168–169, 171
Adherence, 96
  anticoagulant
    assessment of, 38
    characteristics of anticoagulants, 38, 39
    discontinuation rates, 39
    for DOACs, 38, 39
    interventions, 39
    once-daily *vs.* twice-daily doses, 40
    patient adherence, 39, 40
    shared decision making, 39
    suggested questions, 38
    for warfarin, 38, 39
  assess medications, 63
  with warfarin therapy, 46
Adjuvants, 233
American Academy of Orthopaedic Surgeons (AAOS), 124
American College of Chest Physician (ACCP), 123, 124, 261, 264
Andexanet alfa, 298
Anticoagulant adherence
  assessment of, 38
  characteristics of anticoagulants, 38, 39
  discontinuation rates, 39
  for DOACs, 38, 39
  interventions, 39
  once-daily *vs.* twice-daily doses, 40
  patient adherence, 39, 40
  shared decision making, 39
  suggested questions, 38
  for warfarin, 38, 39
Anticoagulation management
  catheter ablation
    patient history, 239
    procedure, 241
    reason for, 242
    thrombotic and hemorrhagic risks, 240–242
    warfarin, 239–242
  mechanical valves
    antithrombotic recommendations, 248–249
    appropriate oral anticoagulant, 246
    Bjork-Shiley tilting-disk valve, 247

Anticoagulation management (*cont.*)
    diagnostic/surgical procedures, 249
    INR goal intensification, 249–250
    medical history, 245
    Medtronic Hall tilting-disk valve, 247
    on-X aortic mechanical valve, 249
    Starr-Edwards caged-ball valve, 247
    St. Jude Medical Regent, 247
    thrombosis, risk of, 246
    valve thrombosis, 246
  oral Xa and IIa inhibitors, 279
  post-procedure, 279
  pre-procedure, 278–279
  warfarin, 279
Antidepressants, 233
Anti-factor Xa assay, 116, 131, 261, 262, 298
Antiphospholipid antibody syndrome (APS)
  bleeding, 256
  chromogenic Factor X levels, 255–256
  diagnosis, 254
  hypercoagulable states, 254
  medical history, 253
  monitoring, 255–256
  thrombophilias, 254, 255
  treatment, 254–255
Antiplatelet therapy, 16, 20, 33, 70, 137–138
Aortic valve stenosis
  anticoagulation, 88–89
  atrial fibrillation, 87–89
  LVEF, 87
  non-valvular AF, 88
  VHD, 88–89
Apixaban, 27, 28, 96
  ACS, 171, 172
  CAD, 138
  CKD, 145–148
  ischemic stroke, 16
  mixed P-gp/3A4 inhibitors, 214, 217
  P-gp, 203, 204
  recurrent VTE, 154, 155, 157
  VTE, 77
    prophylaxis, 123–125
    recurrent, 154, 155, 157
APS. *See* Antiphospholipid antibody syndrome (APS)
aPTT. *See* Activated partial thromboplastin time (aPTT)
ASCVD. *See* Atherosclerotic cardiovascular disease (ASCVD)
Aspirin
  CAD, 69–71
  DAPT, 175
  DES, 137–140
  elderly patients, 20
  GI hemorrhage, 25, 26
  mechanical valves, 250
  monotherapy, 10
  pharmacodynamic drug interactions, 208, 211
  VTE, 124
Aspirin plus clopidogrel combination therapy, 10
Atherosclerotic cardiovascular disease (ASCVD), 209–210
Atrial fibrillation (AF)
  anticoagulant adherence, 37
  aortic valve stenosis, 87–89
  CAD, 70–71
  catheter ablation, 239–242
  chronic pain management, 231
  drug-drug interactions, 221
  elderly patients, 19–22
  GI hemorrhage, 25, 26
  intracranial hemorrhage, 31–33
  ischemic stroke, 15–17
  mitral valve stenosis, 82–84
  OAC, 168
  renal dysfunction, 53–56
  stable chronic kidney disease, 43–47
  stroke prevention therapy, 7, 10
  variable renal function, 61, 62
  and VTE, 75–78
Azole antifungals, 196

B

Bare metal stent (BMS), 137, 175, 177
Bjork-Shiley tilting-disk valve, 247
Bypass grafting. *See* Coronary artery bypass surgery (CABG)

C

CABG. *See* Coronary artery bypass surgery (CABG)
CAD. *See* Coronary artery disease (CAD)
Cancer-associated venous thromboembolism, 113–115, 117, 118, 270, 273, 274
Catheter ablation
  patient history, 239
  procedure, 241
  reason for, 242
  thrombotic and hemorrhagic risks, 240–242
  warfarin, 239–242
CHA_2DS_2-VASc scoring system, 15, 20, 21, 33, 38–40, 54, 56, 70, 71, 78, 81, 82, 84, 88, 174, 188, 190

Index   307

in elderly patients, 20–21
in GI hemorrhage patient, 26
stroke prevention therapy, 8–9
stroke risk, 54
Chromogenic anti-factor X assays, 298
Chromogenic factor X assay, 255–256
Chronic kidney disease (CKD)
   apixaban, 145–148
   dabigatran, 145–148
   DOAC usage, 55–57
   dosing recommendations, 145
   edoxaban, 145–148
   patient history, 53–54, 143
   rivaroxaban, 145–147
   stroke and bleeding risk, 54
   warfarin, 56–57, 144–148
Chronic pain management
   acetaminophen, 232, 234–236
   adjuvants, 233
   interventional, 231
   NSAIDs, 232–233
   opioids, 233
   patient history, 231
   venlafaxine, 233, 235, 236
Cimetadine, 196
Ciraparantag, 298
CKD. *See* Chronic kidney disease (CKD)
Clarithromycin, 47, 196, 198, 199, 202, 204
Coagulation assay monitoring, 296–297
Cockcroft-Gault equation, 15, 26, 37, 53, 55, 145
Coronary artery bypass surgery (CABG)
   bridging therapy, 188
   DOACs interruptions, 189
   elective, 188
   heart valves, 188
   idarucizumab, 190, 191
   patient history, 187
   urgent/emergent, 189–191
   warfarin, 188, 189, 191, 192
Coronary artery disease (CAD)
   antiplatelet in, 138
   antiplatelet therapy, 70
   antithrombotic therapy, 70
   atrial fibrillation, 70–71
   DOACs, 70–71
   echocardiogram, 69
   medical history, 69
   VKA, 70–71
Critical illness. *See* Intensive care unit (ICU)
CYP1A2 inhibitors, 196, 222–224, 226
CYP3A4 inhibitors
   DOACs, 197
   drug inhibitors of, 196

   patient history, 195
   P-gp, 197, 202–205
   warfarin, 196–199
CYP2C9 inhibitors, 63, 196, 222–224, 271
Cytochrome P450, 196, 222, 233

D

Dabigatran, 27, 28, 96, 290, 291
   ischemic stroke, 16–17
   mixed P-gp/3A4 inhibitors, 215, 217
   P-gp, 203, 204
   recurrent VTE, 154, 155
   VTE, 77
Dabigatran overdose
   bleeding complications, 296
   deep vein thrombosis, 295
   DOAC half-life based on renal function, 300
   hemodynamic stability, 296
   lab monitoring, 296–298
   oral anticoagulant reversal agents, 298–300
   patient management, 300
   time since ingestion, 296
DAPT. *See* Dual-antiplatelet therapy (DAPT)
DES. *See* Drug eluting stent (DES)
Diet, 3
Diluted thrombin time (dTT), 291, 297
Direct oral anticoagulants (DOACs), 260, 291
   advantages, 270
   anticoagulant, 296, 298
   aortic valve stenosis, 88, 89
   APS, 255
   bleeding complications, 296
   CABG, 189
   CAD, 70–71
   CKD, 55–57
   CYP3A4 inhibitors, 197
   half-lives based on renal clearance, 300
   hemodynamic stability, 296
   mitral valve stenosis, 82, 84
   mixed P-gp/3A4 inhibitors, 215–216
   PCCs, 298–299
   P-glycoprotein, 203–204
   pharmacodynamic drug interactions, 210
   stable moderate chronic kidney disease
      benefits and risks, 48
      degree of renal elimination, 45
      discontinuation or avoidance, 44
      dose reduction, 46
      drug–drug interactions, 46, 47
      patient affordability, 48
      routine monitoring, 48

Direct oral anticoagulants (DOACs) (cont.)
supportive care, 298
variable renal function
dose selection, 62
management, 62–63
outpatient follow-up, 64
therapeutic activity measurement, 62
VTE, 76
absorption and metabolism of, 155
dosage, 154
risk reduction, 156
warfarin
adherence, 96
apixaban, 96
conversion, 97
dabigatran, 96
edoxaban, 97
FDA-approved indications, 94
renal function assessment, 96
rivaroxaban, 97
safety and efficacy, comparison, 94, 95
self-monitoring, 96
Distance-based management, 102–104, 106
DOACs. *See* Direct oral anticoagulants (DOACs)
Door to needle time, 183
Drug-drug interactions, 3
Drug eluting stent (DES)
anticoagulant, choosing, 136–137
CAD, 138
DAPT, 137–138
patient history, 135–136
triple therapy, 140
Drug interactions
CYP 3A4 inhibitors
DOACs, 197
drug inhibitors of, 196
patient history, 195
P-gp, 197, 202–205
warfarin, 196–199
P-gp
CYP3A4 inhibitors, 197, 202–205
DOAC, 203–204
inhibitors and inducers, 202
mediated drug interactions, 202–203
patient history, 201
transport system, 202
warfarin, 203
pharmacodynamic
bleeding risk, 208–209
clinical risk-benefit considerations, 209–210
COX-1, 208, 209, 211
DOAC, 210

low dose aspirin, 208, 211
mechanism, 208–209
NSAIDs, 208, 209, 211
patient history, 207
with warfarin, 208
pharmacokinetic
vs. anticoagulation therapy, 225
cholestyramine, 226, 227
CYP450, 222
CYP1A2 inducer, 226
distribution, 222, 223
metabolism, 223–225
patient management, 225
vitamin K oxide, 222, 223
Dual-antiplatelet therapy (DAPT), 137, 138, 169, 170, 173–175, 178

E
Edoxaban, 97
ischemic stroke, 16, 17
mixed P-gp/3A4 inhibitors, 215, 217
P-gp, 203, 204
recurrent VTE, 154, 155
VTE, 77
Elderly patients
atrial fibrillation, 20
CHA_2DS_2-VASc risk stratification score, 20–21
HAS-BLED score, 21
intracerebral hemorrhage, 20
recurrent GI bleeding, 20
VKA, 20
warfarin, 21–22
Enoxaparin, 261
ICU, 129–132
pregnancy, 261, 265, 266
TKA, 123, 124, 126
VTE, 116, 117

F
Factor Xa inhibitors, 146, 147, 296, 298
Fibrinolytics, 181–185
Fluconazole, 195–197, 223
Fondaparinux, 4, 76, 112, 113, 122–125, 298

G
Gastric bypass surgery, oral Xa and IIa inhibitors, 278–280
Gastrointestinal (GI) hemorrhage
apixaban, 27, 28
ARISTOTLE trial, 27

Index 309

aspirin, 26
CHADS₂ score, 26
CHA₂DS₂-VASc score, 26
clinical trial data, 27
dabigatran, 27, 28
edoxaban high dose, 27, 28
edoxaban low dose, 27
ENGAGE-AF-TIMI trial, 27
HAS-BLED score, 26
patient history, 25–26
RE-LY trial, 27
risk of recurrence, 26
rivaroxaban, 27
ROCKET-AF trial, 27
warfarin, 26–27
GCS. *See* Graduated compression stockings (GCS)
Gemfibrozil, 196, 223
Graduated compression stockings (GCS), 128, 131

H
HAS-BLED scoring system, 136–137
    bleeding risk, 54
    in elderly patients, 21
    in GI hemorrhage patient, 26
    stroke prevention therapy, 9–10
Heparin, 4

I
ICH. *See* Intracranial hemorrhage (ICH)
ICU. *See* Intensive care unit (ICU)
Idarucizumab, 32, 291, 296, 298
Independent Diagnostic Testing Facility (IDTF), 104, 105
Intensive care unit (ICU)
    enoxaparin, 129–132
    neurological disorder, 131–132
    sepsis
        anti-Factor Xa levels, 131
        bleeding risk, 128, 129
        hematocrit, 130
        hemoglobin, 130
        obesity, 130
        pharmacologic agents dosage, 129–130
        platelets, 130
        risk factors, 128
        serum creatinine, 130
    urosepsis, 132–133
Intermittent pneumatic compression (IPC), 32, 122–125, 128, 131, 132

International normalized ratio (INR), 3, 19–22, 43, 45, 65, 84, 93, 102, 168, 169, 188, 201, 207, 232, 234, 255, 264, 295
International Society on Thrombosis and Haemostasis (ISTH), 27
Interventional pain management, 234
Intracranial hemorrhage (ICH), 291, 292
    anticoagulant reinitiation
        in MVR replacement patients, 33
        in previous lobar ICH patients, 33
        in prior ICH patient, 33
    idarucizumab, 32
    patient history, 30–31
    rapid reversal of anticoagulation, 32
    recurrent ICH prevention, 32
    VKA therapy, 32
Ischemic stroke
    apixaban, 16
    dabigatran, 16–17
    edoxaban, 16, 17
    patient history, 15
    rivaroxaban, 16
    warfarin, 16

K
Khorana score, 273

L
Left atrial appendage (LAA), 83
Left ventricular ejection fraction (LVEF), 87
Low molecular weight heparin (LMWH), 4, 62
    adjusted-dose, 262, 265
    anti-Xa level, 261, 262
    cancer-associated VTE
        advantages, 270–271
        dalteparin, 273
        treatment, 270
    critically ill patient, 129–131
    dosing recommendation, 261
    enoxaparin, 261
    INR, 264
    intermediate-dose, 262
    pregnancy, 260
    prophylactic doses, 262
    renal clearance, 261
    THA/TKA, 123–124
    therapeutic dosing, 263, 266

M

Major bleeding
  anticoagulant reversal strategies, 290–292
  aPTT/TT/dTT testing, 291
  blood pressure management, 290
  idarucizumab, 291
  normalized hemostasis, 290
  resuming anticoagulation therapy, 291
Malignancy, VTE, 112, 113, 115
  chemotherapy agents, 271
  duration, 274
  edoxaban *vs.* dalteparin, 270
  Khorana score, 273
  malnutrition, 272
  management, 273
  optimal duration, 270
  patient history, 269
  primary thromboprophylaxis, 272
  recurrent VTE, 273
  VKA, 270
Mechanical valves
  antithrombotic recommendations, 248–249
  appropriate oral anticoagulant, 246
  Bjork-Shiley tilting-disk valve, 247
  diagnostic/surgical procedures, 249
  INR goal intensification, 249–250
  medical history, 245
  Medtronic Hall tilting-disk valve, 247
  on-X aortic mechanical valve, 249
  Starr-Edwards caged-ball valve, 247
  St. Jude Medical Regent, 247
  thrombosis, risk of, 246
  valve thrombosis, 246
Medtronic Hall tilting-disk valve, 247
Minor bleeding
  bleeding severity, 284
  clinical decision chart, 285–286
  hemodynamic stability, 284
  invasive diagnostic/interventional procedure, 285
  ongoing and further bleeding, 284
  oral vitamin K administration, 285
  thromboembolic risk, 284–285
Mitral valve stenosis
  AF, 82–84
  anticoagulant, choice of, 82
  antithrombotic therapy, 82–84
  medical history, 81
  risk factors, 82
  valvular interventions, 84
Mixed P-gp/3A4 inhibitors
  apixaban, 214, 217
  dabigatran, 215, 217
  DOACs, 215–216
  drug interaction management, 217
  edoxaban, 215, 217
  inhibitors and inducers, 216
  patient history, 213
  renal function, 214–218
  rivaroxaban, 214, 217, 218
Moderate chronic kidney disease. *See* Chronic kidney disease (CKD)

N

Non-ST segment elevation myocardial infarction (NSTEMI), 135, 167–169, 176, 187, 190, 201
Non-valvular atrial fibrillation, 16–17

O

On-X aortic mechanical valve, 249, 283
Opioids, 233
Oral anticoagulant reversal options, 299–300

P

Patient education, 39, 105
Patient self-management (PSM), 102–105
Patient self-testing (PST), 102–107
PCI. *See* Percutaneous coronary intervention (PCI)
Percutaneous coronary intervention (PCI), 168–170, 174, 175, 177, 181–184
Perioperative bleeding, 189
P-glycoprotein (P-gp)
  CYP3A4 inhibitors, 197, 202–205
  DOAC, 203–204
  inhibitors and inducers, 202
  mediated drug interactions, 202–203
  patient history, 201
  transport system, 202
  warfarin, 203
Pharmacodynamic drug interactions
  bleeding risk, 208–209
  clinical risk-benefit considerations, 209–210
  COX-1, 208, 209, 211
  DOAC, 210
  low dose aspirin, 208, 211
  mechanism, 208–209
  NSAIDs, 208, 209, 211
  patient history, 207
  with warfarin, 208
Pharmacokinetic drug interactions, warfarin *vs.* anticoagulation therapy, 225

cholestyramine, 226, 227
CYP450, 222
CYP1A2 inducer, 226
distribution, 222, 223
metabolism, 223–225
patient management, 225
vitamin K oxide, 222, 223
Phenytoin, 221–225
POCT. *See* Point-of-care testing (POCT)
Point-of-care testing (POCT), 102, 104
Post-percutaneous coronary intervention (PCI)
  bleeding risk, 174
  DAPT duration, 175
  double *vs.* triple therapy, 175
  ischemic risk, 174
  patient history, 173
  pharmacotherapy regimen, 174–175
  STEMI, 181–184
  triple therapy, 174–178
  warfarin, 174–176, 178
Pregnancy-associated venous thromboembolism
  clinical considerations, 261, 262
  DOAC, 260
  due date approaches, 263–264
  LMWH, 260–262
  vs. non-pregnancy, 260
  risks, 260
  UFH, 260
Primary thromboprophylaxis, 272
Prothrombin complex concentrates (PCCs), 291, 298–299
Provoked venous thromboembolism, 112, 114, 118, 136, 152, 153, 177, 293
PSM. *See* Patient self-management (PSM)
PST. *See* Patient self-testing (PST)
Pulmonary embolism (PE), thrombolytic therapy
  advantages and disadvantages, oral anticoagulation, 162
  discontinuation of, 160–161
  DOACs use after, 161
  massive, 160–163
  oral anticoagulants selection, 161–163
  patient history, 159–160
  sub-massive, 160, 161
P2Y12 inhibitor, 138, 140, 170, 173–175, 208

R
Recombinant factor VIIa, 291
Resuming anticoagulation therapy, 291
Ritonavir, 47, 196, 201–203, 216, 223

Rivaroxaban, 27, 28, 97
  ischemic stroke, 16
  mixed P-gp/3A4 inhibitors, 214, 217, 218
  P-gp, 203–205
  recurrent VTE, 154, 155, 157, 158
  VTE, 77

S
Selective-serotonin reuptake inhibitors (SSRIs), 208, 209, 211, 233
Sepsis, 127–131
  anti-Factor Xa levels, 131
  bleeding risk, 128, 129
  hematocrit, 130
  hemoglobin, 130
  obesity, 130
  pharmacologic agents dosage, 129–130
  platelets, 130
  risk factors, 128
  serum creatinine, 130
Stable moderate chronic kidney disease
  DOAC
    benefits and risks, 48
    degree of renal elimination, 45
    discontinuation or avoidance, 44
    dose reduction, 46
    drug–drug interactions, 46, 47
    patient affordability, 48
    routine monitoring, 48
  patient decision-making capacity, 48
  patient history, 43–44
  rivaroxaban therapy, 48–49
  warfarin therapy
    adherence and control, 46
    benefits and risks, 48
    characteristics, 45
    therapeutic activity, 44
Starr-Edwards caged-ball valve, 247
STEMI. *See* ST-segment elevation myocardial infarction (STEMI)
St. Jude Medical Regent, 247
Stroke prevention therapy
  aspirin monotherapy, 10
  aspirin plus clopidogrel combination therapy, 10
  CHA_2DS_2VASc score, 8–9
  clinical decision making, 10, 11
  HAS-BLED score, 9–10
  medications, 9
  patient history, 7

ST-segment elevation myocardial infarction (STEMI)
  fibrinolytic therapy
    considerations before using, 183
    dosage recommendations, 182
    in emergency, 184–185
    monitoring parameters, 183, 185
  patient history, 181
  PCI, 181–184
Supportive care, 298

T
THA/TKA. *See* Total hip/ knee arthroplasty (THA/TKA)
Thrombin time (TT), 291, 297
Thrombocytopenia, 256
Thrombolysis in myocardial infarction (TIMI), 182
Thrombolytic therapy, PE
  advantages and disadvantages, oral anticoagulation, 162
  discontinuation of, 160–161
  DOACs use after, 161
  massive, 160–163
  oral anticoagulants selection, 161–163
  patient history, 159–160
  sub-massive, 160, 161
Thrombophilias, 254, 255
Total hip/ knee arthroplasty (THA/TKA)
  apixaban, 125
  bleeding risk, 122
  dosing recommendations, 123–124
  enoxaparin dose, 126
  LMWH, 123–124
  postoperative risk, 122
  SC injections, 125, 126
Tramadol, 233–236
Triple oral antithrombotic therapy (TOAT), 137–140
Triple therapy, 140, 174–178

U
Unfractionated heparin (UFH), 260, 265
Unprovoked venous thromboembolism, 111, 114, 115, 118, 136, 139, 151–153, 157, 226, 254, 262
Urosepsis, 132–133

V
Valvular heart disease (VHD), 88–89
Variable renal function
  anticoagulant discontinuation, 65
  CBC monitoring, 62
  DOAC
    dose selection, 62
    management, 62–63
    outpatient follow-up, 64
    therapeutic activity measurement, 62
  dose changes, 65
  hospitalization follow-up, 65
  LMWH, 62
  medication/anticoagulant changes, 65
  rivaroxaban, 64–66
  routine renal function, 62
  warfarin therapy, 62
Venlafaxine, 233, 235, 236
Venous thromboembolism (VTE)
  ACCP and ACOG guidelines, 262, 264
  active, 112, 113
  anticoagulation treatment, duration, 78
  anti-factor Xa concentrations, 116
  atrial fibrillation and, 75–78
  cancer-associated, 113–115, 117, 118, 270, 273, 274
  CKD
    apixaban, 145–148
    dabigatran, 145–148
    DOAC usage, 55–57
    dosing recommendations, 145
    edoxaban, 145–148
    patient history, 53–54, 143
    rivaroxaban, 145–147
    stroke and bleeding risk, 54
    warfarin, 56–57, 144–148
  DES
    anticoagulant, choosing, 136–137
    CAD, 138
    DAPT, 137–138
    patient history, 135–136
    triple therapy, 140
  DOACs, 113
    absorption and metabolism of, 155
    dosage, 154
    risk reduction, 156
  dosing for, 77
  duration, of anticoagulation, 115
  enoxaparin, 116, 117
  ICU
    enoxaparin, 129–132
    neurological disorder, 131–132
    sepsis, 128–131
    urosepsis, 132–133
  incidence, 260
  inferior vena cava filters, 278
  malignancy, 112, 113, 115
    chemotherapy agents, 271

duration, 274
edoxaban *vs.* dalteparin, 270
Khorana score, 273
management, 273
optimal duration, 270
patient history, 269
primary thromboprophylaxis, 272
recurrent VTE, 273
VKA, 270
medical history, 75
medication, 78
oral anticoagulants, 76–77
patient characteristics/preferences, 156
patient history, 111, 151–152
patient-specific factors, 114–115
post-partum period, risks of, 260, 264
pregnancy
clinical considerations, 261, 262
DOAC, 260
due date approaches, 263–264
LMWH, 260–262
vs. non-pregnancy, 260
risks, 260
UFH, 260
provoked, 112, 114, 118, 136, 152, 153, 177, 293
risk factors, 112
THA/TKA
apixaban, 125
bleeding risk, 122
dosing recommendations, 123–124
enoxaparin dose, 126
LMWH, 123–124
postoperative risk, 122
SC injections, 125, 126
therapy duration, 152
thromboembolic *vs.* bleeding risk, 152–153
unprovoked, 111, 114, 115, 118, 136, 139, 151–153, 157, 226, 254, 262
Vitamin K antagonist (VKA), 20, 261, 265
ACS, 169
APS, 254–255
CAD, 70–71
elderly patients, 20
ICH, 32
malignancy, 270
dalteparin's indication, 273–274
enoxaparin dosing, 274
less efficiency, 270
management, 272
mitral valve stenosis, 82, 84
Vitamin K oxide reductase, 222, 223
VKA. *See* Vitamin K antagonist (VKA)
VTE. *See* Venous thromboembolism (VTE)

W

Warfarin, 3
ACS, 168–169, 171
anticoagulation clinic, 102–104, 221
bleeding complications, 296
CABG, 188, 189, 191, 192
CAD, 69–71
catheter ablation, 239–242
CKD, 144–148
CYP 3A4 inhibitors, 196–199
DES, 136–140
DOACs
adherence, 96
apixaban, 96
conversion, 97
dabigatran, 96
edoxaban, 97
FDA-approved indications, 94
renal function assessment, 96
rivaroxaban, 97
safety and efficacy, comparison, 94, 95
self-monitoring, 96
in elderly patients, 21–22
extended interval monitoring, 102, 104
gastric bypass surgery, 279
hemodynamic stability, 296
ischemic stroke, 16
medical history, 93
mitral valve stenosis, 81, 84
nonadherence, 38
parmacodynamic drug interactions with, 208
patient considerations, 102–103
patients and professionals resources, 105
P-gp, 203
pharmacokinetic drug interactions
vs. anticoagulation therapy, 225
cholestyramine, 226, 227
CYP450, 222
CYP1A2 inducer, 226
distribution, 222, 223
metabolism, 223–225
patient management, 225
vitamin K oxide, 222, 223
post PCI, 174–176, 178
provider/clinic considerations, 103–104
PSM, 102–105
PST, 102–107
R-enantiomers, 196, 224
reversal strategy, 292
S-enantiomers, 196, 224
stroke, 10
VTE, 77

Printed by Printforce, the Netherlands